Perspectives on Palliative Care
for Children and Young People

Perspectives on Palliative Care for Children and Young People

A GLOBAL DISCOURSE

Edited by
RITA PFUND
Lecturer in Child Health
Division of Nursing, Midwifery and Physiotherapy
University of Nottingham

and

SUSAN FOWLER-KERRY
Full Professor
College of Nursing
University of Saskatchewan

Foreword by
SISTER FRANCES DOMINICA
Founding Trustee
Helen and Douglas House
Hospice Care for Children and Young Adults, Oxford

Radcliffe Publishing

Oxford • New York

Radcliffe Publishing Ltd
18 Marcham Road
Abingdon
Oxon OX14 1AA
United Kingdom

www.radcliffe-oxford.com

Electronic catalogue and worldwide online ordering facility.

British Library Cataloguing in Publication Data

A catalogue record for this book is available from the British Library.

ISBN-13: 978 184619 333 0

1005994243

The paper used for the text pages of this book is FSC certified. FSC (The Forest Stewardship Council) is an international network to promote responsible management of the world's forests.

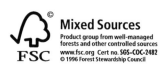

Mixed Sources
Product group from well-managed forests and other controlled sources
www.fsc.org Cert no. SGS-COC-2482
© 1996 Forest Stewardship Council

FSC

Typeset by Pindar NZ, Auckland, New Zealand
Printed and bound by TJI Digital, Padstow, Cornwall, UK

Contents

Foreword

Two decades ago the term 'paediatric palliative care' was not in general use. A few families could recount isolated instances of exceptional support through the illness and death of their child. They usually attributed this to the sensitivity and genuine humanity of one healthcare professional. Joined-up working in this field was scarcely dreamed of. In what is arguably the worst tragedy to befall anyone, at the centre of it all, so many families felt abandoned. Exhausted with grief, they had to fight for the rights of their children and the rest of the family. If it was bad during the children's lifetime, it was so much worse after they had died.

In recent years we have made quantum leaps in developing paediatric palliative care but we can never be complacent. We are always on a steep learning curve, not least because each sick child or young person is a unique individual and his or her family knows their son or daughter better than anyone else in the world. We have so much to learn from them and it is only when we have built a relationship of trust with them that we shall be able to make a meaningful contribution to their well-being.

I hope this book will come to the attention of those healthcare professionals who are privileged to be working with these families. It contains so much wisdom and practical common sense and, most importantly, we hear the words of the children, young people and their families – the real experts. We are confronted on every side by constraints of funding and cut-backs in resources, but we should never let that prevent us from journeying with these families as fellow human beings, for however short a part of that journey, using whatever skills we have to relieve a little of their distress.

Nearly 30 years ago, when we were recruiting a team to work in Helen House, the children's hospice in Oxford, I had a mental checklist I used at interviews. Did this person seem to be a fully paid-up card-carrying member of the human race? Did he or she seem to have an abundance of common sense, compassion and a good sense of humour? Would they feel safe to cry as well as laugh? Was this person going to be a team player, prepared to take appropriate risks, comfortable with him- or herself, with a life beyond work? And then on a good day I would remember to ask about qualifications and experience! Despite the red tape with which we are surrounded today, I still believe those qualities are vital.

In a world of unspeakable suffering each of us *can* make a difference. I believe that this book will help us to do so.

Sister Frances Dominica
January 2010

Preface

With ongoing advances in medical science and technology, we are saving more infants and children than in any previous decade. Children who, in some cases, will survive and live out a normal life expectancy, others will have a life-limiting/life-threatening diagnosis where death may come early and still others will live on well past projected life trajectories, even into adulthood. As you can see there are many different paths a child with palliative needs and their family may travel; however, this new reality means that parents and communities are now facing a growing number of challenges for which neither they nor the healthcare systems are prepared.

It was our intent through this book to offer a forum from which we could encourage a dialogue of these issues. To accomplish this goal we have built from an earlier text by Pfund entitled *Palliative Care Nursing of Children and Young People* (Radcliffe Publishing, 2007), then to provide a broader perspective we invited professionals from around the globe working in paediatric palliative care to share with us their knowledge. And, finally, we have included the most important of perspectives for whom paediatric palliative care services are essentially developed, namely the child and the parents.

As a result of this manuscript, it is our hope that we have been able to stimulate further debate about paediatric palliative care at global, national and local levels; discussions that are translated into actions so that all children and their families – regardless of geographical location, gender, race or socio-economic class – have equal and guaranteed access to comprehensive paediatric palliative care services.

Rita Pfund
Susan Fowler-Kerry
January 2010

About the editors

Rita Pfund is a lecturer (Child Health) at the Division of Nursing, Midwifery and Physiotherapy, University of Nottingham, with extensive experience in palliative care of children and young people. Her previous book, *Palliative Care Nursing of Children and Young People* (Radcliffe Publishing, 2007), offered a reflective insight into this rapidly changing area of service provision. Plans were soon on the way to capture a glimpse of the current state of palliative care of children and young people as experienced by young people, their families and the professionals caring for them in the light of the major developments within palliative care both nationally and internationally.

Susan Fowler-Kerry is a tenured Full Professor and Director of Royal Bank of Canada, Nurses for Kids Program, at the College of Nursing University of Saskatchewan, Canada. As a faculty member she has developed an extensive research programme in the areas of child and youth health, paediatric pain and palliative care. She has been privileged to consult with WHO, and co-edited the monograph, *Cancer Pain Relief and Palliative Care in Children.* Currently she serves as Chair on the University of Saskatchewan International Activities Committee of Council and represents Canada as a member of the International Steering Group of the International Children's Palliative Care Network (ICPCN).

List of contributors

In order to bring together a global writers' community over a comparatively short time span and allow for an exchange of ideas and sharing in each other's good practice, we set up our writers' club over the duration of compiling this book. This allowed the project to take on a life of its own, and soon new contributors were invited to contribute to issues raised and to expand the original brief. These are the members of our writers' club:

CHAPTER 1

Dr Frank Brennan is a Palliative Care Physician in Sydney, Australia. He is also a lawyer. His interests include the legal and ethical dimensions of pain management and palliative care and he has written on the topic of pain management and palliative care as human rights.

CHAPTER 2

Lizzie Chambers is the Chief Executive of ACT (Association for Children's Palliative Care) in the UK and vice-chair of the ICPCN (International Children's Palliative Care Network). Lizzie has been involved in campaigning for the development of children's palliative care services in the UK through her role with ACT and was delighted to be asked to write about the need to develop children's palliative care internationally. There is a need to develop good quality palliative care for every life-limited child or young person around the world. The task is immense and the ICPCN wants to see every country have its own national organisation to champion this need.

Sue Boucher is a qualified teacher with 30 years' experience as a teacher, head of department and school principal. She is a published author of 12 children's books and has co-authored or authored a number of teaching manuals and authored the book *Promoting Early Childhood Development in Paediatric Palliative Care in Africa*. She was appointed to the position of International Information Officer for the International Children's Palliative Care Network (ICPCN) in December 2007.

Sabine Kraft has been Director of the National Association of Children's Hospices in Germany (Bundesverband Kinderhospiz) since 2005 and is a board member of the German children's hospice charity (Bundesstiftung Kinderhospiz). Sabine has a degree in social work and economics and has experience in different kinds of youth work, counselling as well as project management.

Dr Julia Downing is the Deputy Executive Director of the African Palliative Care Association and is an experienced palliative care nurse and educationalist, with a PhD that evaluated palliative care training in rural Uganda, and a Masters of Medical Science in Clinical Oncology. She has been working within palliative care for 17 years, with the last eight being in Uganda, where she was the Director of the Mildmay International Study Centre before joining the African Palliative Care Association. She serves on the boards of several international NGOs in Africa, and is on the steering committee of the International Children's Palliative Care network. She is also an Honorary Research Fellow with the Department of Palliative Care, Policy and Rehabilitation, at King's College London.

Dr Faith Mwangi-Powell is the Executive Director of the African Palliative Care Association, a post she has held since joining APCA in January 2005. Prior to APCA, she worked for two and half years with the Diana, Princess of Wales Memorial Fund, London as an International Advocacy Officer for Palliative Care, and for three years before that as the Director for the Foundation for Women's Health, Research and Development (FORWARD). She is a member of several international boards and advisory committees with regards to palliative care. She comes from a community health background and holds a PhD in women's economic development and fertility-related behaviour.

CHAPTER 3

Jo Rooney is the Children's Services Manager for Barnardo's Sherwood Project in Nottingham. This provides a range of social and emotional support services to families who have a child with a life-limiting condition. She is a Community Children's Nurse who has a background in providing and developing services for children and families in the community, from short break and continuing care services to community children's nursing. As a member of the East Midlands Children's Palliative Care Network (formerly chair) and the East Midlands Children's Palliative Care Board, Jo has an active role in shaping palliative care services for children and young people regionally.

CHAPTER 4

Kirsteen Cowling currently works as a nurse at Robin House Children's Hospice in Scotland. Previously she spent seven years working in Romania with Emanuel Hospice, where she worked alongside an established adult palliative care team, helping them to develop a palliative home care service for children with life-threatening and life-limiting conditions in an area where palliative care was a very new concept.

CHAPTER 5

Dr Lou Millington is a UK-trained GP who spent two years working as a Clinical Consultant at Mobile Hospice Mbarara, a branch of Hospice Africa Uganda. She is now studying for a Masters in Public Health in Developing Countries at the London School of Hygiene and Tropical Medicine and hopes to return to Africa to do further work in palliative care once her studies are completed.

CHAPTER 6

Joan Marston is a professional nurse with 20 years' experience in palliative care. She has established The St Nicholas (now known as Sunflower) Children's Hospice in 1998 in Bloemfontein, Free State, South Africa and is presently the national paediatric portfolio manager for the Hospice Palliative Care Association of South Africa.

She has established the Palliative Care Society of South Africa in 2005 as an organisation for individuals working in palliative care in South Africa. This includes a paediatric portfolio.

Joan is also chair and founding member of the International Children's Palliative Care Network and the African Children's Palliative Care Network.

CHAPTER 7

Dr Sheila Greatrex-White is a Lecturer (Adult Health) at the School of Nursing, Midwifery and Physiotherapy at the University of Nottingham. Sheila has completed her doctoral study in 2004 based on narrative research. She has an extensive publication record and is supervising doctoral students utilising a narrative research approach.

CHAPTER 8

Greg Wilford: 'My name is Greg Wilford. I'm 20 years old and currently studying Media Production at University. I live independently from my parents through the aid of an organised team of carers whom I employ. My reason for wanting to contribute something to this book was really to try and convey a "true" sense of what it really is like to be an individual living with a condition such as the one I have, Duchenne Muscular Dystrophy, on a day-to-day basis; hopefully reflecting on the optimistic and positive aspects – of which there have been many – rather than the dour and morose, where there is tendency to place emphasis in articles of this type. This tone is not through delusion or screening of events, not at all. This is just how it happened to me.'

CHAPTER 9

Anna Gill had to give up a career in nursing on the birth of her son Jamie but remained very active in the voluntary sector. She is now involved at a national level in parent participation and policy making on Ministerial Implementation Groups, as a Trustee of ACT and as a self-employed trainer of both practitioners and parents of disabled children.

Peter Limbrick established One Hundred Hours in the 1990s to develop key worker support for families whose baby has neurological impairment. He works as a writer, trainer and independent consultant to health, education and social services in the UK and Ireland and has developed the Team Around the Child system (TAC) for children who need multiple interventions. Peter publishes the online Interconnections Quarterly Journal (IQJ) and the Interconnections Electronic Bulletin for practitioners who support children and young people with disabilities and special needs. To learn more about Interconnections and his new book, visit www.icwhatsnew.com.

CHAPTER 10

Dr Gordon Martell works in the area of Indigenous education in Canada. He is also involved in local Indigenous issues and community development. The opportunity to learn from his daughter, Sarah, shed light on the values clash in the confluence of a children, illness, cure and cultural experience. Gordon aspires to describe the policy considerations that would mediate the experience of navigating paediatric palliative care for families and children.

Dr Gosia Bryckzynska is a Senior Lecturer (Child Health) Thames Valley University and a nurse ethicist. She edited the first UK textbook on ethical issues in child health nursing in 1989. She has devoted most of her career to teaching, researching and writing about philosophy and ethics related to nursing. She was also the RCN Refugee Nurses Project Coordinator from 2003–05 and RCN International Officer from 2001–06.

CHAPTER 11

Bea Brunton is a bereaved parent and the coordinator for the registered charity PASIC (The Parents Association for Seriously Ill Children), Nottingham University Hospitals. 'Having experienced the "cancer journey" before the death of my son Simon, I feel quite passionate that children, young people and parents/carers should have a voice and be able to work with professionals to ensure the best care possible is provided for as long as it is needed.'

CHAPTER 12

Sally Blower is the sibling support worker at Rainbows Children's Hospice. 'I work one-to-one supporting siblings and also organise group activities. Sibling support groups give the brothers and sisters the opportunity to share their experiences with others in a similar situation and to have fun.'

CHAPTER 13

Jacqueline Newton is a parent. 'This is really just our story and it was a crazy bumpy ride over too soon.'

CHAPTER 15

Linda Ferguson is Full Professor in the College of Nursing, University of Saskatchewan. She is Director of the Centre for the Advancement of the Study of Nursing Education and Interprofessional Education (CASNIE) within the College of Nursing. Her research has focused on education in nursing, in particular on the development of clinical judgement in practice and evidence to support educational methods used in nursing education.

CHAPTER 16

Dr Toni Wolff is a disability paediatrician based at the Child Development Centre in Nottingham. Toni was funded by the Big Lottery Fund to develop children's palliative care services in Nottingham. She has been working with the Nottingham team to develop end-of-life planning tools.

Jackie Brown manages the Children's Bereavement Services Nottingham University Hospitals. She has developed and implemented systems in Nottingham to support families and professionals in discussions of end-of-life care and practical support when a child dies.

CHAPTER 17

Paul Weeding is a Chaplain at the Department of Spiritual and Pastoral Care Nottingham University Hospitals. Paul participated in the working party formulating the local adaptation of the ACT Care pathway.

CHAPTER 18

Ian Woodroffe is a Psychological Support Counsellor for families in Neonatal Services at Addenbrookes Hospital, Cambridge. 'The delivery of care after the death of a baby has been considered – although not always based on evidence. The loss, grief and trauma of a premature birth and the processes that parents have to go through have been less well investigated in the UK. The subject requires more thought and resources for if parents do not process the "trauma grief" the unresolved trauma may effect bonding and the grief journey if the baby dies. I hope the contribution in this publication will further the debate on the subject.'

CHAPTER 19

Dr Mike Miller is a Consultant General Paediatrician. After some years as a Consultant the opportunity arose to work in Paediatric Palliative Medicine at Martin House and around the Yorkshire region. The post was made attractive by the young people's unit (up to 35 years of age). Supporting families to support their children with all the uncertainties of chronic and often complex disability is challenging but rewarding. Even more challenging is supporting and providing opportunities for independence appropriate for age and development.

CHAPTER 20

Jody Chrastek is the Coordinator of Pain and Palliative Care (PPC) for Children's Hospitals and Clinics of Minnesota. Her current areas of responsibility include programme development and coordination of staff and services in the six areas of PPC.

Stacy Remke is a clinical social worker with the Pain and Palliative Care Program at Children's Hospitals and Clinics of Minnesota. She provides clinical leadership to the psychosocial team and coordinates the education and outreach programme, Children's Institute for Pain and Palliative Care (CIPPC).

Dr Stefan Friedrichsdorf is Medical Director, Pain and Palliative Care at Children's Hospitals and Clinics of Minnesota.

Pain and Palliative Care aims to control acute and complex/chronic pain in all of their in- and outpatients in close collaboration with all paediatric subspecialties at Children's Hospitals and Clinics. The team also provides holistic, multidisciplinary care for children and teens with life-limiting or terminal diseases and their families. They see paediatric patients as inpatients, in the interdisciplinary pain clinic, in the palliative care clinic, or in the community/at home.

CHAPTER 21

Paula Dawson is a Lecturer in Child Health at the University of Nottingham, Division of Nursing, Midwifery and Physiotherapy, Derby Centre with 22 years' paediatric nursing experience in clinical, management and development roles in the UK and overseas.

CHAPTER 22

Dr Joanne Griffiths is a Consultant Community Paediatrician in Swansea, with an interest in children's palliative care. She is lead paediatric tutor for the Cardiff University Palliative medicine course, part of the education and training group for paediatric palliative medicine, and organises the South Wales children's palliative care network.

Acknowledgements

Myra Johnson
Communications and PR Manager
ACT (Association for Children's Palliative Care)

Professor Jane Seymour
Sue Ryder Care Professor in Palliative and End of Life Studies
University of Nottingham

Joan Cook
User Involvement Development Worker
Self Help Nottingham
School of Nursing, Midwifery and Physiotherapy
University of Nottingham

Sally Melling
Associate Professor (Child Health)
School of Nursing, Midwifery and Physiotherapy
University of Nottingham

For all the parents on behalf of the children who might never be able to put into words what one child expressed to her parents:

Thank you for giving me 'aliveness'.

(six-year-old child quoted in Sourkes B (1995) *Armfuls of Time: The Psychological Experience of the Child with a Life-Threatening Illness.* Pittsburgh, PA: Routledge; p. 167)

Introducing our discourse

Rita Pfund

The purpose of this book was to introduce readers to a unique discourse between those who are or have lived the paediatric palliative care (PPC) experience with an international, inter-professional group of healthcare professionals who deliver PPC, an approach which challenged the editors both conceptually and methodologically in illuminating the dimensions of this multifaceted relationship. Moving outside the traditional, we utilised the UK strategy (2008) *Better Care: Better Lives*[1] document and its proposed framework to provide a common basis for readers to make informed comparisons and critique. Pathways/guidelines within the current UK context are proposed as a means to ensure the commissioning and implementation of comprehensive paediatric palliative services. As editors we are cognizant that this particular framework should not be considered as a means to an end, but rather an approach based in the current state of research that must continue to be evaluated and revised to improve the current art and science of PPC.

Our methodological approach emphasised a particular notion of experience which analytically linked the lived worlds of young people themselves, parents, siblings and healthcare professionals to existing social structures within PPC. The use of personal narratives from this group of stakeholders provided a vehicle to document knowledge that has typically remained largely anecdotal. Transfer of knowledge and lessons shared will make a significant contribution by expanding our collective understanding about the special practice of PPC. Eliciting narratives of experience from children, parents, siblings as well as those in healthcare allowed us to give this text a different look that can best be described as a collage or montage of interconnected images and representations which connect the parts to the whole. A philosophical research approach that will be very discussed in Chapters 7 and 10.

QUESTIONS WE ASKED

To begin this discourse we have asked contributors:

1 What do colleagues both inside and outside the UK perceive as major barriers limiting service delivery?
2 How does the current United Kingdom (UK) policy impact or potentially impact within your sectors palliative care provisions? Do you currently have a national policy referring to Paediatric Palliative Care (PPC)?

3   What experiences and successes have you had in the implementation of PPC and what lessons could you impart to our readers, so that we do not continue to spend valuable time reinventing the wheel rather than adapting current successes? What made your approach successful, i.e. the right people, policies, lack of constraints, opportunity, and autonomy to make choices, good will, resources, clinical practice guidelines and/or other documents?

4   If you were again challenged with the same task, what would you do differently and/or recommend to our readers?

This book aims to demonstrate how the practice in palliative care for children and young people uses/exploits theory and evidence in order to develop practice further and to advocate for children and young people.

Over the last few years palliative care for children and young people has arrived on the national and international agenda. Endorsed through national strategies and/ or law various models are currently being implemented.

PALLIATIVE CARE – A HUMAN RIGHT

Starting with the premise posed by Brennan in Chapter 1, that palliative care for children and young people is a basic human right.[2]

Brennan summarises the obligation of individual governments towards children's and young peoples' palliative care as:

1   the creation and implementation of paediatric palliative care policies

2   equity of access to services, without discrimination

3   availability and affordability of critical medications, including opioids

4   the provision of paediatric palliative care at all levels of care

5   the integration of palliative care education throughout the learning continuum from informal caregivers to health professionals.

These five obligations are pivotal in the successful delivery of palliative care and therefore are recurrent themes in each chapter.

Contributors have examined these in the context of everyday life, financial considerations and effects on quality of life.

THE TERMINOLOGY

Certainly in a UK context palliative care as a distinct element of care for children and young people originated nearly three decades ago, and is now a recognised sub-specialty in paediatrics.

Yet time after time the difficulty with a clear definition of what is encompassed by the term 'palliative care for children and young people' is highlighted as a hindrance to service provision. How then can we genuinely and effectively adapt concepts such as advocacy and meet our professional and legal obligations to provide palliative care?

Is the term 'palliative care of children and young people' a realistic one, or does it merely lump together a diverse group of children and families, the common denominator being that neither the children or young people will achieve the life expectancy for their country of residence? Whilst there are commonalities of experiences these families face, there will be other diverse and individual issues to deal with.

Does the young adult with Duchenne Muscular Dystrophy transferring to adult services at least in principle share the same needs as the neonate who is unlikely to survive the first few hours after birth? Would each be better cared for in their own specialty that has developed their own pathways for the small but significant number of children who will succumb to their illness? Or is this precisely what the subspecialty of PPC is trying to achieve?

The World Health Organization (WHO)[3] definition, as well as the Association for Children's Palliative Care (ACT) and Royal College of Paediatrics and Child Health (RCPCH)[4] are clear that palliative care of children and young people begins when illness is diagnosed, and continues regardless of whether or not a child receives treatment directed at the disease. Particularly in general children's and adult areas, where children with life-limiting illnesses are not seen consistently, there remains significant confusion and resistance to the acceptance of this definition and principle.

Whilst a barrage of policy statement gives entitlement to palliative care services in some countries, these are often un-enforceable and parents often only find out their entitlement late in the day. Parents are forced to assume the role of key worker or primary caregiver, often attempting to liaise with a staggering number of professionals to ensure that their child is cared for, while at the same time their roles as mum and dad suffer. This is illustrated in Chapters 9, 10, 11 and 13 and raises the question whether to this end palliative care needs more than professionals advocating for families; we certainly cannot add another level of expectation on parents who are often physically, emotionally and spiritually taxed out. Where are the voices of governments and policy makers, given that what is personal is political and that policy is personal? Brennan advances this position, explaining that with rights come obligations, and these are in turn illustrated through practical examples. Section 2 of this book highlights the need for and the access to information, and how service users and carers themselves experience how the special needs of young people are met.

Education of the service providers then becomes an obligation by necessity, which will be explored in Chapter 22, as professionals need a working knowledge of the wider issues in a field that encompasses the active total care of the child's body, mind and spirit, and of course involves supporting and empowerment of the family.

In order to advocate effectively professionals must be prepared to work utilising a broad multidisciplinary approach that includes the family and makes use of available community resources even where these are limited.

THE GLOBAL COMMUNITY

The first section of this book, Chapters 2, 3, 4, 5 and 6, considers the organisation of care globally. The emphasis in this section of the book is to demonstrate differences and similarities of global paediatric palliative care practices. Readers will become aware of common issues and themes that are impacting paediatric services globally, while also recognising that those in the developing and emerging worlds present with different challenges than those faced in the west. Recognising that differences exist, we have attempted to provide a forum that will give readers an opportunity to see the strengths and weakness in the provision of PPC within the global village. A common theme in this context is the focus on community settings, where most children, young people and their families receive the majority of their care. The key message we want to leave our readers with is that even with minimal resources effective palliative care services can exist, and existing programmes can be improved through the utilisation of best practice models of which the ACT Care Pathway[6] should be seen as the 'gold standard'.

Community settings – The home is a place that has been identified over and over within the literature as the preferred place for children to be cared for. In some countries there is quite simply no other option, while in the developed world there continue to be significant challenges, fuelled by myths and misconceptions surrounding the care of children in the terminal stages in the home. Where can hospice care fit into these scenarios and what are the criteria for receiving care there?

Chapter 3 offers a UK perspective, where it is quite acceptable and established practice to care for the terminally ill child in the home and hospice.

Chapter 4 offers the perspective of a resource-limited country of Eastern Europe, where there are no choices about treatment or where to provide care other than the home.

Chapters 5 and 6 discuss the challenges of delivering palliative care in a resource-poor sector. What do palliative care services look like in these contexts? What issues direct the provision of care in these areas, and where are best practice guidelines drawn from?

NARRATIVES AND NARRATIVE RESEARCH

This text places great emphasis on evidence gathered and examined through narratives. Greatrex-White in Chapter 7 contextualises narrative research in terms of the evolving evidence base in children's palliative care: the evidence is in our daily practice, we can put faces to names, and in this book we have given voice to a number of these 'statistics', the really tangible evidence we have and have had for nearly three decades. We must listen to these voices and hear and act on what they say. The second section of this book therefore is written by parents, as well as a young adult and siblings, giving us their very personal and lived experience with life-limiting illness and being the recipients of the services provided. As editors we felt both a moral and an ethical obligation to provide this forum in the book to give them voice and then to provide follow-through where there is an opportunity to meaningfully act on the evidence for specific issues that have been highlighted within commentaries provided by specialists in that area. Readers are challenged and encouraged to reflect on how the specific issues raised by service users and carers can be addressed in his or her own field of work.

PHILOSOPHICAL CONSIDERATIONS AND EVIDENCE

Martell in Chapter 10 encourages the reader to reflect and take stock of the family's experiences. It comes as no surprise that for parents their key consideration is their love for their child. Although palliative care seeks to address a holistic approach, what is the image we hold in our mind when meeting a new patient? Martell offers two perspectives when introducing his daughter. The first follows a pathological approach, the second looks at the whole child. How this is followed through in a wider societal context is enlightening.

A philosophical stance to the points raised is offered by Bryckzynska's commentary in Chapter 10: authentication of narratives allows us to add these very personal stories of families to the evidence base. Whilst a lack of workable statistics as explored in Chapter 23 still hamper the equitable implementation of effective palliative care for children and young people, we also must not hide behind an actual and perceived lack of evidence to guide practice. Brown[5] reminds us that in the children's hospice movement, evidence-based practice is generally understood as the process of finding, evaluating, and applying evidence to the care of life-limited children and their families. Thus there is a significant body of knowledge within children's palliative care as yet not fully exploited, waiting to be validated.

WORKING WITH PATHWAYS

Wolff and Browne in Chapter 16 highlight how palliative care is always about dealing with the unexpected. To manage the care of these children successfully Wolff and Browne illustrate how the ACT Care Pathway[6] customised to reflect the local context[7] and used successfully can make a difference to how both families and professionals experience the challenge of any situation.

For those of us who have been working in the area, the 'unexpected' actually has some common themes, one being the 'planning for emergencies in the end-stages of life – by whom and when'.

What makes this stage most difficult for all involved in the care of these children is the realisation that death is imminent. Emotions are charged and there is the underlying need by all that this period be peaceful and without crisis. To ensure that this goal is met, plans must be developed and discussed so that this final transition period will be one of peace for the child and his/her family.

TRANSITIONS

The term 'transition' has many connotations, but for a great many children and young people and their families receiving paediatric palliative care, this period has too often been described as extremely difficult, fraught with a lot of additional stress and pain. These children and their families are especially vulnerable, because they are quite literally fighting for their child's life. While healthcare institutions and other agencies do not regard transfers as anything out of the ordinary, these situations are not viewed the same way by families.

'Transition' is mainly understood to be the stage at which a child outgrows paediatric services and transfers to adulthood. Wilford (Chapter 8) and Gill (Chapter 9) give us an insight into some of the challenges they have encountered. But there are also different transitions encountered along the journey of a family's life-path, and Newton

(Chapter 13) shares the transitions her family have experienced with us.

We also examined transitions children, young people and their families are subjected to within care settings. Of particular note are the intensive care settings, namely neonatal and paediatric intensive care settings. Places that record the highest numbers of infant and children's deaths, but also these are environments where the emphasis is on aggressive care. Within these highly charged practice settings, can palliative care be effectively administered? In Chapters 17, 18 and 19 practitioners from chaplaincy, neonatology and children's hospice care provide their personal insights and narratives.

FACILITATING LEARNING

Education for professionals is pivotal, but also has to be provided for families and unqualified carers who provide often highly technical care on a day-to-day basis, striking a fine balance to what extent it is acceptable for parents to have the dual role of caregiver and parent.[8] Providing for the educational needs to carry out practical skills is obvious. A seamless team approach here is vital for two reasons: One is to ensure the ongoing clinical support once families do carry out technical care in the community, the other is the fact that if we expect families to provide technical care this needs to be balanced with the provision of respite to allow for a quality of life not just for the sick youngster, but also the family.

Team approaches increasingly need to cater across paediatric and adult services.

Chrastek *et al.* in Chapter 20 demonstrate how effective palliative care teams deliver efficient and effective palliative care through an interprofessional team approach and interdisciplinary teams must be built and nurtured if they are to maintain effective service delivery.

Payne *et al.*[9] tease out some of the tensions that have emerged from examining the state of adult palliative care. The themes they have identified appear to mirror the themes that are emerging in the paediatric field, perhaps in different guises, but have major implications when identifying practice and educational issues:

1 The tension between 'specialist' and 'general' palliative care, and the assumption that 'specialists' in palliative care somehow have a monopoly on the skills and attributes that are required to provide good palliative care.
2 Teamwork – a taxonomy of cross-disciplinary working with 'transdisciplinary' working as the ultimate goal.
3 Complex dynamics of institutional cultures, professional enculturation and territoriality. Like the examples given by Payne *et al.*[9] specialist care providers may have to work across statutory and charitable organisations, across primary, secondary and tertiary healthcare services, and across health and social care services. Similar to their adult equivalent, the community-based paediatric clinical nurse specialist providing care to a specific child and his/her family, may have to work with an NHS-funded paediatric consultant at a local district general hospital, a charitably funded children's hospice, a hospital consultant at a tertiary centre, a health visitor, a social work team, an occupational therapist, a community physiotherapist, a general practitioner, school nurse and teachers, to name just some. As Payne *et al.*[9] point out, the task of coordinating and managing the delivery of appropriate and

timely care is formidable and requires skills in liaison, management, planning and an understanding of how each of these very different organisations and professional groups operate. Whilst the key worker system does go a long way to facilitate this process, it might have repercussions on the issue raised in point one.

4 Like our adult counterparts we have found that health technologies have and are extending life and for many children and families the quality of life. Whilst adult literature is emerging examining the 'trajectories of dying', issues for the younger age spectrum relate to a number of issues, including:
   ➤ confusion of the term 'palliative care needs' as applied to a child or young person
   ➤ need of transition to adult services for young people with conditions not normally encountered by adult services
   ➤ appropriateness of technological interventions at any price – because we can.

5 Whilst many studies around families with children with complex needs have examined the financial impact on these families, Payne *et al.*[9] also identify demographic trends with increased longevity, increased marital breakdown, geographic mobility and more dependence upon female income generation as all likely to impact on the availability of women to offer continued (unpaid) care of family members of any age.

6 As a result of the recent changes to the globalisation of markets, Ling[10] observes that these changes give rise to inequalities, not only within nations but also between countries. There has never been a more important time to demonstrate that the provision of palliative care services not only improves care, but also can save money[10] and that the family unit can no longer be regarded as a coffer for the provision of supports and services for PPC.

LOOKING TO THE FUTURE

To conclude, we have drawn on the salient points from all contributors and provide recommendations for the future of paediatric palliative care because we believe that while paediatric palliative care has its own unique and inherent challenges, these challenges do not detract from the reality that working with children and families is a place of profound privilege.

REFERENCES

1 UK Department of Health. *Better Care: Better Lives.* 2008. Available at www.dh.gov.uk/en/Publicationsandstatistics/Publications/PublicationsPolicyAndGuidance/DH_083106 (accessed 17 February 2010).
2 www.unicef.org/crc/
3 www.who.int/cancer/palliative/definition/en/
4 www.icpcn.org.uk/page.asp?section=0001000100080004&itemTitle=What+is+Children%92s+Palliative+Care%3F
5 Brown E, with Warr B. *Supporting the Child and the Family in Paediatric Palliative Care.* London: Jessica Kingsley; 2007.
6 Elston S. *Integrated Multi-agency Care Pathways for Children with Life-threatening and Life-limiting Conditions.* Bristol: ACT; 2004.

7 Wolff T. *Nottingham Integrated Care Pathway for Children with Life-limiting and Life-threatening Conditions.* Nottingham: Nottingham University Hospitals; 2006.

8 Noyes J, Lewis M. Compiling, costing and funding complex packages of home-based health care. *Paediatr Nurs.* 2007; **19**: 28–32.

9 Payne S, Seymour J, Ingleton C. *Palliative Care Nursing Principles and Evidence for Practice.* Buckingham: Open University Press McGraw Hill; 2008.

10 Ling J. Palliative care in changing economic times. *Int J Palliat Nurs.* 2008; **14**: 523.

SECTION 1

A global overview

Susan Fowler-Kerry

This textbook can best be described as a collage, containing many relevant perspectives which we believe to be worth many columns of statistics. By setting the stage, we provide multiple contexts to challenge the meaning of childhood, a period of time best described as an enigma, the home of all the great questions about life and death, reality, dreams and imagination.

To start it may be useful to consider the place of children within societies' historical and philosophical attitudes and values which are then reflected into the normative dimensions of law, policy or lack thereof. Today it is becoming commonplace to hear politicians and advocates for children's rights stating aphorisms enunciating the value that the state, society and community place on the health and well-being of children and youth – expressions that suggest that children are autonomous, independent individuals, busy discovering their own reality, and that while in this stage of development they might be considered economically 'worthless'; they are, however, emotionally 'priceless'.

Today infant and child mortality rates are a critical gauge from which to judge the economic success of a nation. Death in childhood is no longer solely a private and personal tragedy, but also a sign of the collective failure of the state.[1,2] Today, the experience of childhood should be protected and respected, free from adult worries and responsibilities; a time of learning and play, a period of happiness, health and relative freedom. This belief spurred on a movement to universalise children's rights and a culturally specific perspective of childhood.[3]

As we move into this global recession how we value children will be put to the test. Unfortunately, past practice has shown that a significant down-swing within economic markets and subsequent recessions has often resulted in significant challenges and clawbacks to existing social programmes. The stark reality is that the health and well-being of children and youth will be the basis for economic global recovery and how we treat those most vulnerable, which includes those with paediatric palliative care needs, will also be a lasting testament to our moral integrity as global citizens.

Despite whatever barriers and limitations that exist, both Rita and I are firm in the belief that paediatric palliative care – giving it, administering it, teaching it – should be considered a realm of human enterprise that is often personal, frequently challenging, and always necessary.

This first section provides readers with a unique standpoint from which to see paediatric palliative care from a global perspective. No longer can we live and practise within our contained environments. Rather, taking a tag line from the 'green' movement, we in paediatric palliative care have to *act locally and think globally*. There are lessons to be learned from our collective knowledge and experience in all sectors of this world and through the following chapters we have captured a small picture of the global scene.

We as a global community process the wherewithal to secure a life of health and well-being for every human being on this earth. Living in an era where the human genome has been mapped, organ transplants are commonplace, embryonic stem cells have been successfully grown into organ tissue and we are quickly moving towards cloning of the first human beings, it is clear that there is no lack of knowledge and technology. Yet despite all this combined know-how, millions of children around the world continue to suffer needlessly from the consequences of a life-threatening or life-limiting diagnosis due to limited or no available comprehensive paediatric palliative care services.

In nation states where poverty is the norm, paediatric palliative care services, if available, can do little more than attempt to lessen the severity of symptoms and suffering experienced at the end of life for children and their families with minimal or no resources. Contained within these chapters are some uplifting and extraordinary examples of healthcare professionals refusing to do nothing, developing and implementing some very successful programmes.

In stark contrast to this scenario, wealthy nation states, while not lacking in resources to successfully deliver paediatric palliative care services, continue to wrestle with the moral imperatives resulting from a society that has come to believe that medicine can cure all and postpone death, especially for children, who are considered too young to die – a situation that has limited some children from palliative care services from diagnosis through to death.

REFERENCES

1 Hymowitz KS. *Ready or Not: Why Treating Children as Small Adults Endangers Their Future – And Ours*. New York: Simon & Schuster Inc; 1999.
2 Keating DP, Hertzman C, editors. *Developmental Health and the Wealth of Nations: social, biological and educational dynamics*. New York: Guilford Press; 1999.
3 Heinze E. *Of Innocence and Autonomy: children, sex and human rights*. Burlington VT: Ashgate Publishing Company; 2000.

1

Paediatric palliative care as a basic human right

Frank Brennan

The death of a child with a life-limiting illness is a tragedy. Globally the provision of care for those children and their families remains a neglected area. The adequacy of, and access to, the provision of palliative care for children varies enormously around the world. One modern response to this inadequacy has been to articulate a simple but challenging proposition – that the provision of palliative care for children is a human right. This chapter examines this proposition. It explores the theoretical foundation for this concept, its limitations and its potential as a tool of advocacy for the promotion of better paediatric palliative care services around the world.

THE EXTENT OF THE PROBLEM

Millions of children die each year. Many of those children die from causes secondary to poverty, malnutrition and inadequate supplies of clean water. Others die from a wide range of life-limiting illnesses, for which palliative care could be beneficial.[1] Approximately 130 of out every 1 million children aged 0–14 years develop cancer every year.[2] In developed nations, cancer is the leading cause of death from disease in the 1–14 years age group.[3] In developing countries, most children with cancer do not receive curative treatment. There is significant symptom burden associated with childhood malignancy.[4,5,6]

Infectious diseases such as tuberculosis, malaria and HIV/AIDS have caused widespread paediatric morbidity and mortality. Growing numbers of children and adolescents have HIV/AIDS. They suffer multiple symptoms and the majority will experience pain at some stage in their illness.[7] Children with cardiac, respiratory, renal and neurodegenerative life-limiting illnesses all experience significant symptoms.

The adequacy of the care of those children and the support of their families varies considerably. Around the world paediatric palliative care services remains sporadic. Progress is being made but enormous needs remain. One of the multiple responses to these needs has been, in the context of palliative care generally, to state that the provision of adequate palliative care is a universal human right. Clearly this is a noble sentiment. But beyond advocacy does this statement have a coherent foundation and what practical implications flow from its articulation?

THE CONCEPT OF PALLIATIVE CARE AS A HUMAN RIGHT

In 1992 Margaret Somerville, a leading authority in medical law, framed an argument about pain and suffering in the context of human rights. She concluded 'to leave patients in avoidable pain and suffering should be regarded as a serious breach of fundamental human rights.'[8] In the late 1990s this theme was advanced firstly in the context of pain management and then palliative care more broadly. To Cousins 'the relief of severe unrelenting pain would come at the top of a list of basic human rights.'[9] In a leading text on paediatric pain, the editors stated that 'we believe strongly that the treatment and alleviation of pain are a basic human right that exists regardless of age'.[10] These statements were followed by authoritative declarations by multiple international and national pain associations articulating a right to pain relief.[11] This advocacy culminated in the promulgation of the inaugural 'Global Day Against Pain' in 2004. Co-sponsored by the World Health Organization (WHO), the International Association for the Study of Pain and the European Federation of IASP Chapters, the theme of the day was 'Pain Relief Should be a Human Right'. In the following year the theme of the Global Day was 'The Relief of Pain in Childhood'.

Concurrently the association of palliative care and human rights entered the discourse. Echoing the seminal work of Somerville, a series of national and international declarations were made asserting that the provision of palliative care is a universal right. Each statement refers to all persons, including children. They include a Standing Committee of the Canadian Senate (2000),[12] The Cape Town Declaration (2002),[13] the European Committee of Ministers (2003),[14] the International Working Group (European School of Oncology) (2004)[15] and The Korea Declaration (2005) which emerged from the second Global Summit for National Hospice and Palliative Care Associations.[16] The theme of World Hospice Day in 2008 was: 'Palliative Care as a Human Right'. Concurrently the International Association of Hospice and Palliative Care and the Worldwide Palliative Care Alliance promulgated a Joint Declaration and Statement of Commitment on Palliative Care and Pain Treatment as Human Rights.[17]

To assert that the provision of palliative care to children with life-limiting illnesses is a human right is a powerful statement of advocacy. But beyond advocacy what is the foundation for this assertion? Without foundation it is admirable rhetoric based on a deep need; with foundation it is a much more potent concept that, potentially, leads to practical dividends borne of obligation.

A threshold question is: what are rights? All rights have as their common foundation a crystallisation of 'what is just or good . . . a just claim, whether legal, prescriptive or moral'.[18] Traditionally, a right evokes a correlative responsibility in others to fulfil that right. Possible moral and legal rights to paediatric palliative care shall now be explored.

MORAL FOUNDATION TO PAEDIATRIC PALLIATIVE CARE

The approach and philosophy of palliative care has a long antecedence. The earliest articulations of the responsibility of doctors to their patients with serious illness are not legal but ethical. Hippocrates stated that medicine, in general terms, meant 'to do away with the sufferings of the sick, to lessen the violence of their diseases and to refuse to treat those who are overmastered by their diseases, realizing that in such cases medicine is powerless'.[19] In the 18th century, John Gregory stated: 'It is as much the business of the physician to alleviate pain and smooth the avenues of death, when inevitable, as it is to cure disease'.[20] Similarly, in this century, Sjernsward and Clark opined 'there is a moral responsibility to give those who leave life . . . the same care and attention we give those who enter life'.[21]

Palliative care is a classic example of the bioethical principle of beneficence. Central to the good actions of doctors is the relief of pain and suffering. As Post *et al.* state, 'the ethical duty of beneficence is sufficient justification for providers to relieve the pain of these in their care . . .'[22] The principle of non-maleficence prohibits the infliction of harm. Persistent inadequately treated pain and other symptoms has both physical and psychological effects on the patient. For instance the failure to reasonably treat a child in pain may allow the pathophysiological effect of that pain – including central sensitisation – to occur. The harm, while indirect, is nevertheless, real. As Schechter *et al.* state, 'for humanitarian, physiologic and psychological reasons, pain control should be considered an integral part of the compassionate medical care of children'.[23] Failing to act, where a doctor–patient relationship exists, is a form of abandonment.

Beyond principlism (i.e. an approach founded on the strength of a broader principle), a virtue ethics approach would also yield a clear response. A virtuous doctor would place the investigation, monitoring and treatment of a child with symptoms associated with a life-limiting illness as a high priority. To this end, a virtuous doctor would enquire regularly, respond appropriately and refer wisely if unable to control these symptoms.

Whether one adopts a principlist approach (based on bioethical principles of autonomy, beneficence, non-maleficence and justice) or a virtue ethics approach, the ethics of the medical care of the child with a life-limiting illness has a deep humanitarian core – of compassion in approach, meticulous concentration on symptom control, clarity and sensitivity in communication to the patient and family, guiding all through the tragic journey of serious illness and, potentially, the death of a child. If there is a clear ethical obligation to relieve suffering or act virtuously by doing so, one may argue that from that obligation springs a right. The moral right to palliative care emerges from, and is directly founded upon, the obligation of a doctor to act ethically.

THE FOUNDATION OF PAEDIATRIC PALLIATIVE CARE AS A HUMAN RIGHT

The recognition of human rights has a long antecedence. In the modern era they came to centre stage with the creation of the United Nations (UN) and the promulgation of the UN Declaration of Human Rights and the multiple human rights conventions that followed. In addition human rights are recognised in regional human rights convention and, for some countries, express recognition of human rights under national constitutions. Within that structure what are the foundations of paediatric palliative care as a human right?

INTERNATIONAL LAW

At international law the rights of children to the provision of health services derives from several international covenants.

The Universal Declaration of Human Rights states that: 'Everyone has the right to a standard of living adequate for the health and well-being of himself and of his family, including . . . medical care' and 'Motherhood and childhood are entitled to special care and assistance.'[24]

The International Covenant on Economic, Social and Cultural Rights (ICESCR) articulates the right 'of everyone to the enjoyment of the highest attainable standard of physical and mental health.'[25] The Covenant obliges state parties to deliver on the rights it guarantees to the maximum of their available resources.[26] Rights articulated in the Covenant are seen as aspirational – rights to be achieved progressively over time to the maximum capacity of each signatory nation state. While there is no appeal process, signatory nations are expected to report regularly to a Committee overseeing the Covenant.

The next relevant covenant is the UN Convention on the Rights of the Child (CRC).[27] It applies to all children under the age of 18 years. Article 24 of this Convention states:

1 State parties recognise the right of the child to the enjoyment of the highest attainable standard of health and to the facilities for the treatment of illness and rehabilitation of health. State Parties shall strive to ensure that no child is deprived of his or her right of access to such health care services.
2 State Parties shall pursue the full implementation of this right and, in particular, shall take appropriate measures: . . . (b) to ensure the provision of necessary medical assistance and healthcare to all children . . .

In addition, there are several other Articles in the Convention that have implications, directly or indirectly, for paediatric palliative care. These include a duty on all signatory nations to recognise the dignity of mentally and physically disabled children and to 'take all appropriate legislative, administrative, social and educational measures to protect the child from . . . neglect or negligent treatment . . .'[28] Finally, Article 3 of the Convention states: 'In all actions concerning children . . . the best interests of the child shall be the primary consideration.'[29]

There is no express right to palliative care in these instruments. Nevertheless the WHO defines both 'health' and 'palliative care' broadly. The provision of healthcare occurs in a continuum, which includes serious illness, dying and death. Therefore an argument can be made that a right to palliative care may be implied from the international right to health.

THE CONTENT OF THE OBLIGATION

The international covenants obligate individual nations who have signed them. In the context of paediatric palliative care what are the obligations on governments? These may be gleaned from the conventions themselves and the authoritative Comments made by the Committees overseeing them.

In 2000, the Committee overseeing the ICESCR issued a General Comment on the right to health, stating what it saw as the 'core obligations' of all signatory nations, irrespective of resources.[30] They include obligations to ensure access to health facilities, goods and services on a non-discriminatory basis, to provide essential drugs, as defined by the WHO, and to adopt and implement a national public health strategy. Interpreting this Comment in the context of palliative care generally, including paediatric palliative care, this would oblige nations to ensure a universal access to services, the provision of basic medications for symptom control and terminal care, including analgesics and the adoption and implementation of national paediatric pain and palliative care policies.

In addition to the 'core obligations' the Committee also enumerated obligations 'of comparable priority'.[31] These included: 'To provide education and access to information concerning the main health problems in the community, including methods of preventing and controlling them . . .' and 'To provide appropriate training for health personnel, including education on health and human rights . . .' In the context of palliative care, a 'main health problem' in all countries, this would obligate governments to ensure the education of health professionals in the principles and practice of palliative care and, further, provide access to the general community to information regarding it.

In addition to the above statements on the right to healthcare generally, there have been three other General Comments that are directly relevant to the palliative care of children and adolescents. The first two are included in General Comments made by the Committee that oversees the Convention on the Rights of the Child. General Comment No 4 concerned adolescent health. Here the Committee discussed the special needs of adolescents, reiterated the importance of providing adequate healthcare facilities, goods and services to adolescents and the importance of providing adequate information on health.[32] In General Comment No 3, the Committee stated that adolescents have a right to information about HIV/AIDS as part of an overall right to information. Finally, General Comment No 5 by the Committee that oversees the ICESCR discussed the obligations on individual governments that flow from economic, social and cultural rights for persons with disabilities. These include children and adolescents. Indeed, the Comment cites the Standard Rules, which state that 'States should ensure that persons with disabilities, particularly infants and children, are provided with the same level of medical care within the same system as other members of society.'[33]

Further authoritative guidance on the content of the obligations that flow from the right to health come from statements made by the Committees overseeing these Covenants. Those recommendations were made to individual countries. The Committee overseeing the Convention on the Rights of the Child has recommended that certain countries improve HIV prevention services for children, protect children from HIV-based discrimination and include childrens' rights in HIV strategies.[34] The Committee also made recommendations that certain nations prioritise budget allocations to HIV-affected children[35] and to ensure free-trade agreements do not impede access to low-cost HIV/AIDS medications for children.[36] Another example is a recommendation by the Committee overseeing the ICESCR in 2001 for the Ukraine to provide information on HIV to adolescents.

STATEMENTS BY UN SPECIAL RAPPORTEURS ON HUMAN RIGHTS

In addition to the above, two UN Special Rapporteurs on human rights issues have made explicit statements to the international community linking pain management and palliative care to human rights. In a statement made to the UN Human Rights Council in 2008 the Special Rapporteur on the Right to Health placed palliative care firmly within the obligations that derive from the international right to health: 'Many other right-to-health issues need urgent attention, such as palliative care ... Every year millions suffer horrific, avoidable pain ... Palliative care needs greater attention.'[37]

Similarly the UN Special Rapporteur on Torture in his report to the Human Rights Council in January 2009 stated: 'the de facto denial of access to pain relief, if it causes pain and suffering, constitutes cruel, inhuman or degrading treatment or punishment' and 'all measures should be taken to ensure full access [to pain treatment and opioid analgesics] and to overcome current regulatory, educational and attitudinal obstacles to ensure full access to palliative care.'[38]

In addition, the two Rapporteurs made a joint statement to the Chairperson of the Commission on Narcotic Drugs in late 2008. After reviewing the inadequacies of pain management and Palliative Care around the world, they stated that:

> The failure to ensure access to controlled medicines for the relief of pain and suffering threatens fundamental rights to health and to protection against cruel inhuman and degrading treatment. International human rights law requires that governments must provide essential medicines – which include, among others, opioid analgesics – as part of their minimum core obligations under the right to health ... Lack of access to essential medicines, including for pain relief, is a global human rights issue and must be addressed forcefully ...[39]

These Statements are a major breakthrough. They not only represent the most explicit linkage of human rights with pain management and palliative care made to date by representatives of the UN, but they also provide clinicians and advocates a clear statement of recommendations to present to the health ministries of individual countries.

DO THESE OBLIGATIONS, DERIVED FROM INTERNATIONAL LAW, ACCORD WITH PROFESSIONAL GUIDELINES FOR THE PROVISION OF PAEDIATRIC PALLIATIVE CARE?

This is an important question. If there are tensions between the two, then individual nations, if challenged on their provision of paediatric palliative care, would legitimately point out such differences. A close examination of the two sources – one from international law, the other from the WHO and international palliative care organisations themselves – reveals an identical set of standards.

For paediatric palliative care, further guidance on the minimum standards expected by the international community emerges from two other sources. The first is the WHO; the second, the international palliative care community itself.

The World Health Organization

There are two sources for guidance from the WHO. The first is the WHO definition of paediatric palliative care.[40]

Palliative care for children represents a special, albeit closely related, field to adult palliative care. The WHO's definition of palliative care appropriate for children and their families is as follows; the principles apply to other paediatric chronic disorders.

➤ Palliative care for children is the active total care of the child's body, mind and spirit, and also involves giving support to the family.
➤ It begins when illness is diagnosed, and continues regardless of whether or not a child receives treatment directed at the disease.
➤ Health providers must evaluate and alleviate a child's physical, psychological and social distress.
➤ Effective palliative care requires a broad multidisciplinary approach that includes the family and makes use of available community resources; it can be successfully implemented even if resources are limited.
➤ It can be provided in tertiary care facilities, in community health centres and even in children's homes.

The second is population-wide WHO recommendations on palliative care, which include children and adolescents. They include that all countries should adopt a national palliative care policy, ensure the training and education of health professionals and promote public awareness, ensure the availability of morphine in all healthcare settings and that all countries should ensure that minimum standards for pain relief and palliative care are progressively adopted at all levels of care. Recognising the widely divergent capacities of countries, the WHO set out general recommendations for different resource settings. For countries with low resource settings, home-based care is probably the best way of achieving good quality care. In countries with medium-level resources, services should be provided by primary healthcare clinics and home-based care. In high resource settings, there is a variety of options including home-based care.

International statements by the palliative care community

As indicated above there have been several international statements made, over recent years, asserting that the provision of palliative care is a universal right. Collectively they represent powerful advocacy, statements of intent and objective and provide a sense of the architecture and content of this purported right.

The Cape Town Declaration emerged from a conference of African palliative care trainers held in South Africa in 2002.[41] Conscious of the appalling unfolding tragedy of HIV/AIDS, the poorly-met needs of cancer patients and the inadequacy of governmental response throughout the African continent, the Declaration asserted four main propositions.

1 Palliative care is a right of every adult and child with a life-limiting disease.
2 Appropriate drugs, including strong opioids, should be made accessible to every patient requiring them in every sub-Saharan country and at all levels of care, from hospitals to community clinics and homes.
3 The establishment of education programmes at all levels of the learning continuum . . . for all formal and informal caregivers, including medical and nursing trainees, community workers, volunteers and informal caregivers.
4 Palliative care should be provided at all levels of care: primary, secondary and tertiary. While primary care is emphasised, secondary and tertiary level teams are needed to lead and foster primary level care.

The Korea Declaration emerged from the 2nd Global Summit of National Hospice and Palliative Care Associations (2005).[42] It stated, amongst other points, that governments must include hospice and palliative care as part of all government health policy, integrate hospice and palliative care training into the curricula of health professionals, ensure the availability and affordability of all necessary drugs, especially opioids, eliminate regulatory and legal barriers to opioid availability and strive to make hospice and palliative care available to all citizens in the setting of their choice. The Joint Declaration and Statement of Commitment on Palliative Care and Pain Treatment as Human Rights (2008),[43] an initiative of the International Association of Hospice and Palliative Care Associations and the Worldwide Palliative Care Alliance, enumerated a similar list of ideals. It was the first international Declaration joining palliative care, pain, cancer, AIDS and other related organisations for this same purpose. Finally the International Association for the Study of Pain (IASP) designated the year commencing October 2008 as the Global Year Against Cancer Pain.

Another significant international statement that has clear implications for the provision of palliative care was the Montreal Statement on the Human Right to Essential Medicines (2005).[44] The Essential Drug List provided by the WHO is a model policy guide for the national determination of essential drugs. Relevant to palliative care, that list includes opioids. The Statement emerged from an international workshop of governments, international agencies, civil society groups and academic institutions. The Statement expressly links the international right to health with the universal access to these essential medications.

Towards a transdisciplinary consensus on the content of obligation

Synthesising these sources (the Committees that oversee the international right to the healthcare of children, the WHO and the international palliative care community) a consensus on the content of the obligation on individual governments in relation to paediatric palliative care emerges:

1 the creation and implementation of paediatric palliative care policies
2 equity of access to services, without discrimination
3 availability and affordability of critical medications, including opioids
4 the provision of paediatric palliative care at all levels of care

5   the integration of palliative care education at all levels of the learning continuum from informal caregivers to health professionals.

OTHER FOUNDATIONS IN HUMAN RIGHTS INSTRUMENTS

In addition to the international human rights instruments described above, several regions in the world have charters that articulate a right to healthcare, including for children and adolescents.[45] Regional human rights commissions overseeing these instruments have shown a willingness to find in the right to health a duty on individual governments to provide specific services.[46] That has implications for the provision of all healthcare services, including palliative care.

Another source of human rights are national constitutions. Many of the world's nations have constitutions which enumerate the rights of their citizens to receive adequate healthcare. Several national constitutions expressly protect the economic and social rights of children.[47] One of the strongest examples of a national constitution incorporating the social and economic rights of children is the Constitution of South Africa. Section 28 provides that:

(1)   Every child has the right –
      (c)   to basic . . . health care services . . .
(2)   A child's best interests are of paramount importance in every matter concerning a child.[48]

These rights of children exist concurrently with a universal right of access to health services for all citizens.[49] That universal right includes a responsibility on the South African state to 'take reasonable legislative and other measures, within its available resources, to achieve the progressive realisation' of this right.[50] In *Minister of Health v Treatment Action Committee*[51] the Constitutional Court of South Africa examined the extent of these rights. At the time, the national government restricted the use of nevirapine, a medication whose objective was to prevent the transmission of HIV from mother to infants, to two government hospitals per province as part of a pilot study. The Treatment Action Campaign brought a suit against the South African government alleging that this restriction violated the constitutional right to health of the HIV-positive pregnant women and their children. On the basis of either the general constitutional right to health or the specific rights of children, the Court stated that the policy of restricting the availability of nevirapine was unreasonable and a violation of the government's obligation to take 'reasonable legislative and other measures, within its available resources, to achieve the progressive realisation' of the 'right to healthcare services'. Equally, the Court held that, given the 'incomprehensible calamity' of the HIV/AIDS epidemic in South Africa, the government's plan of moving slowly from limited research and training programmes to a more available programme was not reasonable. This case illustrates that any constitutional right guaranteeing access to healthcare services, including palliative care services for children, will always be circumscribed by the wording of the constitution itself. In the case of South Africa, the Court needed to determine whether it was reasonable or otherwise for the state to make certain decisions on the basis of their national resources.

HOW COULD ARTICULATING THIS RIGHT ADVANCE PALLIATIVE CARE FOR CHILDREN?

Assuming paediatric palliative care can be implied from the universal right 'to the highest attainable standards of health', two questions remain. First, could an individual or group, citing the international Covenants, complain that this right to palliative care in children was not being met? And as a corollary to that, what pressure can UN bodies exert to induce countries to provide adequate palliative care to children as part of their health services?

There is no direct complaint mechanism for rights enunciated in the Covenant on Economic, Social and Cultural Rights. The international community assesses compliance with the Covenant through reports submitted by all nations to the Committee, describing their efforts to implement these rights. This Committee has outlined what it considered to be the 'core obligations' and 'obligations of a comparable priority' of nations in their provision of healthcare, irrespective of their resources.[52]

For the Convention on the Rights of the Child, a Committee was established to examine 'the progress made by State Parties in achieving the realisation of the obligations undertaken' in the Convention.[53] To this end, signatory nations have undertaken to provide regular reports to the Committee of the measures they have adopted to give effect to these rights.[54] Again, there is no direct complaint mechanism but the Committee has a significant moral or persuasive role in the compliance with rights, including paediatric pain management within the universal right to the provision of childhood healthcare. The difficulty remains, as many writers have pointed out,[55] that the Committee does not have an enforcement mechanism beyond the reporting requirements. Effectively, it relies on a combination of constructive dialogue with state parties and moral persuasion.

Two strategies flow from the above. The first is for national and international associations of palliative care and pain management to remind governments of their obligations under the international conventions. The second is for these associations to make submissions to the Committees overseeing both Covenants. Those submissions would seek to highlight the inadequacies of paediatric palliative care management and the critical role of governments in providing policies and programmes appropriate to improve the infrastructure, opioid availability, funding and staffing relevant to paediatric palliative care management. Through that strategy, those Committees could exert moral pressure on countries to fulfil the basic palliative care needs of their paediatric populations.

This avenue of advocacy has commenced. Joint submissions have been made to UN bodies by the IASP, the International Association of Hospice and Palliative care (IAHPC) and the Worldwide Palliative Care Alliance (WWPCA). The first was to the UN Human Rights Council. In 2008 the Council invited submissions on the human rights implications of the HIV/AIDS pandemic. The joint submission outlined the human rights implications of pain management and palliative care for patients, including children, with HIV/AIDS and their families.[56] The second submission was made to the Committee overseeing the ICESCR. In 2008 the Committee prepared a draft General Comment on the issue of discrimination and invited comments. The joint submission described discrimination in the provision of, and access to, both pain management and palliative care to many groups, including children and adolescents.[57]

THE LIMITS OF ADVOCACY BASED ON HUMAN RIGHTS

Advocacy in isolation can be powerful. Advocacy with a solid foundation in both ethics and law may well be irresistible. For the articulation of a right to paediatric palliative care to be anything other than an aspiration, however noble, requires this foundation. Certainly, it is fitting that the international dimension of the problem is matched by, at least as a threshold, international law, which clearly states a universal right of children to the provision of healthcare services. This is a useful point to start, but not to finish. The promotion of a right to palliative care for children and adolescents is an important, but not sufficient, prerequisite for better care. As Hunt stated, rights have the 'capacity to be elements of emancipation, but they are neither a perfect nor exclusive vehicle'.[58] For the palliative care of children to significantly improve, multiple other requirements need to be met. Necessarily this should include comprehensive education of paediatric pain and symptom management to nursing and medical undergraduates, a liberalisation of the availability of opioids in many countries, a cultural shift from opiophobia to opioid acceptance and greater access to services providing for the physical, emotional and spiritual needs of patients and their families.

In basing an argument for the provision of paediatric palliative care on the human right to healthcare, another potential difficulty is the need for context. A child with a life-limiting illness will certainly need adequate pain and symptom management and all the other components of palliative care. But they will need much more. If we are focusing on the comfort of a child with a life-limiting illness, surely that must include water, food, an habitable environment, warmth, bedding and sanitation as much as symptom control. Indeed, it would be artificial to separate a 'right to palliative care' from a general right to health, housing, water and sanitation. All are interconnected. All determine good health, even and including at the end of life.

CONCLUSION

Globally, the provision of palliative care for children and adolescents with life-limiting illnesses remains sporadic, under-resourced and incomplete. The challenge is to move beyond this point. To articulate a right of children and adolescents to palliative care is one tool amongst many. Beyond an instrument of advocacy, that articulation has a significant foundation in ethics and law. A human right to palliative care may be implied from the international right to healthcare. In relation to paediatric palliative care, there is a clear consensus between the obligations that derive from that right and the recommendations of the WHO and the international palliative care community. Nevertheless, the right should not be seen in isolation. Children and adolescents with life-limiting illnesses have many needs – including adequate nutrition, clean water, housing and sanitation. At a broader level, the challenge is for the disciplines of paediatric medicine, law and ethics to combine in not merely promoting, but also providing, compassionate palliative care for children throughout the world.

CASE STUDY

A seven-year-old girl has HIV since birth. Her parents have died of AIDS. With inadequate supervision and family dislocation she has been missing her anti-retroviral medications for some time. She is rapidly becoming more ill. She has multiple symptoms including moderate to severe pain and dyspnoea. The village clinic informs the family 'that nothing can be done for her'. She lives in a country with no formal palliative care services, extremely strict opioids laws and no recognition of palliative care with the national health policy.

N.I.C.E. analysis

Needs
- Understanding of palliative care for children.
- National palliative care and pain policies that include children.
- Access to essential medications, including opioids.
- Education.

Concerns
- Human rights are not universally accepted.
- An argument based on human rights is not the only answer.
- The obligations that flow from international human rights apply to governments and not to individuals.
- Many nations have draconian opioid laws.

Interests
- A growing movement of advocacy employing a human rights discourse to argue for a universal access for palliative care.
- A growing recognition of these needs within the UN.

Expectations
- That the UN will hold nations accountable for breaches of their obligations in providing universal access to paediatric palliative care.
- That individuals/professional associations will use an argument based on human rights to advocate for paediatric palliative care.

From the above analysis please reflect on:
- You are making a submission to the national government to improve access to paediatric palliative care. What argument based on human rights could you employ?
- Specifically what obligations does the government have?
- Which Committees of the UN could a national or international palliative care association approach to make a submission?
- If the country replied 'We have no resources' what would be your response?

- In addition to healthcare, what other basic human rights are essential for the provision of adequate paediatric palliative care for this young girl?

Action plan: next steps

- To include, in making submissions to governments advocating better provision of paediatric palliative care, an argument based on their obligations under international human rights law.
- To advocate for more liberal opioid laws based, in part, on these human rights obligations.
- For international palliative care associations to make submissions to the relevant UN committees overseeing the right to health, including the Convention on the Rights of the Child.
- To help governments to fulfil their international obligations by advice, advocacy and facilitating links.

REFERENCES

1 World Health Organization. *The World Health Report*. Geneva: World Health Organization; 1995.
2 Robinson LL. General Principles of the Epidemiology of Childhood Cancer. Principles and practice of paediatric oncology. 2nd ed. Philadelphia, PA: Lippincott; 1993. pp. 3–10.
3 Ibid.
4 Wolfe J, Grier HE, Klar N, *et al.* Symptoms and suffering at the end of life in children with cancer. *NEJM*. 2000; **342**: 326–33.
5 McCallum DE, Byrne P, Bruera E. How children die in hospital. *J Pain Symptom Manag*. 2000; **20**: 417–23.
6 Hongo T, Watanabe C, Okada S. Analysis of the circumstances at the end of life in children with cancer: symptoms, suffering and acceptance. *Pediatr Int*. 2003; **45**: 60–4.
7 Oleske JM, Czarniecki L. Continuum of palliative care: lessons drawn from caring for children infected with HIV-1. *Lancet*. 1999; **354**: 1287–90.
8 Somerville M. Death of pain: pain, suffering, and ethics. In: *Death Talk: The Case Against Euthanasia and Physician-Assisted Suicide*. Montreal, QC: McGill-Queen's University Press; 2001. pp. 218–30 at 227.
9 Cousins MJ. Pain: the past, present and future of anesthesiology? The EA Rovenstine Memorial Lecture. *Anesthesiology*. 1999; **91**: 538–51.
10 Schechter NL, Berde CB, Yaster M. Pain in infants, children and adolescents. An overview. In: Schechter NL, Berde CB, Yaster M, editors. *Pain in Infants, Children and Adolescents*. 2nd ed. Philadelphia, PA: Lippincott, Williams & Wilkins; 2003. pp. 12–13.
11 The American Academy of Pain Medicine, the American Pain Society, the Joint Commission on Accreditation of Healthcare Organizations (JACHO), the American Geriatrics Society, the Canadian Pain Society, the European Federation of IASP Chapters, the Australian and New Zealand College of Anaesthetists, Faculty of Pain Medicine and the Joint Faculty of Intensive Care Medicine.
12 Standing Committee on Social Affairs, Science and Technology. *Quality End-of-Life Care: The Rights of Every Canadian; Final Report of the Subcommittee to Update Of Life and Death*. Ottawa, ON: Senate of Canada; 2000.

13 Mpanga SL, Mwangi-Powell F, Pereira J, *et al.* The Cape Town Palliative Care Declaration: home-grown solutions for sub-Saharan Africa. *J Palliat Med.* 2002; **6**: 341–3.

14 Council of Europe. Recommendation Rec (2003) 24 of the Committee of Ministers to member states on the organisation of palliative care and explanatory memorandum. Available at: www.coe.int/t/dg3/health/recommendations_en.asp (accessed 20 February 2010).

15 Ahmedzai SH, Costa A, Blengini C, *et al.* A new international framework for palliative care. *Eur J Can.* 2004; **40**: 2192–200.

16 The Korea Declaration. *Report of the Second Global Summit of National Hospice and Palliative Care Associations.* Seoul, Korea: National Hospice and Palliative Care Associations; 2005.

17 Joint Declaration text. Available at: www.hospicecare.com/resources/pain_pallcare_hr/docs/jdsc.pdf (accessed November 2008).

18 *The Macquarie Dictionary.* 2nd ed. Sydney, NSW: The Macquarie Dictionary Publishers; 1992.

19 Hippocrates. The arts. In: Reiser SJ, Dyck AJ, Curran WJ, editors. *Ethics in Medicine: historical perspectives and contemporary concerns.* Cambridge, MA: MIT Press; 1977. p.6.

20 Gregory J. *Lectures on the Duties and Qualifications of Physicians.* Philadelphia, PA: M Carey & Sons; 1817.

21 Stjernsward J, Clark D. Palliative Medicine – a global perspective. In: Doyle D, Hanks G, Cherny N, *et al.*, editors. *Oxford Textbook of Palliative Medicine.* 3rd ed. Oxford: Oxford University Press; 2005. p. 1199.

22 Post LF, Blustein J, Gordon E, *et al.* Pain: ethics, culture and informed consent to relief. *J Law Med Ethics.* 1996; **24**: 348.

23 Schechter NL, Berde CB, Yaster M. Pain in infants, children and adolescents: an overview. In: Schechter NL, Berde CB Yaster M, editors. *Pain in Infants, Children and Adolescents.* 2nd ed. Philadelphia, PA: Lippincott, Williams & Wilkins; 2003. p. 14.

24 United Nations Declaration of Human Rights (1948), Article 25 (1) and (2). Available at: www.unhchr.ch/udhr/ (accessed 17 February 2010).

25 International Covenant on Economic, Social and Cultural Rights. Article 12. Available at www.unhchr.ch/html/menu3/b/a_cescr.htm (accessed 17 February 2010).

26 Ibid.

27 *Conventions on the Rights of the Child* (1989), Article 24. Adopted by the United Nations General Assembly in November 1989 and entered into force in September 1990.

28 Ibid, Article 19.

29 Ibid, Article 3.

30 Committee on Economic, Social and Cultural Rights. General Comment No 14 *The Rights to the Highest Attainable Standard of Health* (Article 12 of the Covenant). 22nd Session April–May 2000 E/C 12/2000/4 para 43.

31 Committee on Economic, Social and Cultural Rights. General Comment No 14 *The Rights to the Highest Attainable Standard of Health* (Article 12 of the Covenant). 22nd Session April–May 2000 E/C 12/2000/4 para 44.

32 United Nations Conventions on the Rights of the Child. General Comment No 4: *Adolescent Health and Development in the Context of The Convention on the Rights of the Child* (2003). Available at: www.unhchr.ch/tbs/doc.nsf/(symbol)/CRC.GC.2003.4.En (accessed 20 February 2010).

33 Committee on Economic, Social and Cultural Rights. General Comment No 5, Article 34.

34 See comments made by the Committee on the Convention on the Rights of the Child on Benin (2006), Senegal (2006), Swaziland (2006), Nigeria (2005), Uganda (2005), Armenia

(2004), Burkina Faso (2002), Mozambique (2002), Ukraine (2002), Kenya (2001), Georgia (2000), Tajikistan (2000) and South Africa (2000).

35 See comments made by the Committee on the Convention on the Rights of the Child on Swaziland (2006), Uganda (2005) and Botswana (2004).

36 See comments made by the Committee on the Convention on the Rights of the Child on Botswana (2004).

37 UN Human Rights Council. Statement by Paul Hunt, Special Rapporteur on the Right of Everyone to the Highest Attainable Standard of Physical and Mental Health. Available at: www. hospicecare.com/resources/painpallcarehr/docs/paulhuntsoralremarks_hrcmarch2008.pdf (accessed 17 February 2010).

38 Report of the Special Rapporteur on Torture and other cruel, inhuman or degrading treatment or punishment, Manfred Nowak. Promotion and Protection of all Human Rights, Civil, Political, Economic, Social and Cultural Rights, including the right to development. Human Rights Council, Seventh Session, Agenda Item 3. A/HRC/10/44. 14 January 2009.

39 Special Rapporteurs on the question of Torture and the Right of everyone to the highest attainable standard of physical and mental health. Letter to Mr D. Best, Vice-Chairperson of the Commission on Narcotic Drugs, December 10, 2008. Available at: www.ihra.net/ Assets/1384/1/SpecialRapporteursLettertoCND012009.pdf (accessed 17 February 2010).

40 World Health Organization. WHO Definition of Palliative Care for Children. Available at: www.who.int/cancer/palliative/definition/en/ (accessed 17 February 2010).

41 Mpanga SL, Mwangi-Powell F, Pereira J, et al. The Cape Town Palliative Care Declaration: home-grown solutions for sub-Saharan Africa. *J Palliative Medicine*. 2003; **6**: 341–3.

42 The Korea Declaration. *Report of the Second Global Summit of National Hospice and Palliative Care Associations, Seoul, March 2005*. Available at: http://docs.google.com/viewer ?a=v&q=cache:wlAAO82I3cYJ:www.eolc-observatory.net/global/pdf/NHPCA_2.pdf+The +Korea+Declaration.+Report+of+the+Second+Global+Summit+of+National+Hospice+a nd+Palliative&hl=en&gl=uk&pid=bl&srcid=ADGEEShW4rid9Rebexl0BPry63oAUxAa5fF Yv-NYzKRV1Zs-y88XUPWBVRft0tMYL2hOInPpb4AFuthiEjd5OuqdMis42PUFdzU ufoi4cAnU9tOcrA2w7xd-8ySDVlmrJNnyiIlvoEBa&sig=AHIEtbSR3dziDQ4aIqyeZo QpkMmnbLwubA (accessed 20 February 2010).

43 Joint Declaration and Statement of Commitment on Palliative Care and Pain Treatment as Human Rights. Available at: www.hospicecare.com/resources/pain_pallcare_hr/docs/jdsc. pdf (accessed November 2008).

44 www.accessmeds.org/Statement.htm

45 European Social Charter of 1961 as Revised in 1996, Article 11 (1966), African Charter on Human and Peoples' Rights, Article 16 (1981) and the Additional Protocol to the American Convention on Human Rights in the Area of Economic, Social and Cultural Rights, Article 10 (1988).

46 For instance see *World Organization Against Torture, Lawyer's Committee for Human Rights and Others v Zaire*. African Commission on Human and Peoples' Rights. Session 19. April 1996.

47 These include Brazil, Columbia, Croatia, Malawi, South Africa and Turkey.

48 Constitution of the Republic of South Africa, section 28.

49 Constitution of the Republic of South Africa, section 27.

50 Constitution of the Republic of South Africa, section 27 (2).

51 Constitutional Court of South Africa 2002 (10) BCLR 1033.

52 Committee on Economic, Social and Cultural Rights. General Comment No. 14 *The Rights to*

the Highest Attainable Standard of Health (Article 12 of the Covenant). 22nd Session April–May 2000 E/C 12/2000/4 par 43.

53 UN Convention on the Rights of The Child. Article 43.

54 UN Convention on the Rights of The Child. Article 44.

55 Freeman M. The End of the Century of the Child? In: Freeman M, editor. *Current Legal Problems*. Vol. 53. New York: Oxford University Press. p. 509; Douglas G. The significance of international law for the development of family law in England and Wales. In: Bridge C, editor. *Family Law Towards the Millennium: essays for PM Bromley*. London: Butterworths; 1997. pp. 91–2, 105–6.

56 International Association for the Study of Pain (IASP), International Association for Hospice and Palliative Care (IAHPC) and the Worldwide Palliative Care Alliance (WWPCA). *Pain Management, Palliative Care and Human Rights in the Context of HIV/AIDS – a submission to the United Nations Human Rights Council.* November 2008.

57 International Association for the Study of Pain (IASP), International Association for Hospice and Palliative Care (IAHPC) and the Worldwide Palliative Care Alliance (WWPCA). *Non-Discrimination in the Provision of Pain Management and Palliative Care in the Context of 'the right to the highest attainable standard of health'* (Article 12 of the International Covenant on Economic, Social and Cultural Rights). *A submission to the Committee for the International Covenant on Economic, Social and Cultural Rights regarding: Draft General Comment No. 20 Non-discrimination and Economic, Social and Cultural Rights (Article 2(2)).* January 2009.

58 Hunt A. Rights and social movements: counter-hegemonic strategies. *J Law Soc.* 1990; **17**: 309–25.

The International Children's Palliative Care Network (ICPCN): a global overview

Lizzie Chambers, Sue Boucher, Julia Downing, Faith Mwangi-Powell and Sabine Kraft

BACKGROUND TO CHILDREN'S PALLIATIVE CARE WORLDWIDE

The global children's hospice and palliative care movement is growing significantly to meet the increasing need for service development worldwide, largely as a result of the HIV/AIDS pandemic. However, in many places around the world, children's hospice and palliative care services are emerging with little or no national support and with no local or regional networks to provide advocacy and coordinated strategies for ensuring the sustainable development of services. There are approximately 20 countries in the world that have children's hospice and palliative care services. The unmet need is immense.

Worldwide it is estimated that at least seven million children can benefit from palliative care. Epidemiological data on mortality and morbidity points to the growing need to focus on improving children's access to palliative care and its integration in paediatric care.[1]

Each year in the United States (US), approximately 500 000 children cope with life-threatening conditions, and 53 000 children die from trauma, lethal congenital conditions, extreme pre-maturity, heritable disorders or acquired illness. Less than 1% of children needing hospice services receive it. In the US, 80% of children under 15 with cancer are cured, but 80% of the world's children with cancer live in low- and middle-income countries where there is a higher risk of death because of late diagnosis or lack of treatment. Palliative care, including end-of-life care, is vital.[3,4]

Figures in England show that the annual mortality rate for children aged less than 19 years with life-limiting conditions is 1.44 per 10 000, and for 20- to 29-year-olds 1.64 per 10 000. The estimated prevalence rate for children and young people likely to require palliative care services in England is 16 per 10 000 population aged 0–19 years.[5]

In Germany a national study was done to show that the majority of children dying from cancer do not have access to comprehensive palliative care services at home, and that there needs to be increased education about palliative and end-of-life care.[6]

With the global surge of AIDS/HIV affecting populations, child mortality figures have increased drastically in developing countries due to mother-to-child transmission (MTCT). According to the UNAIDS/WHO Epidemic Update for 2005,[7] out of the 3.1 million people who died from AIDS, over half a million were children under 15 years of age. It is estimated at the end of 2005, 2.3 million children in the world were living with HIV, and 700 000 were newly infected. For example, child mortality figures have nearly doubled in Botswana and Zimbabwe since 1990. Globally, at least one-quarter of HIV-infected newborns die before the age of one year due to immuno-suppression; up to 60% die before the age of two; and most die before the age of five. It is important to consider that due to limited HIV-monitoring facilities in developing countries, estimates are inaccurate, and actual figures will be much higher. Almost 40% of all admissions to hospice programmes in South Africa from 2005 to 2006 were children and youth under the age of 21.[8,9]

Children's palliative care provision is an area of great need within sub-Saharan Africa. In 2007, more than 1.8 million children under 15 were living with HIV/AIDS and 240 000 dying from the disease in 2007.[9] In terms of cancer, 20% of all cancer cases in sub-Saharan Africa are among children contributing to 25% of total cancer deaths.[1] Consequently, the need for palliative care for children is immense.

KEY ISSUES

Listed below are some of the key issues that need to be addressed to ensure the development of good quality palliative care for all children and young people:

Specific differences between adult and children's palliative care

➤ Children have specific palliative care needs and continue to need education and play.
➤ Children with a life-limiting illness continue to develop physically, emotionally and cognitively, which affects their communication skills and ability to understand their disease and death.
➤ The number of children dying is small, compared with the number of adults, except in sub-Saharan Africa, where AIDS is causing the deaths of large numbers of children.
➤ Many of the individual conditions are extremely rare with diagnoses specific to childhood, although the child may survive into early adulthood.
➤ The time scale of children's illness is generally different from adults; palliative care may last only a few days or months, or extend over many years.
➤ Care for children embraces the whole family. Grandparents, parents and siblings are especially vulnerable and bear a heavy responsibility for personal and nursing care.

Assessment and control of symptoms and availability of medications

➤ There is insufficient research and evidence base on the use of medication to treat pain and other symptoms for children. Most studies have not included children as test subjects due to ethical reasons, and there is therefore limited information available on side effects of drugs and dosage effectiveness.[10]

➤ Pain in children is under-assessed and under-treated because healthcare professionals do not have access to necessary analgesics or are not adequately trained in their administration.[11,12]

➤ Children need appropriate pain and symptom management during the course of their illness. Studies have concluded that a vast majority of children with cancer need regular pain medication while in terminal care, whether it is administered orally or intravenously at home. Suffering from pain was more likely in children whose parents reported that the physician was not actively involved in providing end-of-life care.[13,14]

➤ Potentially life-saving drugs for children living with HIV and AIDS are simply not yet available in many parts of the world. Formulations of anti-retrovirals for children remain rare. Many that do exist are unpleasant and can affect children adhering to their treatment. Palliative care must be provided concurrently with treatment where treatment is available, and is vital where treatment is not available.[3]

➤ HIV progresses to AIDS much more rapidly in babies than adults, increasing their risk of dying in their very first years due to immunosuppression. With most children having no access to treatment for HIV/AIDS, it is challenging to prevent infection and death of children in resource-limited settings, and palliative care will have an increasing role in improving the quality of life of these children as well as the length of their life.[15]

Misconceptions about children's palliative care

➤ Families should not have to choose between life-prolonging care and palliative care, when they can go hand-in-hand. There exists an assumption that palliative care should not be considered until all curative options are exhausted, when in fact palliative care should be seen as significantly improving a child's quality of life. It should be integrated with curative treatment, and throughout the course of the illness regardless of the child's outcome.

➤ In some countries healthcare professionals never acknowledge death in children. The cultural denial of the fact that children actually die prohibits the development of children's palliative care services.

➤ The taboo around child death, without an open and honest approach in dealing with death and without adequate children's palliative care options, means that families are often forced to make inappropriate and ill-informed decisions to attempt aggressive curative treatments.

➤ Increased high-technology interventions are often not appropriate for those in less well-developed countries who need to develop access to basic healthcare services. Initiatives in developing countries should be community-orientated and sustainable.

Workforce issues

➤ A lack of trained personnel worldwide makes scaling-up palliative programmes difficult with limited resource capacity.

➤ Adult hospice and palliative care personnel may be able to provide expertise in end-of-life care for adults, but often have no paediatric expertise. Many of the conditions that are common in paediatrics are virtually unknown in adult palliative care. This decreases access for families and their children to health benefits such as home-based pain and symptom management, which should be individualised for specific family needs.

Children's palliative care is a small but growing speciality of children's care. The UK is often regarded as the world leader in this field, but many other countries, both in the industrial and developing world, are developing palliative care services to meet the needs of children and families in a wide variety of social, economic and health environments. It is critical that health professionals involved in these services have access to support, information resources, guidelines on best practice and the opportunity to network with similar services throughout the world. Similarly professionals in the UK and the developed world have a lot to learn from colleagues in the developing world about innovative approaches. Below are contrasting experiences of children's palliative care provision from Western Europe and from Africa.

A WESTERN EUROPEAN EXPERIENCE: GERMANY

In 1982 the first children's hospice in England opened. Fifteen years later in Germany, the first children's hospice at home service became operational and the first purpose-built children's hospice opened its doors. Today in 2009, there are about 65 children's hospice at home services and eight purpose-built children's hospices, where a child and family can stay from the time of the diagnoses onwards, either for respite care or end-of-life care. Special facilities for young adults are also being developed, the first of which opened in 2008.

In 2002 the National Association of Children's Hospices (NACH) was founded as a charity. Today it is recognised as the umbrella organisation of the children's hospice movement in Germany and has been accepted by politicians and the health insurance authorities.

The objectives of the NACH are to provide:

➤ an information centre to the public, affected families, volunteers, professionals, politicians, health funds and donators

➤ training courses for professionals and volunteers

➤ public funding for children's hospice services

➤ public awareness about the work of children's hospice services

➤ coordination and networking of child hospice initiatives and organisations

➤ setting and monitoring of quality standards in children's hospice services

➤ networking with paediatric palliative care organisations on a national and international level.

Sustainable funding for children's hospice services remains a big issue in Germany. There is a different funding mechanism for children's hospices services provided in the hospice building and those provided at home. Statutory (public) funding is based on an adult hospice funding model, using social security codes for each individual, and as such the specific needs of children's hospices were not well integrated. The funding model stipulates that funding is provided for hospice care delivered in purpose-built hospices and by specific hospice at home services. Regulatory statutes had to be negotiated nationally, with statutes for purpose-built hospices coming into effect in 2002 and then statutes for at-home hospices. This was a great breakthrough for the hospice movement. But it still left a considerable gap in funding to be raised through donations. Children's hospices still need a specialised lobby to ensure that their services are fully covered by the statute and that they receive funding. The funding model remains focused on end-of-life care (90% of cases) with only 40% of children's hospice service running costs coming from statutory funding sources.

The funding situation is even more complicated for children's hospice at home services as funding is based on the number of insured people in each region, the total number of hospice cases and the number of volunteers. In reality, this system means that the more hospice at-home services, cases and therefore the more volunteers there are, the less funding is provided. This is a flawed system which implicitly leads to competition and concern about new children's hospice services being established. In general, children's hospice at home services only receive funding towards the costs of their employed staff, and no contribution to other running costs.

Paediatric palliative care services

As well as the children's hospice at home services in Germany, there are also special palliative care community children's nursing services which depend on the health insurance system to cover their funding. In purpose-built hospices specialised professionals are employed to cover the whole field of palliative care while the at-home services cooperate with these special community children's nurses. Volunteers in purpose-built hospices support in all different kind of areas and are a major part of the workforce.

Standards in children's hospices

Germany's children's hospice movement has its roots in England and therefore the standards of ACT are applied in most organisations. Organisations also use the IMRaCCT standards (developed by the Steering Board of the EAPC task force for children and adolescents palliative care in the home) and the ICPCN Charter (developed by the Steering Board of the International Children's Palliative Care Network). Standards for children's hospices in Germany have been developed from these documents by the members of the National Association of Children's Hospices in Germany. The Association is now developing a set of measures for benchmarking the quality of children's hospice services. An expert scientific board has been set up to decide on the process for inspecting and reporting on the quality of an organisation and whether they should be awarded the official 'Seal of Approval' of the National Association of Children's Hospices. It is anticipated that this seal will have to be renewed every three years.

Education and training

Palliative care training in Germany is rooted in the mandatory training regulations of the social security code statutes. These have not yet been adapted to the special needs of children, although it is recognised that there is a need to develop specialist training in paediatric palliative care and there is now specialist training leading to a paediatric palliative care qualification. This training is open to all professionals working in paediatric palliative care and the demand is high. There is also a training need for those professionals who have qualifications in general palliative care but no specialisation in paediatric care. The NACH has worked in partnership with the University for Social Work in Freiburg and the Freiburg University Children's Clinic to develop specialist paediatric 'top-up' training, which began in 2009.

Training for volunteers working in the sector has so far not been centrally coordinated and standardised, with courses being developed by individual organisations. A modular curriculum framework has now been published by NACH which can be adapted to regional needs. This curriculum means that all members of the NACH have a nationally recognised and accepted training certificate for volunteers.

AFRICA

Although the development of palliative care in Africa dates back 25 years in Zimbabwe, the concept of palliative care in many countries in Africa is still relatively new. Currently there are about 21 African countries that have no known palliative care service provision.[16] In other countries palliative care is largely being provided from centres of excellence and with minimum integration into the mainstream healthcare system. Consequently, for the majority of Africans, both adults and children, who currently endure progressive, life-limiting illnesses, access to culturally appropriate, holistic palliative care (that includes effective pain and symptom management) is at best limited, and at worst non-existent.[17] Responding to this need, the Cape Town Declaration in 2002 declared that palliative care (and pain and symptom control) is the right of every adult and child with life-limiting illness[18] and since then tremendous progress has occurred in palliative care development across the continent.

Traditionally children have been relatively neglected by palliative care service development, despite the fact that they may well have already experienced parental and sibling deaths and be facing their own mortality.[19] This neglect is attributable to many challenges that hamper the provision of palliative care to children. These challenges include: lack of trained personnel and a fear amongst health professionals in providing care to children; restricted access to children's formulations for essential medicines; limited access to treatment such as chemotherapy and anti-retroviral therapy (ART), (and where it is available it is often found only in major cities); a lack of understanding of the needs of children with life-threatening illness; and financial challenges that may mean carers have to make difficult decisions about who should benefit from limited resources.

Over recent years, there has been growing awareness of the need for children's palliative care and the difference that it can make to the quality of children's lives. This has resulted in significant developments around children's palliative care across the region.

Indeed, children's palliative care is now seen as an essential part of care provision in many places and it is recognised that children's palliative care should be integrated into all palliative care education programmes. This is an effective approach because it is often the same nurse who has responsibility for delivering care to adults and children, particularly in rural areas where there are no specialist children's hospitals or palliative care services. In conjunction with the general training, it is important that some health professionals are provided with a more specialist children's palliative care training to enable them to provide support and mentorship to others.[19]

Across Africa, children's palliative care services can be found in many countries and these programmes often provide the basis upon which training and mentorship to other individuals and organisations take place. Examples of such programmes include: Umodzi Palliative Care Service for Children at Queen Elizabeth Hospital, Blantyre, Malawi; the children's palliative care programme at Hospice Africa Uganda; The Mildmay Paediatric Care Centre in Uganda; children's palliative care services that have been integrated into existing services in Zambia, e.g. at Jon's Hospice; Island Hospice in Zambia; along with numerous programmes in South Africa. An appraisal of children's palliative care in sub-Saharan Africa is currently underway, which is addressing issues such as the context for care provision; the interface and potential for children's palliative care to improve patient outcomes in cancer and HIV/AIDS particularly with reference to anti-retroviral therapy; and identifying and appraising existing descriptions and evaluations of paediatric palliative care projects in sub-Saharan Africa.[8] This appraisal is similar to a previous appraisal looking at adult palliative care which found that there was a wealth of experience within the region but a dearth of evidence of what is being done.[17]

Training for care providers on children's palliative care is vital for ongoing service development within the region. Various training courses exist across the region ranging from introductory training courses on children's palliative care to more specialised children's palliative care training (e.g. the Masters programme in South Africa on children's palliative care), specialised palliative care training such as the BSc in palliative care at Makerere University which has a children's component within it. Currently work is underway, funded by the Diana Princess of Wales Memorial Fund to develop a Children's Palliative Care Curriculum aimed at improving the quality of life of African children with life-limiting illnesses and their families through improving knowledge, skills, attitudes and behaviours of health professionals working in the African context.[15] It is anticipated that this curriculum can be adapted according to the specific situations within countries and may be available at different levels, e.g. certificate, diploma, degree or Masters. Resources for children's palliative care within the region are also being developed, some of which are already available. These include: the Clinical Guide to Palliative Care in sub-Saharan Africa;[20] The Toolkit for Children's Palliative Care in Africa;[21] Children's Palliative Care in Africa;[22] and a clinical pocket guide for children's palliative care. These are supplemented by a variety of other resources and training manuals that are available on children and palliative care within the region.

While there are a great a deal of resources being developed across Africa, the issue of national policy for palliative care in general, and more specifically palliative care in children, is an area that still needs to be developed. Reviews have been undertaken in various countries with regards to what policies and guidelines are available, what needs to be changed/written and establishing the process for ensuring that these policies and guidelines are implemented. A small number of countries within the region have well defined national policies and standards for palliative care, but the majority do not, and even getting access to essential medications for palliative care, especially children's formulations, is a challenge. The African Palliative Care Association (APCA) is about to undertake a review of national policy in eleven countries across the region, looking at policies and guidelines for palliative care including those for children. This builds on work that APCA has been doing in addressing access to essential palliative care medications, for both adults and children, across 18 African countries. It is anticipated that this review will continue to support developmental work around the policy issues for both adult and children to improve access to palliative care in the region.

Standards for children's palliative care exist in a few countries, e.g. South Africa, and within the broader context of home-based care in palliative care in countries such as Zimbabwe. Organisations such as Family Health International (FHI) and the Hospice and Palliative Care of South Africa (HPCA) have developed their own standard operating procedures (SOPs) for children's palliative care and these are used widely within individual organisations. Generic palliative care standards are being developed for the region through a collaborative process by APCA. These standards address the provision of care at the different levels of the health service delivery system, including community-based organisations, healthcare facilities, hospitals and specialist palliative care service providers. Integral to these standards are the standards of care for children's palliative care. These standards should be finalised by mid-2009 and will then be available, with mentorship, for adaptation and implementation in different countries across the region.

Research and monitoring and evaluation within children's palliative care in Africa is an area that needs to be developed further. As is the case in many aspects of palliative care across the region, much is being done, but there is little documentation or evidence to support the work. A validated outcome measurement tool for palliative care in adults – the APCA Africa Palliative Outcome Scale (POS)[23,24] was developed in order to measure the outcomes of palliative care within the region. The need to develop a similar outcome tool for children has been identified and a literature review addressing outcome measures in children has been undertaken. The development of APCA African Children's POS has just started and it is expected that it will be developed across a range of countries and settings, and will be developed alongside other indicator guides to help service providers to utilise the tool in order to assess and improve outcomes of care for children.

Children's palliative care is a challenging area in Africa, due to the immense need for services across the region. Much has been done and much is happening within the development of services to improve the quality of life of children with life-threatening conditions and their families.

THE INTERNATIONAL CHILDREN'S PALLIATIVE CARE NETWORK (ICPCN)

Background to the network

The idea for an International Children's Palliative Care Network (ICPCN) originally arose at the meeting of national hospice and palliative care associations (now the Worldwide Palliative Care Alliance (WPCA)) in The Hague in 2003. It was recognised that it was important to ensure that the voice and experience of paediatric palliative care was heard alongside that of adult palliative care and that structured and coordinated approaches were taken to lobbying for children's and adult palliative care at an international, pan-national and national level.

The ICPCN was founded in 2005 as a collaborative partnership in order to connect these services while at the same time raising awareness of children's palliative care across the globe. The original founders of the network were concerned that while the concept of children's hospice and palliative care had been in evidence since its early days in the United Kingdom (UK) in 1982, there were still fewer than 30 countries worldwide that had embarked on a similar path to ensure that the unique palliative care needs of children and young people were met. Added to this, many of the countries with existing adult palliative care services failed to acknowledge that children had special needs and needed specialist paediatric expertise.

The founders of the ICPCN saw the need for a network whose strength would lie in the sharing of knowledge, good practice and expertise to enable and support agencies around the world to develop a range of dedicated children's palliative care services. They recognised that although every country was unique in its scale of provision, motivation and capacity to provide palliative care to children, it was possible for each to contribute and learn from the other. For instance, developing countries often have innovative projects in order to provide palliative care to children.

The founders also realised that in order to make a difference in the lives of children and the families of those children afflicted with life-limiting and life-threatening illnesses and who die without any form of palliative care, it was imperative to form a strong and globally recognised organisation that would not only advocate for children's palliative care on an international scale, but would be a 'virtual place' where information for both existing and developing children's hospice and palliative care services could be found and shared.

The ICPCN Vision

To achieve worldwide the best quality of life and care for children and young people with life-limiting illnesses, their families and carers, through networking, advocacy, information sharing, education and research.

At the 2nd Global Summit for National Hospice and Palliative Care Associations held in Seoul, South Korea in March 2005, the following statement was released:

> Children and adolescents with life-limiting conditions have very specific palliative

care needs which are often different to those of adults. If these children's and adolescents' physical, emotional, social, spiritual and developmental needs are to be met, the carers require special knowledge and skills. We ask that the voice of these children and adolescents is heard, respected and acknowledged as part of the expression of hospice and palliative care world-wide.

Members of this original group were from 15 different countries and some members now form the core of the Steering Group that is the governing body of the ICPCN today, all of whom volunteer their time and their skills to keep this vision alive.

The objectives of the ICPCN

Since its formation in 2005, membership of the ICPCN, which is open and free to both organisations and individuals, has grown rapidly and to date is representative of 36 countries worldwide. The ICPCN aims to facilitate communication and sharing of resources, information and research, working in partnership with other organisations and raising awareness of the needs of life-limited children and young people and the need for global development of children's hospice and palliative care.

The four core objectives of the ICPCN are:

1 information provision
2 advocacy
3 research and education
4 networking.

Information provision

The ICPCN have produced a range of international information resources including:

➤ up-to-date website
➤ quarterly newsletter
➤ international service directory
➤ policy documents
➤ position papers, best practice papers, briefing papers.

The ICPCN website has become a trusted source for news, information on new developments, document downloads, dates and information on relevant conferences and available training in the field of palliative care for children and has been visited by thousands of people over the past year.

Quarterly newsletters are published and disseminated to members and national organisations. These newsletters deal with research issues relevant to the field and articles that highlight advances and challenges experienced in both developed and developing countries around the world. Members are sent important information, reminders of upcoming events and conference abstract submission dates on a regular basis.

Advocacy

The ICPCN steering group members have presented at all the major international palliative care conferences since 2007 thus raising awareness of children and young people's palliative care issues in the international palliative care arena. The ICPCN Charter was published in 2008.

Every child's right to palliative care: the ICPCN Charter

According to the United Nations (UN) Convention on the Rights of the Child, every child and young person has the right to the enjoyment of the highest attainable standard of health. Governments are also required to do everything in their power to ensure that they enjoy full and holistic development. Children have the right to be protected against abuse, neglect and all forms of ill-treatment.

In the spirit of the UN Convention, the ICPCN developed a Charter which sets out the international standard of support that is the right of all children living with life-limiting and life-threatening illnesses worldwide, and their families.

The Charter calls for all such children to receive appropriate palliative care – care whose main purpose is to relieve suffering, whether physical, spiritual or emotional, and to promote quality of life.

> A child who dies without receiving adequate pain control and symptom management has suffered abuse and an untreated HIV positive child is suffering neglect.
>
> Joan Marston, Chair of the ICPCN.

Palliative care encompasses the entire family. It should begin at the time of diagnosis and continue alongside any curative treatment aimed at the disease. Should curative treatment fail, it is maintained through death and into bereavement for as long as it is needed.

The Charter calls for palliative care to be provided within the child's home or within an environment that is child-friendly. This care should be offered by professionals and caregivers who have undergone training in palliative care specific to the needs of children.

To date the Charter has been translated into 21 different languages, and can be downloaded from the ICPCN website at www.icpcn.org.uk.

The ICPCN Charter of Rights for Life-limited and Life-threatened Children and Young People

The ICPCN Charter has been adapted from and fully endorses the ACT Charter for Life-limited Children, Young People and Families.

1. Every child should expect individualised, culturally and age appropriate palliative care as defined by the World Health Organization (WHO). The specific needs of adolescents and young people shall be addressed and planned for.
2. Palliative care for the child and family shall begin at the time of diagnosis and continue alongside any curative treatments throughout the child's illness, during death and in bereavement. The aim of palliative care shall be to relieve suffering and promote quality of life.
3. The child's parents or legal guardians shall be acknowledged as the primary

caregivers and recognised as full partners in all care and decisions involving their child.

4. Every child shall be encouraged to participate in decisions affecting his or her care, according to age and understanding.

5. A sensitive but honest approach will be the basis of all communication with the child and the child's family. They shall be treated with dignity and given privacy irrespective of physical or intellectual capacity.

6. Every child or young person shall have access to education and wherever possible be provided with opportunities to play, access leisure opportunities, interact with siblings and friends and participate in normal childhood activities.

7. The child and the family shall be given the opportunity to consult with a paediatric specialist with particular knowledge of the child's condition where possible, and shall remain under the care of a paediatrician or doctor with paediatric knowledge and experience.

8. The child and the family shall be entitled to a named and accessible key worker whose task it is to build, co-ordinate and maintain appropriate support systems which should include a multidisciplinary care team and appropriate community resources.

9. The child's home shall remain the centre of care whenever possible. Treatment outside of this home shall be in a child-centred environment by staff and volunteers, trained in palliative care of children.

10. Every child and family member, including siblings, shall receive culturally appropriate, clinical, emotional, psychosocial and spiritual support in order to meet their particular needs. Bereavement support for the child's family shall be available for as long as it is required.

Research and education

A programme of expertise-sharing through the awarding of scholarships and bursaries has been launched, focusing initially on paediatric palliative care leaders in resource-poor countries.

An ongoing project has been launched to gather and publish information on the website on what education and training is available worldwide in the field of paediatric palliative care, which will also serve to highlight the existing gaps.

What does the future hold?

ICPCN will continue to develop information and support to enable organisations to lobby for the inclusion of children's hospice and palliative care on the agendas of their national governments and to encourage non-government organisations to include children's palliative care within their development programmes.

The ICPCN will continue to be the voice for children who cannot always speak for themselves and its Steering Group is committed to advocacy work with the ultimate aim of making palliative care recognised as a basic human right for every child and family faced with the distress and the challenges that accompany the diagnosis and progression of a life-limiting or life-threatening condition.

The ICPCN is a part of the Worldwide Palliative Care Alliance (WPCA) where it represents the voice of children. It is administered from the Cape Town offices of the Hospice Palliative Care Association of South Africa and is coordinated by an International Information Officer.

N.I.C.E analysis

Needs
- More resources for development of children's palliative care.
- Better networks between service providers and those lobbying for change.
- More robust evidence/advocacy for children's palliative care.

Interests
- Growing membership of ICPCN.
- Worldwide Palliative Care Alliance formed to raise profile of adult palliative care.
- Children's palliative care is become established as a specialty.

Concerns
- Children and children's palliative care not a high priority for governments.
- Lack of capacity/resources.
- Advocacy work is for most practitioners an 'add on' to their daily work.

Expectations
- More successful advocacy for children's palliative care.
- Practitioners will be more informed.
- There will be international development of children's palliative care.
- Children and families will receive better care and support.

1. What is already known about these concerns?

There is increasing awareness of the need for a more informed and coordinated approach to developing children's palliative care services globally. ICPCN has been established to further promote this.

2. Misconceptions contributing to barriers of delivering care.

The differences between adult and children's palliative care are not always well understood. Children often have very different illness trajectories and live for many years with a life-limiting condition, often into adulthood. Children's palliative care is not just about end-of-life care, but is an approach to care that is important across the whole care journey of a child or young person with a life-limiting or life-threatening condition. There is a perception also that parents/carers can provide the bulk of the care for a sick child, but it is not appropriate or acceptable to place this huge burden of care on their shoulders.

3. Advantages/disadvantages with the required changes highlighted.

ICPCN has been set up to try overcome some of the challenges of advocating for children's palliative care and this is a great boost to the lobbying that we can all do in our own countries. The disadvantage is that at the moment ICPCN is under-resourced and lobbying and advocacy work is not a high enough priority when those passionate about children's palliative care are overwhelmed with delivering care directly to children and families. The establishment of national umbrella bodies to undertake advocacy work in each country is a good way forward, but is expensive and will take time.

4. How ready are the various parties involved for change?

There is willingness from many practitioners around the world to create more sustainable services for children with life-limiting and life-threatening conditions, as evidenced by the growing membership of ICPCN.

5. Are there any barriers to this change?

The challenge is to make decision-makers and funders of services aware of the need for change and investment in children's palliative care and basic resources such as drug availability in developing countries. There is only a relatively small workforce in relation to children's palliative care and a small number of medical specialists.

6. What is the most effective way of communicating with the people who can affect change?

Advocacy is a lengthy and ongoing process which can be described as 'structured nagging'. It is often a case of repeated letters and face-to-face meetings with key influencers to bring about change. It is important that a cohesive approach is made in each country so that decision makers are given clear and repeated information about the change and investment that is required. Clear data and evidence is important as are examples of how effective the proposed solutions can be. ICPCN aims to support countries in developing such evidence and providing the tools that can be used to bring about real and lasting change for children's palliative care services across the world.

Action plan: next steps
- Join ICPCN – contribute information, share expertise and learning, get involved.
- Sign up to the ICPCN Charter and share this with as many people as possible.
- Contribute to the development of robust lobbying materials in your own country and share with ICPCN.
- Further development of national umbrella bodies in each country for children's palliative care.
- ICPCN to secure funding for its further development.

REFERENCES

1 Cancer Research UK. *Children in the Developing World Bear the Burden of Cancer*. Press Release. 14 February 2003. Available at: http://info.cancerresearchuk.org/news/archive/pressreleases/2003/february/39505 (accessed 10 March 2009).
2 Romer AL. The children's international project on palliative/hospice services (ChIPPS): An interview with Marcia Levetown. *Innovations in End-of-Life Care*. 2000; **2**. Available at: www.edc.org/lastacts (accessed 17 February 2010).

3 Kumar S. Poverty shouldn't mean poor quality palliative care. Available at: www.id21.org (accessed 4 March 2006).

4 Himelstein B, Hildne, J, Boldt, A, *et al.* Pediatric palliative care. *NEMJ.* 2004; **350**: 1752–62.

5 ACT. *A Guide to the Development of Children's Palliative Care Services.* 2nd ed. Bristol: ACT; 2003.

6 Friedrichsdorf SJ, Menke A, Brun S, *et al.* Status quo of palliative care in pediatric oncology – a nationwide survey in Germany. *J Pain Symptom Manag.* 2005; **29**: 156–64.

7 UNAIDS/WHO. *AIDS Epidemic Update: December 2005.* Geneva. Available at: www.unaids. org/epi/2005/ (accessed 20 February 2010).

8 Harding R. *The Status of Paediatric Palliative Care in Sub-Saharan Africa: an appraisal.* Protocol Version 1. London: KCL; 2008.

9 UNAIDS. *Report on the Global AIDS Epidemic.* Geneva: UNAIDS; 2008.

10 Cooley C, Adeodu S, Aldred H, *et al.* Paediatric palliative care: a lack of research-based evidence. *Int J Palliat Nurs.* 2000; **6**: 346–51.

11 Jennings AL, Davies AN, Higgins JPT, *et al.* Opioids or the palliation of breathlessness in terminal illness. *Cochrane Database Syst Rev.* 2006; **1**: CD002066.

12 Simons JM, Macdonald LM. Pain assessment tools: children's nurse's views. *J Child Health Care.* 2004; **8**: 264–78.

13 Wiffen PJ, Edwards JE, Barden J, *et al.* Morphine by mouth is an effective pain-killer for cancer pain. *Cochrane Database Syst Rev.* 2006; **1**: CD003868.

14 Wolfe J, Grier HE, Klar N. Symptoms and suffering at the end of life in children with cancer. *N Engl J Med.* 2000; **342**: 326–33.

15 Amery J. *Diana Princess of Wales children's palliative care courses*: Curriculum document. 2009.

16 Wright M, Clark D. *Hospice and Palliative Care in Africa: A review of developments and challenges.* Oxford: Oxford University Press; 2006.

17 Harding R, Higginson IJ. Palliative care in sub-Saharan Africa: an appraisal. *The Lancet.* 2005; **365**: 1971–7.

18 Mpanga Sebuyira LM, Mwangi-Powell F, Pereira J, *et al.* The Cape Town palliative care declaration: home-grown solutions for sub-Saharan Africa. *J Palliat Med.* 2003; **6**: 341–3.

19 Mwangi-Powell F, Ddungu H, Downing J, *et al.* Palliative care in Africa. In: Ferrel B, Coyle N, editors. *Oxford Textbook of Palliative Nursing.* Oxford: Oxford University Press; 2009.

20 Gwyther L, Merriman A, Mapanga Sebuyria L, *et al.* *A Clinical Guide to Supportive and Palliative Care for HIV/AIDS in Sub-Saharan Africa.* Uganda: APCA; 2006.

21 HPCA. *A Toolkit for Children's Palliative Care Programmes in Africa.* South Africa: HPCA; 2008.

22 Amery J. (in press) *Children's Palliative Care in Africa.* Oxford University Press, London.

23 Powell RA, Downing J, Harding R, *et al.* Development of the APCA African palliative outcome scale. *J Pain Symptom Manag.* 2007; **32**: 229–32.

24 Harding R, Selman L, Agupio G, Dinat N, *et al.* Validation of a core outcome measure for palliative care in Africa: the APCA African Palliative Outcome Scale. *Health Qual Life Outcomes.* 2010 Jan 25; **8**(1): 10. [Epub ahead of print].

3

Organisation of care in the UK

Jo Rooney

SETTING THE SCENE

Alisha was the second child born to Mohammed and Nasreen, a couple who were born in the UK but whose parents were immigrants from Pakistan during the 1970s.

Nasreen's pregnancy had been uneventful and Alisha was born at 36 weeks by normal delivery. However, during the birthing process Alisha passed meconium, and there was a possibility that she had aspirated, so she was transferred following delivery to the neonatal unit for 24 hours' observation. During her stay in the neonatal unit, Alisha's intake and outputs were monitored and she was feeding normally. However, over the course of her admission the number of wet and dirty nappies increased, following assessment there was evidence that Alisha was becoming dehydrated.

The diarrhoea became profuse, though there was no evidence of infection, and despite intravenous fluids Alisha remained dehydrated. It was determined that Alisha, now three days old, should be transferred to a specialist hospital for further tests and a surgical opinion.

It was in my role as Community Children's Nurse Coordinator in Alisha's local hospital that I became part of Alisha's care. At this point in time Alisha was five months old and her discharge from the specialist hospital to her home was being considered. Alisha still did not have a definitive diagnosis and the healthcare team could not provide her family with any concrete insights about her future health needs. Rather, in the lack of any diagnostic label, her future could only be discussed using conjecture, rather than knowledge or research evidence.

From my initial assessment I saw a very happy and contented little girl, who was engaged in her environment, looking around and laughing. There was no family present. However, I soon observed that her development was delayed, such as her gross motor skills; she could not roll over, her head control was poor, but she could pass objects from hand to hand. She cooed and babbled and demonstrated appropriate social responses to stimuli. From both observations and measurements, Alisha was small for her age with a mildly distended abdomen, and obvious signs of jaundice in her eyes and skin.

Alisha was a challenge to the healthcare team, since she still did not have a diagnosis that would assist with the management of care. But this type of situation is not uncommon to those of us who work in paediatrics.

Alisha was able to take feed orally and enjoyed her bottles, she was offered small amounts of a specialist feed six times a day. However, she absorbed insufficient nutrition or hydration through oral feeds as it caused her to have profuse diarrhoea. Alisha's nutrition was provided by parenteral nutrition via a tunnelled central line.

It was confirmed that Alisha had some degree of liver damage, which might have been a side effect from the parenteral nutrition, despite concerted efforts to monitor her biochemical status. In addition, Alisha developed several other complications such as repeated infections both bacterial and viral, plus her bottom was sore and bleeding due to the profuse diarrhoea.

FAMILY AND SOCIAL CONSIDERATIONS

Alisha had an older brother, Zakim, who was two years old and exhibited normal traits for growth and development. Mohammed, who had limited English language skills, worked in a catering business, which often involved long hours, thus making it a challenge for him to visit his daughter while in the hospital. Nasreen was in her mid-twenties and had not worked outside the home since she had her first child. Nazreen had the support of a large extended family living close to her. In particular, her sister, with whom she shares a close relationship, had had a child, who died suddenly at age five due to liver failure. This child's death was very distressing to both the immediate and extended family.

They lived in their own home and Mohammed could drive and had his own car.

INTRODUCTION

This chapter will look at the issues in relation to the organisation of care in the UK. However, it is limited to England and will not include a commentary on the strategy or development of services in Scotland, Wales and Northern Ireland. This is due to the fact that it is a perspective based on the experience of developing a palliative care service including end-of-life care in one area of England. However, I hope that some of the thoughts and issues will have relevance for others to improve the experience for children and their families.

I'm trying to capture the voice – my voice – of a professional trying to provide the care that will help this child and family, against a background of conflict, both philosophical and system-based. Conflict may seem like a strong, emotive word to use, but there was discord amongst the professionals not only philosophically but also about financial costs; there was contradiction and inconsistency in the messages we gave the family, divergence from theories of care to the lived experience and tension between the care the family needed and that which could be provided.

The development of services for life-limited children, children with complex healthcare needs, disabilities and long-term health conditions has varied considerably across the UK over the last 15–20 years. The discussion below is an illustration of this.

MODELS OF CARE

The models of service such as Community Children's Nurses, Diana Teams[1] and Disability Nursing Teams have developed piecemeal in this time. They have different client groups and differing eligibility criteria yet often they include children and young people who could be described as having palliative care needs.

Very few services have been commissioned following a local needs assessment, developing an understanding of the local population or client group and how that might change in 2, 5 or 10 years' time. Many have grown out of the enthusiasm and dedication of individual professionals. This form of service development can lead to gaps in service provision but also duplication and overlap in services. This has implications in terms of the costs; what is not provided can lead to increased needs for other services in the future and duplication is wasteful of limited resources. Services developed in this way are unable to adapt to changing needs and also there are limitations in the service that can be provided, from issues regarding supplies (medical consumables) to hours of service provision.

The range of models of service provision is more easily understood by examining those services provided in neighbouring areas. Within 40 miles of each other there are three children's community nursing services linked to three hospitals. All the hospitals have paediatric inpatient services; all the services have areas of urban deprivation and large rural catchments.

The first of the district general hospitals has no community nursing service; the needs of families with complex medical needs are met by the inpatient facility locally, a specialist hospital, school nurses or health visitors. Support and care is not provided to the family in their home; families either become very self-sufficient or struggle. This model has no easy access to telephone support or out of hours support. Care is often provided at a considerable distance from their home, which leaves families with little choice if their child's condition becomes terminal and they wish to die at home.

Less than 20 miles away, the second of the district general hospitals has a community nursing team which has traditionally had a strong emphasis on care to children with disabilities and has been based outside of the hospital. They provide a Monday to Friday service between 8.30 am and 5.00 pm, plus a 24-hour on call service to all their families, seven days a week. Families can call about any issue at any time of the day or night. However, this is not a large team, it has about seven nurses on a combination of full-time and part-time hours. The families have a link between the medical staff in both the hospital and the community; they have support in their own homes and build a relationship with a team, which allows them to make choices about the care of their child.

The third service is a service based within the hospital, and has a team of nine nurses, again on a mix of both full- and part-time hours, they provide an on-call service from 8.00 am to 8.00 pm, seven days a week, and 24-hour on call when a family choose to care for their dying child at home. The team provide strong liaison between the families and the multidisciplinary team in the hospital and services in the community, including non-health agencies such as social care. The families have support in their home and again build up a relationship with a team.

Within a small geographical area it can be seen how services to families vary considerably. This is due to the history of development of these services based on little accurate information of the population they might serve, often developed to enable children to be discharged home, meeting the needs of the hospital rather than the needs of a family. There are obvious limitations of no service compared with the advantages of either of the other teams. Team 2 has had a community in-reach relationship with their local hospital, which has advantages to the third team that has operated as a hospital outreach service, where the needs of the acute service may be divergent from what the families need from a service. Team 3 do not provide 24-hour on-call unless a child is dying or in the short-term special circumstances. However, they feel they provide strong support and training to families to allow them to feel able to provide the care needed or to make decisions about their child's care when circumstances change overnight. However, there are issues related to eligibility criteria: an acute-based service will accept those children who have a nursing need – in crude definition this has been described by some practitioners as children who have a tube – a disability team will accept children with a disability where there are no definite nursing needs offering support and advice to families from diagnosis to advice on behaviour management. Both these criteria run the risk of excluding a large proportion of children and young people who may have a life-limiting condition.

These are just a few indicators of how services have developed very differently; however there are some services in other areas of the UK which have developed in a systematic way, who have clear criteria which encompass children with healthcare needs, disability and those children who have a life-limiting condition who may not fit into either category at the point of diagnosis, but it is recognised that the family have a need for support on many different levels from the beginning and that early involvement from a team which can meet those needs is important in families feeling supported on their journey. The UK strategy 'Better Care: Better Lives'[2] identifies some of those elements as nursing, psychology, sibling support and bereavement based on the good practice examples that are available.

There was a development of children's community services following the Big Lottery Palliative Care Initiative (formerly the New Opportunities Fund) in 2003.[3] This was a UK Government initiative, utilising money from the National Lottery to develop home-based palliative care services for children. Many areas, which were successful in their bids for funding, developed new services or expanded their existing provision, however many of these projects have not continued once the funding ceased. This is a recurring difficulty where organisations are not held to account for the services they provide. Organisations who received funding made a commitment that this would be continued once the grant had ended but there has been no central government enforcement of this. The short-term nature of some of these projects could be seen as a failure of this programme. However this time limited funding and the increase in services it provided has raised expectations in professionals and parents of the service that is possible but has also raised the profile of an area of care for children, which has been described as a 'Cinderella' service. It is this raising of the profile and developing an understanding of children's palliative care amongst professionals from many different spheres which is vital to the development of services.

Craft and Killen[4] found a lack of understanding of what children's palliative care involved, most assuming it was just about end-of-life care. They found this lack of understanding and lack of recognition of children's palliative care as a specialism have added to its Cinderella status.

The needs of children and families have been recognised through the many Government strategy documents and initiatives over the last five years, from the National Service Framework,[5] 'Aiming High for Disabled Children'[6] to 'Healthy lives, brighter futures'.[7] There has been increasing pressure, through the independent review,[4] by professionals involved in caring for children with a life-limiting condition or complex needs for standards of service provision to be set.

The National Service Framework's[5] Standard 8 asserts that children and young people who are disabled or who have complex healthcare needs receive coordinated, high quality child and family-centred services which are based on assessed needs, which promote social inclusion and, where possible, which enable them and their families to live ordinary lives.

It gives clear directions for the development of services within this document which would meet the needs of children and families who have a wide range of needs including palliative care. However, it does not put in place mechanisms by which these standards will be managed or make the provision of these services a statutory responsibility. The 'core offer' as outlined in 'Aiming High for Disabled Children', which includes children with palliative care needs will be monitored through a National Indicator (NI54)[8] which will be based on the experiences of parents on the services they receive. How effective this will be, as a measure and monitoring tool to raise standards of services, can be questioned, as it is a subjective tool, which will be affected by parental expectations, education, background and life experiences, and where they are on their journey with their child, have they had previous difficulties with services, have they recently been given a diagnosis or if their child's needs are becoming more complex will effect their perception of the services they receive. That is not to say it is not real, not valued and also important to collect, however as a stand alone measure on which to judge the complexity of services which can be required for a child with palliative care needs or complex healthcare needs it seems limited in its scope and raises issues regarding its validity.

However, while still arguing that recognition and development of children's palliative care as a specialism is vital to increasing the profile of the needs of children and their families for improved services, it is important to look outward at developments in other disciplines and how they could also be used to impact on the development of service provision to children.

Recent government initiatives such as *Better Care: Better Lives*, The Child Health Care Strategy[2] and the development of a continuing care policy for children are specifically aimed at children and young people, but developments in primarily adult services should not be ignored. For example, the Liverpool Care Pathway for the Dying Patient (2008)[9] and the Gold Standards Framework (2005)[10] as the learning and developing philosophy which underpin these could translate into positive benefits for children and young people with palliative care needs and especially around end-of-life issues. Developing all service providers to think holistically about the needs of the dying and their families can only lead to better services. If we can find a common language for the approach and the care across service providers including improving the involvement of primary care, then care to the whole family will be improved.

The Gold Standards Framework[10] has been developed by the Royal College of General Practitioners and the NHS End of Life Care Programme. Its aim is 'to develop a practice or locally based system to improve and optimise the organisation and quality of care for patients and their carers in the last year of life'. It is a standard for all those approaching the end of their life, regardless of diagnosis, stage or setting. The Liverpool Care Pathway (LCP)[9] and the Gold Standards Framework (GSF)[10] have had a major influence in the development of the Department of Health's End of Life Care Strategy.[11]

The LCP is designed to provide a guide and template to the delivery of care to the dying, to complement the skill and expertise of the practitioner using it. The practitioner can use the pathway guidance but it also gives the opportunity to document the reasons for decisions why in this individual care plan to deviate away from the pathway. It is argued that it is 'a means of empowering health professionals by winning time in a climate of "busyness" to enable best practice in the last hours/days of life. The LCP is a vehicle through which best quality of care for the dying is made measurable, explicit and visible.' By achieving a positive impact on those involved with its use, patients, carers and staff, it is argued that it can bring about a change in culture within organisations. Matthews *et al.*[12] described how they were adapting the LCP for use with children with a stated aim of facilitating the delivery and recording of optimum care for all dying children and their families. Evaluation of this was not available to the author at this time.

As a community practitioner I worked with a team of very dedicated paediatricians, but their contracts were either hospital-based or they had no remit to work outside of 'normal working hours' 9–5 Monday to Friday. In reality this left the community nursing team having to develop frameworks to support out of hours care for children dying at home. This included proactive planning for symptom control, ensuring medicines and equipment were in place in the home before they were needed based on clinical assessment of the child, and providing information and training to the family about what to expect in order to develop their confidence that something could be done. Another strategy that needed to be considered in end-of-life care at home was how to manage the child's death and the formalities and legalities, which needed to be observed once the child died. This was fairly straightforward during the working week but needed planning for out of hours care. It would have been easier to have a paediatrician on call but this was not available and in my experience I would have to argue it would have been an unnecessary and expensive resource. Through working proactively with the family with honesty about the possibilities (including symptom control), the services that can be provided, and the procedures that are necessary, plus a skilled community nursing team on call, the paediatrician would have been needed only to pronounce the child dead and to write a death certificate. It is not always easy to engage the general practitioner – they rarely see a child at end of life – however, when they had a clearly defined role and understood their part in the family's care, it was unusual to find a family doctor who would remain uninvolved. Working with the family's primary care team, the general practitioner, the out of hours services, even the practice receptionists, it was possible for them to provide an active service to families at end of life. The increasing development and understanding of the LCP[9] and GSF[10] in primary care can only make engagement with children's care easier, especially if we can share a common language and aims. Therefore would it not be better to look at these developments in a positive light and to take the elements from this which can be used with children and young people, rather than becoming isolated and insular in our developments, systems and approaches, which makes true community working harder and also places more hurdles in the process of transition to adult services.

When considering the model of service development in *Commissioning Children's and Young peoples Palliative Care Services*,[13] these are the elements which are also inherent in the LCP and the GSF, and the raising of standards and developing pathways for adults – which includes all services, from general practitioners to out of hours services such as NHS Direct and ambulance services – will lead to a pathway which can more easily and more readily be adopted to end-of-life care for children. Whilst specialism and specialist services are needed, this may not always be possible locally and therefore local practitioners need a core pathway and standard, which they have the skills to deliver. Why is the ideal of a specialist service for all not what is being advocated here?

1   Over-reliance on specialists can lead to a de-skilled workforce, loss of confidence from the staff and the family.
2   There are practical considerations which make this an impossible standard for all local areas to provide access to specialist knowledge and support for staff is a more realistic aim. Remote rural locations or areas with low numbers of children and young people would be difficult to cover with their own specialist team, whereas a community-led service with access to specialist support would allow families to have the choice in caring for their child at home.

There has been extensive work by many on developing pathways such as the ACT Care Pathway[14] which others then adapt. However, the ACT pathway is a very theoretical document which sets standards for care and service delivery. Its use by local service commissioners and providers is surely not merely to adapt the paperwork but to facilitate the commissioning of services to meet the standards and to develop the processes and organisational structures to facilitate this. In other words, to populate the theory with the services and processes which can meet those standards.

LIVING WITH THE UTILISATION OF THE ACT GUIDELINES: RELATING THEORY TO PRACTICE

To best exemplify how practice guidelines work in reality, I made a decision to discuss this as real experience, to discuss the difficulties and issues that I experienced as the Community Children's Nurse involved with this child and family, from discharge planning to when she died, using a case study approach. It is therefore an experiential account, which will discuss the issues for the child, family and the nurse as I observed them. Where possible I will relate this to the ACT Care Pathway[14] and the standards it sets and discuss the process as a lived example. There are many articles and strategy documents by many different authors and groups and they are all based on the experiences of those families who live through the death of their child, either through their own voices or the voices of those who work with them. This chapter will hopefully add to that evidence and professional dialogue, as I have used them to consider my own practice and develop the care to families in whatever role I take on.

I have spent time considering this scenario both as the situation unfolded and subsequently, and I can only assure you that this has been a reflective process from which my practice has grown and developed.

ACT CARE PATHWAY[14]

Could we consider Alisha to be a child with palliative care needs?

Was her condition life-limiting or life-threatening? Does this make a difference to the process and planning for discharge?

Due to the nature of the treatment required to keep her alive, Alisha was obviously a child who was technology-dependent and therefore because this was a necessity in the interventions to maintain life she was always considered to be a child with a life-threatening condition but not a child with palliative care needs.

Alisha's condition meant she fitted into group 1 of the ACT/RCPCH palliative care categories[15] as she had a life-threatening condition for which curative treatment may be feasible but can fail, where access to palliative care services may be necessary when treatment fails. Examples for this category are conditions such as cancer or irreversible organ failure.

However, life-threatening does not equate comfortably in the mind with palliative care, which often implies to many, both lay people and professionals, that there is no further treatment and we are 'giving up' or have 'failed'.

During the conversations that I had with both Nasreen and Mohammed in relation to taking Alisha home it was apparent that they were aware that Alisha's condition was severe, but were not prepared to talk about her dying even as a possibility. When thinking about this case and others especially, I have concluded that while families can hear and understand the fact of a condition having the potential to cause their child to die, families live with that possibility but they cannot keep on living with it as a probability. They live with the knowledge of the possibility but in actuality by not acknowledging it, they were also living with the hope that it would not happen.

This is illustrated by the decision Alisha's parents made before discharge from the specialist hospital not to go forward with an assessment for liver and bowel transplant and were clear that they understood the full implications of this, and were unwilling to enter further discussion.

I cannot truly understand the many emotions and processes a parent who has a child with a life-limiting condition may go through. I understand that they have many fears, partly of their loss and grief of their child dying but also of how that may be, their fear of the process of dying, sometimes expressed as fear that their child will suffer or be in pain and that this is not the right time, or that they are 'giving up too soon'. Parents can confront their own fears, we cannot force this on them, they can make decisions such as the one that Alisha's parents made, but be unable to acknowledge the possibility of her death.

This was an acceptance of the possibility of their child's death and admission that this was in fact the likely scenario. However, this understanding became distorted by the messages they were hearing from the medical team.

Discussions about how they wished to manage Alisha's care were clouded by their wish and hope to do the right thing, and therefore when they were given instructions about managing Alisha's care at home they didn't question these as they were still living with hope. A hope based on their need as parents and their strong faith that, whatever they decided, it would be as Allah wished.

COMMUNITY CARE IS DIFFERENT FROM HOSPITAL CARE

In my experience, going home to care for a technology-dependent child is based on a balance of the care required and the risks that are inherent in that care.

A balance of providing adequate care that is manageable in the home situation. It is always possible to take a child who is technology-dependent home to be cared for but it must be balanced by maintaining a home and not merely transporting the hospital environment with all its attendant burdens and negative aspects into the home. This is even more so in a scenario in which the child is unlikely to live. If the purpose in taking the child home to be cared for at this time is to improve the quality of life for the child by experiencing normal family life, then it is important that this is enabled without placing the expectation of 'perfect' care on the parents and family.

We know as professionals, we know as human beings, that life is not certain, that the pathways are not always straight or clear-cut, and the same is true when a child has a palliative condition; we cannot always know the timeline or the progression of the disease. This even more likely when we have no name to give to the condition that the child has. ACT[14] concedes that some children require constant medical attention and may frequently be in the hospital setting, whereas others may be managed in the home environment. In this situation the dilemma was when to move from one form of care to the other. How do we discuss this with families, so that it is a real concept and belief without constant reiteration? Some families could not live with this as a real possibility every day.

The plan to discharge Alisha went ahead without recognition by the specialist medical team that this was a palliative care scenario. Their expectations of the care that the family could give at home were high, as was their expectation of the local nursing team, in terms of the interventions and observations they requested.

It became palliative care when the balance of treatment was such that it was not significantly prolonging life and to do so was actually reducing the quality of life.

When talking to parents it is hard to find the words to express what we mean in a way which does not sound harsh. Balanced with this is a parent's desire for their child to live. Parents may not be able to say clearly the words 'let my child die', but by the choices and decisions they make in the knowledge of what the likely outcome may be, in this case the parents found several ways of telling us they were ready as long as we were prepared to hear them. The first was their decision to not go forward with the transplant assessment, the second occasion was at home and whilst talking about Alisha's blood results. She had very low platelets at this time and was therefore at significant risk of developing a catastrophic bleed, especially in light of her worsening liver failure and probable portal hypertension. Nasreen's biggest fear was that Alisha would suffer a distressing death from an episode of bleeding like that of her nephew. She knew this was a possibility with her low platelet count, but she stated that she did not want to take Alisha back into hospital, even locally. I had already explored the possibility of platelet transfusion at home and this was not considered feasible given the distance from the hospital and the life of platelets once defrosted. The specialist centre had asked for routine full blood counts at least twice a week, even though I had discussed with them Nasreen's wish not to take Alisha into hospital, a wish she had made plain as the days went by, through her refusal to attend either hospital for review. When Nasreen again made this very specific request for no further hospital treatment, I made the decision to discontinue taking bloods for a full blood count. Nasreen questioned why I had stopped these, as she knew they had been requested by the hospital. She asked if I was giving up on Alisha, I explained that I had stopped an investigation because it was one that we were not going to act on, that it would not affect the care that we gave Alisha because we could only give blood or platelets in the hospital. This had already been explored with the family and they did not wish Alisha to go into the hospital for this. But if they had changed their minds about this then we could agree together how to go forward. Nasreen sat quietly for a while and I sat with her. I knew it was a difficult time as Nasreen was forced to face again the reality that her child was going to die and to question: were the decisions she and Mohammed made the right ones?

I mentioned earlier the expectations of care placed on everyone by the specialist medical team because they did not recognise Alisha's care as palliative, they did not seem to hear the messages they were being given by the family or understand the nature of caring for a child at home, even though I had repeated communication with both the nurses and the specialist paediatrician on the team. They said there was no hope, no further treatment but they asked for tests and observations that were distressing to Alisha and would not be acted on.

I left Alisha's house questioning the decision I had made and the care we were providing because Nasreen had questioned me. However, I also left knowing we had had an open conversation about the future for Alisha and knowing that they had made decisions about her care with full knowledge of the implications of those decisions. I subsequently discussed Alisha's care with her local paediatrician and at length with the specialist, who after speaking to Nasreen again agreed with the decision that had been made.

Alisha was at home for about five weeks before she died, and for much of that time she was a happy baby who enjoyed people who talked to her and made silly noises. She became increasingly unhappy on handling as her abdominal distension became worse, her skin improved as long as she remained on Dioralyte (a solution of electrolytes and sugars) orally and via her nasogastric tube. Alisha liked to take a bottle, she enjoyed being fed, unfortunately any formula gave her diarrhoea which caused her skin to blister. Nasreen discontinued formula feeds which she only felt able to tell me after several days, as the regime had been suggested by the specialist hospital and she felt I would insist on her maintaining these. Oral morphine was prescribed for pain relief and it was explained that this should be given regularly, but also if they thought Alisha had any discomfort between her routine doses. It took several days for the family to begin to give regular pain relief, but once it became clear that Alisha was happier being held when she had pain relief, Nasreen was happy to do this, as she had had few opportunities during Alisha's life in which to hold her.

Nasreen was anxious that Alisha should be part of her family's religious celebration (Eid), and we talked about how this could be managed, as this was not at Alisha's home. The plan therefore was that Alisha would not start her parenteral nutrition until later in the night on that day, after the family had returned home, but Nasreen was anxious that Alisha might become dehydrated or uncomfortable. I arranged to phone during the afternoon to talk to Nasreen and if necessary I would visit in the early evening.

Nasreen and Mohammed had been given access to the team 24 hours a day, seven days a week at this time as it was apparent that Alisha would not live for much longer, though she continued to amaze the nursing team with how alert and playful she was for most of the time. The signs that we could see were her increasing jaundice and distension, which gave a false impression of health as her limbs were becoming more wasted, she was in pain even if she did have regular pain relief (which we needed to increase over this period), and her respiratory rate was increasing and appeared to require more effort.

In the evening of Eid, I saw Alisha with Nasreen, and Alisha's extended family at her grandparents' house. Alisha was asleep and had apparently been asleep for most of the afternoon.

I observed Alisha while I talked to Nasreen and her sisters, she appeared unsettled though she did not wake and her breathing was more laboured, I explained to Nasreen that I thought Alisha's condition wasn't as good as it had been the day before but that I could not say how long Alisha had left. We discussed how they could contact the team during the night and who was on call overnight. As a team we did this regularly with families, ensuring they knew there was someone on call and who it was. Over the weeks that Alisha had been at home, when she had needed routine care the whole team had met Alisha and her family, building a relationship between the team and the family in a short space of time. On this night it was myself who was on call.

The family used the paging service at 2.00 am, I called the number given and spoke to Nasreen, she was very distressed and upset. Alisha's breathing had become very laboured, though from the description Nasreen gave it did not sound as though she had Cheyne-Stokes respiration. Nasreen was very distressed, so I advised giving Alisha some morphine via her nasogastric tube and that I would be with them as soon as I could.

When I arrived, Nasreen was upstairs in Alisha's bedroom with her sister and her husband. Alisha's breathing was very slow and laboured. She was not conscious. Nasreen picked her up when I arrived and she became slightly agitated but settled quickly in Nasreen's arms. While we were talking Alisha's breathing changed; the gaps between breaths got longer and she had several long gaps between breaths, which I had already explained to Nasreen would be one of the indicators that she would not have long to live. It was apparent Alisha would not survive through the night. Nasreen sat crying in the bedroom holding Alisha. Mohammed was present, as was Nasreen's sister, who held her while she cried. The room was softly lit and I sat with them in silence for a while. Nasreen took a breath and asked if we could stop the IV feed, which I did while she held Alisha. Nasreen gently rubbed Alisha's chest and called her name every time she did not take another breath. Nasreen spoke to Mohammed and her sister and they both left the room for a while. We did not talk but sat in silence, it was apparent from the noises downstairs that other family members were arriving. Several female relatives came into the room and sat with Nasreen. Some were crying, others asked questions, but there appeared to be an acceptance in the room of what was happening. Nasreen asked if the nasogastric tube could be removed. I explained I was unwilling to do this in case Alisha needed more pain relief, but Nasreen felt she wanted her daughter's face free of the tape and tubes which had been across it for much of her life. We compromised by giving Alisha another dose of morphine and allowing some time for this to take effect before removing the tube. Alisha's breathing was steadily getting worse. There were obviously a lot of family members in the house as they came upstairs to touch Alisha and went away again. Nasreen was calm and composed, she asked if I would leave, which I accepted, and we again went through the necessary procedures for when Alisha died, who needed to be called but also that she could call again if she needed to.

I left Nasreen holding Alisha with Mohammed next to her, surrounded by her family. Alisha died at 6.30 am.

The family did not call the nursing team but they followed the instructions, which we had discussed several times, and the out-of-hours General Practitioner visited and pronounced Alisha dead. Alisha was buried later the same day.

It is difficult to say that the ACT Care Pathway[14] was followed. A multidisciplinary approach was initiated to facilitate Alisha's discharge home, but there was not the adoption of a palliative care philosophy by the specialist team, though they discussed and sought acknowledgement from the family that Alisha had a life-threatening if not life-limiting condition. However, I look at the final element of the pathway and feel that without using this, Alisha's care met the fifth and final standard, 'every child and family should be helped to decide on an end-of-life plan and should be provided with care and support to achieve this as closely as possible.' Having as central to our approach and philosophy as professionals the child's needs across all domains – physical, social, psychological and spiritual – balanced with the needs of the family enables this standard to be met. However, where the pathway can be useful is explaining the variety of needs and services required to professionals outside of the field of children's palliative care.

APPENDIX: SOME OF THE ISSUES IDENTIFIED DURING ASSESSMENT IMPACTING ON PLANNING DISCHARGE HOME

➤ Parental knowledge and skill to administer TPN (total parenteral nutrition) at home. Alisha was to come home on five nights of TPN, which was to be given over 12 hours, to commence at 8.00 pm and to finish at 8.00 am.

➤ Issues pertaining to the home environment – the bedrooms were all up a narrow steep stairway.

➤ Difficulty in providing the right facilities for hand hygiene if control measures were put in place.

➤ Need for an adult to occupy Zakim, or Zakim playing in his room with a stairgate across the doorway to prevent him placing his hands on the sterile equipment and also to prevent him becoming injured.

➤ Parental capacity to manage on a day-to-day basis with the emotional and physical demands of caring for a sick child at home. Alisha's mother was her main care provider both in the hospital and when she was discharged.

➤ The family were very anxious to take Alisha home as they found it difficult to spend much time with her in the hospital due to Mohammed's work. Zakim became bored and irritable in the hospital and there was the dilemma of finding child care. Nasreen also struggled to come on her own to somewhere unfamiliar on public transport, though she was unwilling to discuss the reasons.

➤ Could I accept lower standards for Alisha's care at home because of her poor prognosis? Alisha's care was based in the management of risk and good practice principles in relation to administration of TPN and central-line care.

N.I.C.E. analysis

Please reflect on the issues raised in this chapter in relation to your own practice.

Needs

- Understanding across professions in paediatric and primary care of palliative care for children.
- Honesty with families enabling them to make informed choices.
- Staff with skills in communication.
- Staff given support with the emotional labour of working in palliative care.

Interests

- Identification of the needs of children and families across the wide range of palliative care conditions rather than the narrow focus of condition specific services.
- Development of services to support across the spectrum of conditions rather than services commissioned and provided in a condition specific manner.
- Providing proactive care, incorporating clear and honest communication, that will lead to the most effective care.
- Using limited resources (staff, time, money) effectively.

Concerns

- Children who undergo unnecessary distress from treatments and interventions, which will offer little benefit to them.
- That the current political interest and high profile of paediatric palliative care will wane with no concrete improvements in the provision of services.
- Staff's fear of working with children and families due to emotional distress at children dying.

Expectations

- Increasing acknowledgement of the need for children's palliative care.
- Improved collaboration through better communication.
- Providing coordinated services for children with complex health and palliative care needs.
- An experienced and skilled workforce.

Reflecting on the scenario described, the issues arose from several of the areas identified in the 'Needs' section. The need to support staff with the emotional labour comes from the recognition that personally I have moved away from direct care with families partly because of this lack of support.

Action plan: next steps

To ensure staff that work with families are provided with the necessary support through formal supervision structures, with access to therapeutic support if needed. Supporting staff is one mechanism to ensure a skilled workforce. Staff with experience, knowledge and skills are the most valuable resource in any service.

Improve the understanding and perception of paediatric palliative care and how this needs to work alongside families with honesty and working with their hope. In order to achieve this there needs to be a workforce who are skilled and experienced, including communication skills.

REFERENCES

1 Davies R. The Diana community nursing team and paediatric palliative care. *Br J Nursing.* 1999; **8**: 506–11.
2 UK Department of Health. *Better Care: Better Lives.* 2008. Available at: www.dh.gov.uk/en/ Publicationsandstatistics/Publications/PublicationsPolicyAndGuidance/DH_083106 (accessed 17 February 2010).
3 www.biglotteryfund.org.uk/er_eval_palliative_report_yr3.pdf
4 Craft Sir A, Killen S. *Palliative Care Services for Children and Young People in England.* An independent review for the Secretary of State for Health. London; 2007.
5 www.dh.gov.uk/en/Healthcare/NationalServiceFrameworks/Children/DH_4089111
6 www.everychildmatters.gov.uk/socialcare/ahdc/
7 www.dh.gov.uk/en/Publicationsandstatistics/Publications/PublicationsPolicyAndGuidance/ DH_094400
8 www.everychildmatters.gov.uk/socialcare/ahdc/coreoffer/
9 www.mcpcil.org.uk/liverpool-care-pathway
10 www.goldstandardsframework.nhs.uk/
11 www.dh.gov.uk/en/Publicationsandstatistics/Publications/PublicationsPolicyAndGuidance/ DH_086277
12 Matthews KE, Gambles M, Brook L, *et al.* Developing the Liverpool Care Pathway for the Dying Child. *Paediatr Nurs.* 2006; **18**: 18–21.
13 Department of Health. *Commissioning Children's and Young peoples Palliative Care Services.* 2005. Available at: www.dh.gov.uk/en/Publicationsandstatistics/Publications/ PublicationsPolicyAndGuidance/DH_4123874 (accessed 17 February 2010).
14 Elston S. *Integrated Multi-agency Care Pathways for Children with Life-threatening and Life-limiting Conditions.* Bristol: ACT; 2004.
15 Association for Children with Life-Threatening or Terminal Conditions and their Families and the Royal College of Paediatrics and Child Health. *A Guide to the Development of Children's Palliative Care Services.* Bristol: ACT; 2003. p. 6.

4

Organisation of care in Romania

Kirsteen Cowling

INTRODUCTION

Emanuel Hospice is in Oradea, Romania. It started in 1996 providing palliative home care to adults with terminal cancer. In 1999, I, a British paediatric nurse, joined the team to help them develop the services for children. There were many obstacles and challenges to overcome in setting up this new service. In this chapter I will use a case study of an exceptional young patient to illustrate how we addressed some of these challenges to set up a successful service for children living with life-threatening and life-limiting conditions in Oradea and the surrounding area. Permission has been given by her parents for us to share her story.

BACKGROUND

Romania is a former communist country, located in South-East Central Europe – as far east as you can go without dropping into the Black Sea. It shares a border with Moldova, Ukraine, Hungary, Serbia and Bulgaria. It is approximately 237 000 sq km, making it the ninth largest territory and the seventh largest population (with 21.5 million people) among the 27 European Union member states (Romania joined the EU in 2007).[1]

According to the CASPIS study (the Romanian anti-poverty commission),[2] some 6.5 million Romanians live in poverty, of whom 2.4 million live in extreme poverty and another 1.2 million cannot afford basic food rations.

Oradea, where Emanuel Hospice (EH) works, is found in Bihor county in the north west of the country, close to the Hungarian border. It is the eleventh largest city in the country and has a population of 206 614, while the total county population is 600 223.[3] The ethnic breakdown of the county is:

➤ Romanians – 67.6%
➤ Hungarians – 26%
➤ Roma – 5%
➤ Slovaks – 1.2%
➤ Germans – 0.2%

Bihor county has the highest registered incidence of cancer in the country – 1800 new cancer cases/year and 1300 cancer related deaths/year (no paediatric figures available). The paediatric population of the district is approximately 100 000.

BARRIERS LIMITING SERVICE DELIVERY

Palliative care is still a relatively new concept in Romania. When the hospice began there was very limited knowledge/awareness of palliative care, both by professionals and laymen. So this was one of the first barriers to overcome and necessitated diplomacy and education as we sought to share the philosophy of palliative care with professional colleagues and explain how we could help them to provide better care for their patients.

When the hospice began there was no concept of community nursing, medical care stopped on discharge from hospital. When patients no longer responded to treatment, they were discharged to the care of the family, with little or no support or advice. Over half the population of the county live in a rural setting, making access to adequate medical care difficult. In many of the villages there is limited access to a doctor – there may be a clinic for a couple of hours every two weeks, or they may have to go to a neighbouring village. GPs rarely do home visits. There was no state provision for community care, no information, advice or backup – this is where the EH provides an invaluable service.

When I was trying to research and establish the need for a children's palliative care service it was very difficult to get any clear statistics. There was an element of suspicion from local authorities when we asked about paediatric morbidity/mortality statistics and they were reluctant to share these. In the hospital there were poor/incomplete patient records and no reporting system in place for specific diagnosis (i.e. cancer) – making it difficult to identify those who would benefit from palliative care (each doctor knows his/her own patients but there was no reporting system, i.e. cancer database). This has now changed and a paediatric cancer database has been established. However, there is still no reporting system for other life-threatening and life-limiting conditions.

There is very tight legislation regulating the prescription of morphine and until 2006/7 only oncologists were allowed to prescribe it. The law is now changing to allow other doctors (who have undergone suitable training) to prescribe. However, there is still a lot of fear and lack of experience in using morphine, particularly in children.

Another barrier to the development of palliative care services, which is pretty universal to most areas, is the lack of resources: funding, trained personnel and equipment. When resources are limited and local authorities are struggling to provide adequate primary healthcare then palliative care and funding for extra personnel or training needs are a low priority. I'm happy to say that even this is now changing in Romania and as a result of many years of lobbying and probably their entry into the EU, palliative care is now on the national agenda and local authorities are being encouraged to develop palliative care provision in the hospitals (primarily adult services). Legislation does not yet cover domiciliary palliative care.

There have been many obstacles and challenges to setting up the hospice, but with God's grace, over the past 12 years we have found favour with the local authorities and have established good relations with local professionals. Since 1996, EH has provided specialised palliative care to adults with advanced cancer and, since 1999, to children with life-threatening or life-limiting conditions.

HOW DOES UK POLICY IMPACT? IS THERE A NATIONAL POLICY FOR PAEDIATRIC PALLIATIVE CARE?

When EH started there was little awareness/recognition of need for palliative care and no legislation for home care services. Now there is legislation covering general home care services but this does not yet cover specialist palliative care services. There is a national policy currently being drawn up for palliative care (which hopefully will include paediatrics).

Prior to 1996 there were no domiciliary adult palliative care services available in Bihor District. With funding provided by a UK charity, EH was founded and became the second adult hospice in Romania. Since then, several other palliative care services have been developed throughout the country.

Recognising the need for paediatric palliative care services and their own limited resources and knowledge, EH invited myself, a British paediatric nurse, to join the team to develop the children's services. Thus, in 1999 the paediatric programme began.

In setting up the children's services we referred to the ACT document *A Guide to the Development of Children's Palliative Care Services*[4] and set our admission criteria to include any life-threatening or life-limiting condition, using the four groups listed in the document as a guideline. This document proved an invaluable resource for us, which we referred to regularly, particularly in the early days. Unfortunately the care pathways[5] which were also developed by ACT, were not available to us when we started and we have only recently become aware of them.

PROMOTION OF PALLIATIVE CARE/EDUCATION

As part of our ongoing commitment to the promotion of palliative care, EH has funded several nurses from the paediatric hospital to attend palliative care conferences and courses at the National Education Centre for Palliative Care in Brasov. Since the establishment and development of the paediatric services in Oradea a number of EH staff have been trained by the National Education Centre for Palliative Care in Brasov as trainers, so as well as providing hands-on care to patients they are also actively involved in the education of other professionals, providing courses locally in Oradea, in collaboration with the National Education Centre.

Emanuel Hospice has been active locally and at a national and international level in promoting the need for the palliative care services. Myself and the hospice director Marinela Murg were privileged to be included in a team of palliative care professionals who drew up a document outlining 'national standards for developing palliative care services' in Romania, which were completed and presented to the Romanian health minister in 2002. Marinela was also a member of the Council of Europe's 'committee of experts' for the development of palliative care recommendations for all EU member states. 'The recommendation of the Council of Europe expert committee on the organisation of palliative care was formally adopted by the Committee of Ministers on 12 November 2003 as the recommendation Rec (2003) 24 "on the organisation of palliative care". The decision to adopt this report is indicative of the commitment of member states to develop palliative care services to the highest possible standards."[6]

SUCCESSES AND LESSONS IN IMPLEMENTING PALLIATIVE CARE

As I have already said, palliative care is still a relatively new concept in Romania, and yet there have been many changes in the past 12 years, with a growing interest in the development of palliative care services throughout the country. The development of the Emanuel Hospice is very much a work in progress. Nevertheless, many of the lessons learned in this setting may be utilised in other regions of the world.

While the need for services in Oradea was great, the development of the programme did not occur quickly. The programme started first by identifying and establishing contacts with local paediatricians and specialists at the local Children's Hospital. The development and nurturing of community resources are perhaps the most important steps in the success of any hospice programme. The programme's first patients were oncology patients identified by a paediatric haematologist at the Children's Hospital.

Initial contact was made while the child was hospitalised. If the parents consented, the child was then followed up by the hospice team once the child returned home. This approach has been successful and continues today. However, the programme has since expanded its services to include other children and their families with life-limiting conditions in addition to those with cancer, using the four groups listed in the ACT document as a guideline.

Another factor contributing to the programme's success is that expansion of the services has not occurred before adequate resources were in place to manage the additional caseload. There are currently two full-time nurses and a part-time social worker providing direct care for children. However, the overall team is larger since they share accommodation and administrative support with the adult services.

When we began to develop the children's services we started with oncology patients, due to the personal background and knowledge of the nurse setting up the service and due to the relative ease of identifying patients.

The paediatric team work in close collaboration with the oncology unit and provide support to families from diagnosis (there are no other support services available in Romania and no information). We began by developing a relationship with the paediatric oncologist, regularly visiting the ward and discussing the merits/need for palliative care and meeting any patients/families currently on the ward. Through time the oncologist came to trust us and our motivation and began to introduce us to all new patients with a haemato/oncological diagnosis. We regularly visit them in hospital then follow up at home as required. The level of support offered varies depending on the response to treatment and is tailored to individual needs of the family. Approximately half of the oncology patients enter remission and are subsequently discharged from the hospice. For those children who do not respond favourably to treatment the level of support is increased as required and palliative care is provided at home until the death of the child. In the rest of this chapter we will demonstrate our model of care by sharing the traumatic journey of a courageous young girl from diagnosis to her subsequent death. Some of the pictures are of a graphic nature and may be disturbing, but illustrate the reality of the situation this family and our team faced.

INITIAL CONTACT

'S' was two years old when diagnosed in July 2000 with embrionic rhabdomyosarcoma of her right nasal fossa. Our first contact with the family was in January 2001 when we were asked by the paediatric oncologist in Oradea to contact the family to discuss the need to continue treatment, which was interrupted by the parents due to a family crisis.

During that first visit it was evident that S had relapsed and we convinced her mum to return to the hospital so S could be seen by the oncologist in Oradea. She then referred S to the larger teaching hospital in Cluj (three hours away), who recommended the chemo protocol to be given by the local hospital. Unfortunately the tumour was very aggressive and did not respond to the curative treatment and S was discharged home to the care of her family 18 months after our first contact. From that point her principal treatment became purely palliative.

As her condition deteriorated we increased the frequency of visits according to her needs. Whilst S underwent chemotherapy in Oradea children's hospital the hospice team were involved in providing psychosocial support to her and her family. She was regularly visited by the team who provided distraction by way of play and built a trusting relationship with her. We also provided support and information for mum regarding treatment, side-effects and expected outcomes – due to time and personnel restraints there was limited opportunity to ask questions of hospital personnel and no

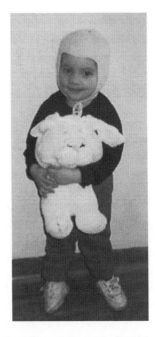

FIGURE 4.1 January 2001 when S was first admitted to Emanuel Hospice

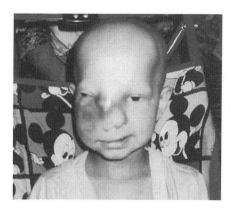

FIGURE 4.2 August 2002, S discharged from oncology – care became purely palliative

literature was available. Transport was also accorded on a number of occasions from the village to the hospital to ensure she continued treatment. When S was transferred to Cluj for radiotherapy and further chemo the team maintained telephone contact with the family.

MEDICAL CARE

While still undergoing chemo a submandibular tumour became evident (1 October) and within a month two growths the size of an egg were evident. Her right eye was pushed out of its socket and the skin around her eye was discoloured brown/black. S was referred back to Cluj for radiotherapy as it was not available in Oradea and had to travel three hours to another county. She was admitted to hospital for the duration of her treatment, which had financial and social implications for the family. (Mum had to pay for her bed/food) and the other four children were at home; the eldest daughter at 13 years of age took care of them, including the two-year-old.

After radiotherapy there did seem to be some improvement but it was obvious from the facial features that the tumour was still evident. Chemotherapy treatment continued until August 2002; however the tumour began to grow over her right cheek bone and S complained of headache. Within a couple of weeks the tumour had extended over to the left cheekbone and she could no longer breath nasally, had right) ochular oedema and became blind in her right eye. She had little appetite and became mildly agitated.

While S was still undergoing treatment, mum consulted a homeopath/naturalist who recommended a radical dietary regime, involving raw fruit and vegetables, no sugar and no cooked or refined foods. This was very challenging for the team, as we sought to support the family in their decisions, but at the same time encourage them to allow S the foods she liked/wanted, especially as her condition deteriorated.

As the tumour advanced and broke down, S's appearance changed radically. At the tender age of four she was very aware of the physical changes taking place and was very self-conscious when out in public and didn't like mum to stop and talk to anyone in the street. Her siblings accepted her visual appearance and were fully involved in her care.

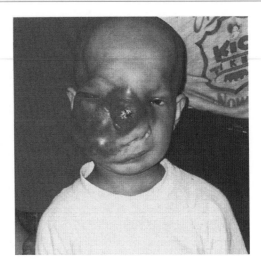

FIGURE 4.3 Rapid growth, just two weeks since discharge from hospital

To help develop the therapeutic relationship and trust with S and the hospice staff we minimised the number of staff members involved in her care. S expressed a great deal of joy when she heard the car horn outside her house.

Eighteen months after our first contact, S was discharged from the oncology hospital in Cluj to the care of her family as she was no longer responding to curative treatment – treatment became purely palliative (August 2002). Once discharged home there was rapid progression and breakdown of the tumour and S was visited almost daily by the hospice team.

Within a couple of weeks of discharge the tumour had extended over to the left cheekbone, a fistula formed on soft palate and S found it increasingly difficult to eat anything, she took a fluid diet through a straw or from a teaspoon. Mucous secretions became purulent. In Romania, the most commonly used drugs for pain control are pentazocin and pethidine instead of morphine. There is still a lot of reticence among professionals to use morphine and, as already stated, until recently only an oncologist had the right to prescribe morphine. Remarkably S's pain was controlled sufficiently initially by regular ibuprofen and paracetamol. As the tumour progressed her analgesia was changed to oral tramadol drops 5–10mg twice a day. Two weeks prior to death, all movement became painful and tramadol increased to 12.5mg three times daily. Hyoscine was given for secretions.

The tumour developed several small bleeding points, which S's mum treated with home 'diathermy' using a magnifying glass and the sun with good effect. The tumour developed a mildly offensive odour and oozing exudate – twice daily dressings were carried out, by hospice in the morning and mum in the evening. S sat up in a chair for dressings and supported her head with her hands.

We used what materials we received in donations or what we could access locally and didn't always have the 'ideal' treatment available. One of the challenges for us was the 'naturalist' regime and the completely different approach to treatment, including

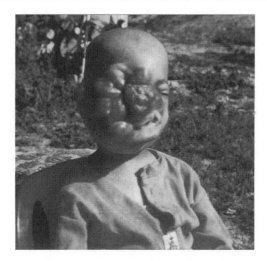

FIGURE 4.4 September 2002, home 'diathermy' using the sun's rays

dressings. It was challenging for us professionally, not knowing the effect of the alternative dressings, but in discussion with S's mum we reached a compromise where she allowed us to carry on with the 'medical' dressings in the mornings and she changed them in the evenings using a completely different regime recommended by the 'naturalist' doctor, using aloe vera, herbal plants, crushed and applied and covered with cabbage.

By the end of September S was completely blind, her upper teeth were enveloped in the tumour and one or two fell out. She was on a fluid diet through a straw. She became drowsy, hypotonic, peripherally shut down, tachycardic and skin dehydrated. The sight of S moved us profoundly, raising sentiments of affection, compassion and suffering in our hearts. Throughout this time we were thankful to be able to bring comfort and ease her suffering by offering nursing care, love and compassion.

S was still conscious and talking with her mum the day before she died. S died peacefully at home in the care of her family two months after she was discharged from the oncology unit. The team had explained to mum prior to this what to expect so she was prepared and able to reassure her husband about what was happening. Caring for S presented many challenges but we consider it a privilege to have shared the journey with this amazingly resilient family.

PSYCHOSOCIAL AND SPIRITUAL SUPPORT

More than half the population live in a rural setting including our young patient who lived in a village 20 miles from town. With limited public transport, no family car, one wage earner and five children there were many challenges to overcome. The family of seven lived in two rooms, with no running water or indoor sanitation or bathing facilities.

S was admitted to Cluj for several weeks at a time, which had financial and social

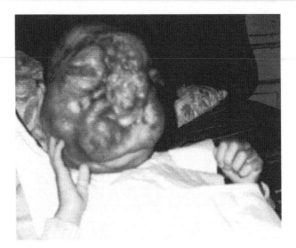

FIGURE 4.5 October 2002, two weeks prior to death

implications for the family. Mum had to pay for her bed/food in hospital. Dad had to work or lose his job, which meant the eldest child at 13 years of age took care of her three younger siblings, including the 2-year-old – there was no extended family available to provide support.

The team were able to advise the family about benefits they were entitled to and assist with the bureaucracy involved in obtaining them.

As well as help with paperwork we also offered practical material aid, including food and clothing for the family and occasionally financial assistance.

During this difficult time we came alongside the family and offered them emotional and spiritual support and prayed and shared scripture with them during our visits. Spiritual care is recognised as an integral part of the hospice ethos, providing support for the 'whole' person. While we are a Christian hospice, under the authority of a local church, we provide non-discriminatory care to any person eligible despite ethnic or religious background. We do not have other religions in our area, rather, various Christian denominations. Care is individualised, responding to the varied needs of families, facilitating contact with their own local priest/minister when required. The family had a very strong faith and throughout S's illness they hoped and prayed for a miraculous healing, but as her condition deteriorated both parents expressed that they accepted God's will for their daughter's life, whatever that may be.

BEREAVEMENT SUPPORT

Staff counselled parents in preparation for S's death. As a result of the total support provided to the family they felt able to cope with her at home and provide the care she needed in familiar surroundings rather than in the hospital.

Members of the team attended the funeral and continued to visit the family regularly, to offer ongoing bereavement support for the first year following her death. During one of those visits S's mum told us how she was comforted by her two-year-old

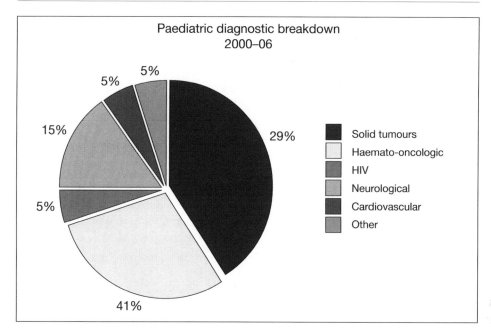

FIGURE 4.6 Diagnostic breakdown of children cared for by EH

son, who observing her crying told her 'mummy don't cry, maybe Jesus needed a little girl in heaven'. As Christians, the family hold onto the hope of seeing her again. The family maintained contact with the hospice even four years later. Two of S's siblings attended summer camp, providing distraction, fun and peer support.

SUMMARY

To date EH has provided professional palliative care services to approximately 1000 adults and 160 children and their families, of which 70% of the children had an onco-logical diagnosis and 30% non-oncological.

The development of paediatric palliative care services can present many challenges. Prior to the establishment of any hospice programme it is critical to assess the needs of the community to determine whether there is a need for an ongoing service (as far as this is possible). Should a need for services be identified, the first ingredient for success is a commitment by an individual or group to undertake the challenge.

Good public relations with the community including existing health services is the second most important ingredient. This process is ongoing and time-consuming, but necessary for the programme to develop successfully.

Finally, with limited resources available, it may be useful to consider developing paediatric programmes that complement existing adult services. This relationship may allow for sharing of supplies, personnel and other resources necessary to launch the programme, as was the case in Oradea.

Once you have the vision and the team, it's important to set some clear guidelines for the service you want to provide and clarify your criteria for eligibility. In Romania there are many medical and social problems and without clear criteria for eligibility it would have been very easy to be inundated and overwhelmed by needy people in the community seeking help. The ACT document *A Guide to the Development of Children's Palliative Care Services* was an invaluable resource for us to be able to do this. While it is always difficult to turn people away, especially when there is a very obvious need, we found that having very clear eligibility criteria from the outset helped us address this difficult issue when it arose. It also helped us keep focused on the integrated family-centred care, which is central to paediatric palliative care, and not become too medicalised nor purely a social service, but to look at the holistic needs of the individual families and adapt their care accordingly.

I find it difficult to comment specifically on the care pathways as I have not used them. However, I am sure these would be an equally useful tool in helping to ensure families get the integrated care they need and deserve from the point of diagnosis to ongoing bereavement support. It is always good to have a clear outline of what needs to be done and to be able to refer to others' expertise. Since I first became involved with ACT in 1999 I have been very impressed with the organisation and the quality of their publications. They are true champions of paediatric palliative care.

The road to a successful paediatric palliative home care service in Oradea has not been easy, but hopefully our lessons will provide some assistance for others who are interested in developing similar programmes.

N.I.C.E. analysis

Please reflect on the issues raised in this chapter in relation to your own practice.

Needs

- Increase awareness of palliative care.
- Palliative care education.
- Trained palliative care personnel.
- More palliative care services nationwide.
- Recognition of need for paediatric as well as adult palliative care.
- National policies to be developed and implemented for domiciliary palliative care.
- Training/education on use/prescribing of opiates.
- Funding for service provision.

Interests

- Growing interest in palliative care locally and nationally.
- Hospitals developing interest in palliative care.
- National policies being developed for hospital palliative care units.

Concerns

- Focus on adult services, paediatric palliative care not being specifically addressed.
- No policies for domiciliary palliative care.
- Lack of knowledge/confidence in use of opiates.
- Suspicion and competition rather than cooperation/collaboration between different service providers.

Expectations

- Increasing numbers of providers trained in paediatric palliative care.
- Transparency and better cooperation between service providers.
- Palliative care education added to national curriculums.
- Development of national policies to cover comprehensive service provision (not just hospital inpatient units).
- National funding to include community PPC services – not just hospitals.

From the above analysis please reflect on:

- While there is growing awareness of palliative care in Romania and gradual development of services and policies, both are patchy. Policies cover hospital services but don't address community palliative care. Services have developed randomly where there have been personnel with an interest rather than as part of a national strategy, although that is now changing.
- Over the last few years some charities have been established in response to changing legislation and available funding. This has led to inconsistent service provision in some areas as they are funding-driven rather than needs-driven.
- There is still a lot of fear and lack of experience in use of morphine, particularly with children, which has an impact on good symptom control.
- Suspicion and sense of competition hinders collaboration to the detriment of patient care.

Action plan: next steps
- Continue collaborating with national committee developing policies.
- Continue providing palliative care education to local professionals.
- Advocate for inclusion of palliative care in national medical/nursing curriculums.
- Advocate for implementation of new opiate legislation.
- Lobby for recognition of community palliative care services, not just hospital services.
- Need to promote transparency and good communication between service providers and policy makers.

REFERENCES

1 www.wikipedia.org/wiki/romania
2 www.relieforromania.co.uk
3 www.wikipedia.org/wiki/romania
4 Association for Children with Life-threatening or Terminal Conditions and their Families and the Royal College of Paediatrics and Child Health. *A Guide to the Development of Children's Palliative Care Services*. Bristol: ACT; 1997.
5 Elston S. *Integrated Multi-agency Care Pathways for Children with Life-threatening and Life-limiting Conditions*. Bristol: ACT; 2004.
6 www.coe.int/t/dg3/health/Source/CDSP(2004)59_en.doc

5

Organisation of care in Uganda

Lou Millington

INTRODUCTION

Paediatric palliative care was something of a black hole to me until very recently. As a UK-trained GP my only palliative care experience had been with adults and was well within my 'comfort zone'. Almost overnight, said 'comfort zone' was obliterated as I took up a post as a palliative care consultant for a hospice in Uganda. It was not difficult to identify the biggest unmet need: paediatric care, primarily Burkitt's lymphoma and HIV/AIDS. The learning curve was steep initially but soon plateaued – I knew well enough what we did do; my concern became what we didn't do, which is where this module fits into the picture. What I wanted to gain most of all from this course was an idea of what I should be aiming for, the 'gold standard' that we could aspire to, that I could measure and audit our services and performance against.

With no NICE (National Institute for Clinical Excellence) or NSFs (National Service Frameworks), no Children's Act or Charter, no apparent accountability within the field of medicine in Uganda and no appointed clinical director to act as my line manager ensuring good quality of care is an ongoing concern of mine. I realise that I must continually monitor my own standards of care and teaching to ensure that I am still delivering my best and enabling colleagues to do the same. There is so much that needs to be done here; one of the difficulties lies in trying to see what is achievable and there is a danger that after spending some time working here one becomes resigned to the poor standards of care, lack of resources and minimal staffing levels and begins to tolerate it. There seems to be a relatively fine line between accepting what cannot be changed and failing to try to change what possibly can. Reading about the pathways and frameworks that are being introduced and implemented in the UK in paediatric palliative care has inspired me to try to make improvements in the services that we offer here, rather than accepting what we do as 'not bad given the circumstances'. With careful thought and planning, communication and cooperation between different services and ongoing teaching and support, improvement and expansion of the paediatric palliative care services is no longer something that I just dream about; little by little it's becoming a reality.

THE UGANDAN PICTURE

Uganda was the first country in sub-Saharan Africa to register a drop in adult national HIV prevalence. Its epidemic, however, remains serious. An estimated 6.7% of adults (15–49 years) were living with HIV in 2005 – approximately 1 million.[1] Infection levels are highest among women (7.5% compared with 5.0% among men). With a population growing as rapidly as that of Uganda (which had a total fertility rate of 6.7, according to the 2006 Demographic and Health Survey,[2] a stable HIV incidence rate means that an increasing number of people acquire HIV each year.[3]

In November 2007 the Ugandan Ministry of Health issued statistics showing that over 100 000 children are living in Uganda with HIV/AIDS.[4] Of these children, 47 000 require anti-retroviral treatment (ART) but only 8000 are receiving it.

BACKGROUND TO THE CASE STUDY

Mobile Hospice Mbarara (MHM) was set up 10 years ago, 5 years after the main branch of Hospice Africa Uganda (HAU) was started in Kampala, to offer home-based palliative care to the south-western region of Uganda. Patients with cancer and/or HIV are accepted onto the hospice programme for pain and symptom control, psychological/spiritual/emotional/social support, end-of-life care and (in the case of Burkitt's lymphoma patients only) provision of chemotherapy. The majority of referrals are received from Mbarara Regional Referral Hospital (MRRH) but referrals are readily accepted from other health centres, community volunteers, traditional healers and self-referral from patients themselves. Patients are seen in a clinic setting at the hospice, on home visits (up to a 20 km radius from Mbarara), in the hospital and on 'outreach' clinics which take place on a monthly basis and involve hospital-based and roadside clinics 70–100 km from Mbarara. The clinical team consists of a palliative care consultant, a medical officer, two clinical officers and three nurses. The clinical officers and nurses have all completed a nine-month palliative care training programme which qualifies them to prescribe morphine in Uganda, in keeping with the Ugandan Ministry of Health protocol. The hospice is supplied with a selection of drugs from the *World Health Organization Model List of Essential Medicines* (March 2007)[5]. Morphine is imported as a powder and reconstituted into solutions of 1 mg/mL, 10 mg/mL or 20 mg/mL. The vast majority of the drugs are only available as oral preparations; subcutaneous, IM or IV administration are seldom used.

The following case study is typical of the HIV-positive children referred to the Mbarara hospice programme (*see* Appendix 1).

CASE STUDY: NATHAN

Nathan was 11 years old when he was referred to the hospice by a doctor at the nearby regional referral hospital for pain and symptom control. He had first become unwell three years previously, whilst living out in his village, with unexplained weight loss, recurrent fevers and diarrhoea. He was seen several times at his local health centre (run by an enrolled nurse) where he was treated for malaria, worms and brucellosis on numerous occasions but saw no improvement in his condition.

He started to develop abdominal distension and pain a year ago, which was associated with night sweats and malaise and was taken to a local hospital where he was diagnosed with abdominal tuberculosis and commenced on anti-TB treatment, which he completed six months earlier. However, his general health continued to decline, with ongoing fevers, anorexia and weight loss, and two months prior he developed bilateral cervical lymphadenopathy and two dark lesions on his hard palate. At this stage he was referred to Mbarara regional hospital where a biopsy of one of his oral lesions revealed Kaposi's sarcoma (KS) and an HIV test was positive. He was commenced on ART and was awaiting chemotherapy for his KS.

Nathan had lost his father and mother to AIDS-related illnesses, and two brothers to undiagnosed illnesses over the past eight years. He had three older brothers remaining and a younger sister (Rose, aged eight) who had been unwell for the past few months, but had not yet had any investigations.

Nathan and Rose lived with their oldest brother, Moses, his wife and their one-year-old baby. His carer whilst he was in hospital was his 16-year-old brother, Peter, who explained that he was the only person available to look after Nathan as both of the older brothers had to continue farming in order to support the rest of the family. The extended family had abandoned them many years ago when their parents became sick and were diagnosed with HIV and none of them were still in touch with Nathan or his siblings. He hadn't been to school since his illness started three years ago but Peter admitted that even if Nathan was well enough to attend there was no money to support his or his sister's education.

Nathan had been told about his HIV diagnosis but not about the Kaposi's sarcoma. With time his diagnoses were explained more fully and treatment was discussed with both Nathan and Peter. Both had a good understanding and a firm grasp of his various medications, how and when to take them, when his chemotherapy was due and side-effects to be aware of. Nathan's village was almost 200 km away and it was agreed that he was too unwell to make the return journey repeatedly for his ART follow-up and chemotherapy cycles so he and Peter remained on the ward for the duration of his treatment. Both brothers found this a huge struggle; financial upkeep was a constant issue, including buying meals and water and paying for investigations and drugs. Peter's wage from the plantation was also greatly missed by the rest of the family.

And Nathan started to feel quite homesick, admitting one day that he really missed his younger sister and baby nephew and was looking forward to going home and playing with them in the fields near his home.

Nathan tolerated his first two cycles of chemotherapy, but there was no reduction in the lymphadenopathy or oral KS lesions. Before receiving the third dose he became acutely unwell with a high fever, oral candidiasis, profuse diarrhoea, dehydration and anorexia. He was diagnosed with neutropenic sepsis and commenced on intravenous antibiotics and fluids and nasogastric feeding.

After five days of treatment his pyrexia and diarrhoea had subsided but he remained lethargic and his oral intake was minimal. He began to look pale and a full blood count revealed a haemoglobin of 6.5 g/dL so he was transfused two units of blood and the paediatricians decided to withhold his next dose of chemotherapy for a few extra days. Sometime during this period Peter noticed three dark spots that had appeared on Nathan's legs, which were confirmed as further Kaposi's sarcoma – neither the ART nor the chemotherapy were halting the growth and spread of the cancer and all of the time Nathan was growing weaker and more debilitated as a result of both the disease and its treatment.

Discussions were held with the paediatricians who wanted to send Nathan to Kampala for second-line chemotherapy, and Nathan and Peter who said that they could not afford to pay for the treatment, the cost of upkeep in Kampala or even meet the transport costs, and the hospice team who felt that the priority was establishing what Nathan and his family wanted and trying to support this and offer whatever help was available. If Nathan was discharged home he would not be able to access any HIV, palliative care or paediatric services, yet despite the input from all three specialities in hospital his condition was continuing to deteriorate and he and his brother made a compelling argument for allowing him to go home and 'let God's will be'. Telephone contact was made with Moses (Nathan's eldest brother and main carer) through someone in the village who worked in the hospital and he was persuaded to come and discuss Nathan's care and the possibility of taking him home.

After initial resistance from the paediatricians, with further consultation they agreed that discharging him was the best course of action for Nathan and that at this stage in his illness the ART and chemotherapy were of no benefit to him. The hospice team spent some time with Nathan, Peter and Moses discussing what to expect over the weeks following discharge and how to handle various eventualities. All three brothers were aware that Nathan was dying and that the priority of care now was to keep him as comfortable as possible and to provide support to him and his family. With mentoring and support from the hospice team Nathan's hospice worker brought up the subject of dying and death with him and spent some time exploring his fears and concerns.

The family was provided with a package of medications including morphine, bisacodyl, diazepam, metoclopramide, hyoscine and some powdered nutritional supplements. The older brothers were also given advice on feeding, hydration, hygiene, pressure sore prevention, treatment of constipation, and end-of-life care. There was no mobile telephone coverage in the village but once a week Moses travelled to a nearby town to sell produce so an arrangement was made for him to telephone the hospice from the town to give them his number so that they could then call him back and receive an update on Nathan's condition and give any advice as needed.

Following Nathan's discharge Moses contacted the hospice by telephone a month later as arranged, he reported that Nathan had died two weeks after returning home, quite peacefully, surrounded by his brothers and sister in the family home. Rose had since had an HIV test, which was negative, but had been diagnosed with tuberculosis and commenced on treatment. The family were very grateful for the care that they had received from the hospice staff.

DISCUSSION

This case could be about many thousands of HIV-positive children in sub-Saharan Africa and it illustrates some of the major obstacles that are faced by them and their carers.

Wishful thinking – development of paediatric pathways and care plans

Nathan's care was neither sophisticated nor elaborate and at times the barriers faced by him and his family to obtaining good clinical paediatric and palliative care were considerable. However, certain aspects of his care were planned for and did indeed occur as intended. In a resource-poor setting such as this one, co-coordinating care without sufficient health-service infrastructure can be a major challenge and yet communication, cooperation and planning are achievable and often successful. As stated in the UK-based ACT Care Pathways:[6]

> a pathway aims to link children and families with community services, hospital-based services, social services, education and the voluntary sector in one joined up planning process ... (the Framework) can be used to develop local care pathways suitable to the needs of the children and can incorporate available local skills and resources. The planning of local pathways should facilitate co-operation and co-ordination between professionals and services to produce a holistic approach to the care of children and families. The vital point is that the care pathway should be jointly owned by all those involved in its design, implementation and review.

Within Europe the importance of co-coordinated paediatric palliative care has been recognised by the EAPC,[7] which emphasises in its IMPaCCT report that 'the care coordinator should act as the main link, providing continuity, ensuring that the care provided is consistent with the needs of the child and family'.

Currently no such pathways or frameworks exist within Uganda and palliative care, in particular paediatric palliative care, is in its infancy and still a very limited service. However, proposals are afoot within the Mbarara region to launch a basic care plan according to the local resources and hospice capabilities, which would take the child from diagnosis through to end-of-life care (see Appendix 2).

Staff support

The hospice paediatric team currently consists of two nurses, one trained in paediatrics and the other in palliative care. Due to the emotionally difficult nature of the job it has been proposed that they work very much as a pair; reviewing patients together and sharing responsibility for coordinating follow-up. They also have close liaison with the clinical consultant, a weekly case conference, journal club and clinical supervision meetings (with in-depth case debriefs and reviews of ongoing medical education needs), monthly clinical team meetings and staff meetings and an annual appraisal.

There has been little research into burnout in palliative care health workers in resource-poor settings but the causes are likely to be similar to those identified in the west: high workload, poor institutional support, struggling to practice according to personal philosophy of care, a sense of putting in more than they receive and role conflicts.[8] In fact, due to the stark lack of resources, staffing and education, and the high numbers of children dying from cancer and HIV/AIDS-related illnesses, the incidence of burnout may be even greater in this setting and therefore it is even more crucial that measures are in place to reduce the risks of this. A modified version of Niebuhr's Serenity Prayer[9] has been a useful teaching/discussion tool for the staff; 'The goal is to eliminate stressors that can be eliminated, master stressors that cannot be eliminated, and develop techniques for recognition and modification of stress response.'

MILLENNIUM DEVELOPMENT GOALS AND HIV/AIDS IN AFRICA

In 2000 the United Nations (UN) General Assembly devised the Millennium Declaration with a number of Millennium Development Goals (MDGs),[10] these included eradicating extreme poverty and hunger, achieving universal primary education, reducing child mortality, combating HIV/AIDS, malaria and other diseases and providing access to affordable essential drugs.

In 2005, at the UN World Summit, the 191 member nations agreed to a 'scaling up of response to HIV/AIDS', yet despite these commitments AIDS has become the primary cause of death in Africa.[11]

A declaration by the UN General Assembly in 2006 expressed 'grave concern that half of all new HIV infections occur among children . . . 2.3 million children are living with HIV/AIDS today, and the lack of paediatric drugs in many countries significantly hinders efforts to protect the health of children'.[12] Further commitment was made to addressing as a priority the vulnerabilities faced by children affected by and living with HIV; providing support and rehabilitation to these children and their families; promoting child-oriented HIV/AIDS policies and programmes and increased protection for children orphaned and affected by HIV/AIDS; ensuring access to treatment and intensifying efforts to develop new treatments for children; and building, where needed, and supporting the social security systems that protect them.

As Steinbrook (2004) reminds us: 'the challenge of the epidemic is that despite the increases in funding, global attention, and political will, more infections and more deaths continue to occur' and he goes on to describe the HIV treatment coverage rates in many countries as 'dismal'.[13] It is estimated that of the 680 000 children who currently need access to life-saving treatment, less than 8% received it.[1,14]

In the 2006 WHO report on Child and Adolescent Health Development,[15] the plight of children living in communities affected by HIV/AIDS was discussed in depth. It stated that:

> the difficulties experienced by children, caregivers and families living in communities affected by AIDS are increasing dramatically as the epidemic matures and deaths increase.[16] Under these conditions, the worst affected children experience multiple losses. They lose: their health and vitality, through infection, inadequate nutrition, and poor health care; their economic support through the constriction and collapse of livelihoods resulting from the illness and death of breadwinners and other adults in the extended family previously engaged in economic support and subsistence activities; their parents and other primary caregivers to illness and death; their families, as they are parted from caregivers and siblings because of distress mobility and migration; their connections to social institutions as a result of stigma in the community and withdrawal from school because of poverty, lack of supervision, and work obligations in the home, and their human right to development in an environment that meets their basic needs for health, education, care and protection.[17,18,19,20,21]

The MDG African Steering Group highlights that Africa as a whole is off track for meeting the MDGs on reducing child mortality, improving maternal health and combating infectious disease and suggests scaling-up intervention in Africa in order to provide comprehensive access to HIV/AIDS treatment by 2010.[22]

CHILD PROTECTION AND ISSUES SURROUNDING STIGMA

An inter-agency report headed by UNICEF highlights that children who have lost one or both parents in sub-Saharan Africa often live in households that are headed by older caregivers (usually female) who have low levels of education and are thus unlikely to have a regular source of income. This may result in orphans receiving inadequate care and food.[23]

Children and adolescents affected by AIDS are also at risk of heading their own households, and while it appears that the number of child-headed households has remained small,[24] they are a particularly vulnerable group. Children may head households to avoid sibling separation and property grabbing.

The report also discusses the stigma that children and adolescents affected by AIDS may face due to HIV in the family, their own HIV status, HIV-related poverty, or the loss of their parents and being labelled orphans. It goes on to say that this stigma can prevent children and families from seeking help or prevent others from offering them assistance; it can also prevent equal access to financial opportunities and block the development, approval or implementation of protective legislation and policies, increasing children's risk of experiencing violence and abuse. Breaking the silence surrounding HIV infection and promoting open discussion are key to addressing stigma and discrimination and helping children gain access to basic protections, services and financial opportunities. This requires that harmful attitudes and behaviours be recognised and named.

PAEDIATRIC PALLIATIVE CARE IN AFRICA

It is widely acknowledged that in the majority of poorly-resourced countries, despite the fact that there are many children suffering from diseases that are incurable or curable but without the necessary treatment available, the concept of palliative care has yet to become accepted and taken up readily. It is estimated that only 0.08% of children requiring it receive effective palliative care and more than 90% of children with cancer and other life-limiting illnesses receive only local remedies.[25] To some extent, this situation relates to the overwhelming need to provide emergency care within poorly funded health systems. Palliative care is still considered a luxury, not only by the general public but also by health professionals struggling to work in an already overburdened health system. In many developing countries there is a severe shortage of trained health professionals, a grave lack of resources and an often erratic and extremely basic supply of drugs. Commonly all efforts and energy are poured into tackling the treatable diseases or the opportunistic infections associated with AIDS because this is where the expertise and resources lie. Palliative care, and in particular paediatric palliative care, requires specialist training, support and mentoring. Health systems need to be in place to provide continuity of care for the patients as well as to ensure a good standard of care is being delivered and ongoing support is available for the health workers.

Home-based palliative care has been shown to be the most cost-effective model for resource-poor settings and certainly within the Ugandan context is more culturally acceptable to most. However, it is not without its hindrances – access to care is a major difficulty where transport infrastructure is so underdeveloped, covering a large radius for home visits is not practical yet often patients are too unwell or too poor to travel to a treatment centre themselves. Terminally ill children are often placed in acute care facilities, but they may receive inappropriate care in these facilities because they must compete for resources with patients who are more acutely ill.

Norval *et al.* in Goldman *et al.*[26] assert that an HIV/AIDS diagnosis in a child creates difficulties beyond the physical sickness, because of the associated guilt and the possibility or likelihood that more family members are infected, sick or dying. The child and parents are often ill-prepared for the coming death because of late diagnosis, the reluctance or inability of health workers to discuss death with patients, the unpredictability of the disease progression and denial. Where parents and/or caregivers are aware of or suspect a child's imminent death, they may react by withdrawing emotionally. This contrasts sharply with needs at the end of life: for physical comfort, physical touching, emotional closeness and spiritual health, all of which can have a major positive impact on the quality of remaining life. In the African setting, there are complex belief systems and rituals surrounding death and dying, and these systems may be different for a child and an adult.[26]

CONCLUSION

Children have the right to good quality healthcare, including HIV/AIDS treatment and palliative care services. Globally, but particularly in resource-constrained settings, the terminal care needs and services for children with life-threatening illnesses are poorly understood and poorly developed (*see* Appendix 3).

Delivering basic HIV/AIDS care, anti-retroviral treatment and terminal care to HIV-infected children and their parents requires planning to ensure more than episodic contact with the healthcare system, at both the institutional and community levels. Continuity in provider and services is essential for ensuring optimal quality of life for the child and family.

At the Kampala Declaration and Agenda for Global Action meeting (2008), government leaders, ministers of health and other national leaders committed to providing 'all people, everywhere with access to a skilled, motivated and facilitated health worker within a robust health system'.[27] The question is, what needs to be done to put pledges such as this into action?

A recent letter from the heads of the World Bank, UNICEF, the WHO, the Global Health Programme and many more key international organisations to the government head attending the G8 Summit in Japan, has called for 'strengthening the health systems to deliver integrated services to communities, then train new healthcare workers – and provide the money to pay them. Commit to new, long-term predictable financing, and link this investment to quantifiable results including fewer maternal, newborn and child deaths, less childhood under-nutrition, fewer HIV, malaria and TB infections, and expanded access to treatments'. In its recent report the African Steering Group for the Millennium Development Goals states that achieving these goals, and other internationally agreed development goals in Africa holds the promise of saving millions of lives, ending the scourge of hunger and malnutrition, and ensuring that Africa's children are empowered through education and good health to lead productive lives. They voice their hope that world leaders will take up these recommendations and commit to implement them.[22]

The WHO recognises that 'children have not, to date, received due attention in the global effort to prevent, treat and ameliorate HIV/AIDS' in its 2006 report on Child and Adolescent Health Development. It also acknowledges that 'deepening poverty is compromising national development achievements as well as any hope of meeting the Millennium Development Goals'. It goes on to say that 'in the face of the scale and anticipated duration of the AIDS epidemic, there is widespread consensus that strengthening systems to support children is the best option for achieving population level improvements in children's health, their psychosocial well-being and their educational development. This is consistent with a right-based approach to child well-being . . . the health sector is well placed, by utilizing its systems approach and an infrastructure that reaches into most affected communities in developing countries, to lead multisectoral responses that facilitate the holistic care and protection of children living in communities affected by HIV/AIDS'.[28]

Children's HIV/AIDS and palliative care needs ongoing advocacy to keep it in the limelight and on the agenda for ongoing review and discussion. Children's issues featured strongly on the programme for AIDS 2008 in Mexico and it is hoped that thanks to pressure from many of the large international aid organisations it will also receive coverage at the G8 summit in Japan – what happens as a result of these two events remains to be seen.

APPENDIX 1: FURTHER HIV/AIDS INFORMATION
HIV/AIDS in children in sub-Saharan Africa – the size of the problem
UNAIDS estimated that 41 million people were infected with HIV worldwide in 2003, 70% of whom were in sub-Saharan Africa (SSA) and 60% of whom were women, and infection rates are still rising. In 2004 UNICEF estimated that 20 million people around the world had died from AIDS, more than three-quarters of who were from SSA.[3]

Almost 3 million children under the age of 15 are estimated to have HIV worldwide, 90% of which are in SSA. In the developing countries approximately 1600 children are infected daily by HIV positive mothers. In 2002, there were 700 000 new paediatric infections in SSA and 580 000 paediatric HIV-related deaths (this equates to 2000 deaths per day, compared with 500 per year in the United States or Europe). There is a 75% mortality rate by five years of age for children with HIV/AIDS in resource-poor countries. In sub-Saharan Africa AIDS is the cause of approximately 70% of deaths in the under-fives. However, globally, AIDS accounts for 0.01% of the mortality rate in this age group.[25]

More than 14 million children under the age of 15 have lost one or both parents to HIV, the vast majority being in SSA. By 2010 the number of children orphaned by AIDS is expected to exceed 25 million globally, and the number of vulnerable children will greatly surpass that estimate.[30] The number of children infected with HIV will also increase significantly, and half of these children will most likely die before their first birthday.[31] It is estimated that fewer than 200 000 children worldwide have access to Anti-Retroviral Treatment (ART).

According to the UNAIDS 2007 Uganda report the overall mortality rate for children under five is 137/1000.[4] Orphans account for 13% of all under 18-year-olds (7% of the country's total population) and 20% of orphans have neither mother nor father.[32] mother-to-child transmission (MTCT) accounts for 21% of all HIV infection (25 000 children per year are born HIV-positive), and 54% of children infected with HIV die before they reach the age of two;[33] whereas the median survival age in the west was 11 years, prior to the introduction of highly-active anti-retroviral therapy, HAART.[34]

APPENDIX 2: PROPOSED PAEDIATRIC PALLIATIVE CARE PATHWAY: MBARARA REGIONAL REFERRAL HOSPITAL (MRRH) – MOBILE HOSPICE MBARARA (MHM)

➤ Child with suspected cancer and/or HIV referred from community health centre or local hospital to MRRH.
➤ Child investigated and diagnosed with cancer and/or HIV at MRRH.
➤ Child and family informed of diagnosis.
➤ Referral made to MHM, with consent of patient and family, prior to discharge from hospital.
➤ Child accepted onto MHM palliative care programme and introduced to the hospice paediatric team.
➤ Joint care of the child between MRRH and MHM during hospital stay.
➤ MRRH to make follow-up arrangements if child receiving any active treatment for disease, e.g. chemotherapy, ART.
➤ MHM paediatric team to make discharge arrangements regarding any palliative treatments and ensure follow-up within community (home visit if within 20 km radius of Mbarara, hospice appointment if well enough to travel, Outreach Clinic monthly, liaison with community health clinic or worker, Community Volunteer visit if available, telephone follow-up if possible).
➤ MRRH and MHM staff to communicate with each other if any change in child's condition.
➤ MHM team to identify end of life when appropriate and communicate this with MRRH and any community workers involved in child's care.
➤ Initiate end-of-life pathway (await modified adult's version).

APPENDIX 3: THE COST OF INTERNATIONAL AID AND THE MDG PROJECT

The international aid input required to achieve these goals is US$72 billion per year (US$25–30 billion of which would need to be spent on health). In 2004 the actual amount of overseas aid was US$29.3 billion. In 2000, as part of the Abuja Declaration, African governments pledged to give 15% of their budget to health, and 20% to education (Dar es Salaam, Conference of Education Ministers, 2002). One of the difficulties faced by African countries is the uncertainty surrounding foreign aid – without knowing how much they are going to receive over a number of years they cannot plan and budget for the expansion and improvement of services such as health and education in order to meet these MDGs.[22]

Serenity Prayer – Reinhold Niebuhr

God, give us grace to accept with serenity the things that cannot be changed, courage to change the things that should be changed, and the wisdom to distinguish the one from the other.

N.I.C.E. analysis

Please reflect on the issues raised in this chapter in relation to your own practice.

Needs

- Further advocacy for paediatric palliative care in all resource-poor countries through lobbying governments, increasing awareness, local, national and international pressure groups, etc.
- Wider and deeper recognition of paediatric palliative care in resource-poor settings on national, district and local levels (government, ministry of health, district health authorities, individual hospitals and clinics).
- Training for health professionals in all specialties on basic palliative care principles.
- Specialist training in paediatric palliative care for health professionals involved in paediatrics.
- Funding for training (governmental, non-governmental, charity).

Interests

- Recognition of existence and validity of palliative care as a medical specialty and immense need for it within the setting of HIV infection in resource-poor countries.
- Introduction of a palliative care degree course at Makerere University, Kampala, set up jointly by the university and Hospice Africa Uganda.
- Increasingly international palliative care conferences are being held in developing countries and many such countries now hold their own national or regional conference looking specifically at the needs of their populations and how they can be met with what they have available.
- Recognition by international HIV-based NGOs and charities for the need for provision of palliative care alongside interventional care for HIV patients.

Needs (continued)

- Expansion of hospice care within Uganda (and all resource-poor nations).
- Strengthening of hospice infrastructure ensuring ongoing support and mentoring for clinical staff.
- Encouragement of ongoing evaluation of standards of care, both at an individual and an organisational level.
- Development of national guidelines and frameworks for paediatric palliative care.
- Development of local pathways, guidelines and care plans for paediatric palliative care.
- Further input through UN and Millennium Development Goals project to reduce HIV transmission, improve HIV testing and treatment for children.
- Improving AIDS-orphan support and services (social, health and education).
- Increase number of doctors and nurses in rural settings so that access to good healthcare is improved.
- Ongoing training of health professionals by Hospice Africa Uganda to allow them to prescribe oral morphine in the community.
- Improve drug availability in hospitals and health centres through improving healthcare systems and infrastructure and ongoing advocacy at national level.
- Introduction of some degree of accountability and responsibility within the healthcare profession (appraisal, significant event analysis, complaints procedure, regulatory bodies, disciplinary proceedings, etc.).

Interests (continued)

- Ongoing pledges from the UN that the MDGs of reducing child mortality, combating HIV/AIDS and providing access to essential drugs will be reached.

Concerns

- Lack of available funding for training and provision of palliative care in countries where resources are already extremely stretched.
- Lack of funding to provide essential drugs.
- Lack of expertise in palliative care to provide training, support and mentoring or to develop national guidelines and pathways.
- Difficulty retaining staff in under-resourced and poorly supported settings.
- Ongoing stigma surrounding HIV/AIDS.
- Long-standing misconceptions held by medical professionals surrounding palliative care and in particular morphine use.
- Belief that palliative care is a luxury that the developing countries cannot afford.
- Cultural beliefs surrounding disease, cancer, HIV and dying.
- Rights of children are not officially recognised or protected.

Expectations

- Improved awareness of palliative care at all levels; governmental, in health professionals and within communities.
- Recognition of the importance of palliative care in resource-poor settings and commitment by ministries of health to make it a priority and address it as an area of need.
- Increased funding for hospices and palliative care services.
- Increased number of palliative care practitioners and hospices, thereby improving access to good quality palliative care.
- Development of national guidelines regarding children with cancer and HIV and of local paediatric palliative care pathways, thereby improving paediatric palliative care delivery.
- Increased referral to hospices through raised awareness of the specialty and its function.
- Improved drug availability due to increased funding and improved healthcare system infrastructure.
- Improved HIV maternal transmission rates, child mortality, testing and treatment rates.
- Advocacy for and recognition of children's rights.
- Further development of services providing support for AIDS orphans with increased access to local organisations providing financial, social and educational support.

From the above analysis please reflect on:
- Relief from pain is a widely accepted human right but in a setting where people die from preventable diseases every day due to lack of education, poor access to healthcare, lack of trained personnel and lack of resources, how can governments and health professionals be convinced that palliative care provision should also be on the agenda?

- In countries where children's rights are largely not respected or even considered, how can you ensure that paediatric palliative care patients have their own voice, have choice over their treatment and some autonomy over their care?
- In such a setting as that in Uganda, where the paediatric palliative care workload is high, few paediatricians recognise palliative care as a worthy or useful discipline, there are limited specialist-trained professionals, mentoring and support is minimal and there are numerous cultural issues to contend with, what measure can be put in place to prevent burnout, to improve staff retention and reduce the 'brain drain' of highly trained medical personnel to the better resourced, more developed nations?

Action plan: next steps
- Continue to advocate for palliative care in resource-poor countries and to use the model of Hospice Africa Uganda to encourage governments to look at developing the same model in their countries and to send their health professionals to HAU for training in palliative care if it is not available in their own country.
- Where palliative care services already exist, strengthen them by ensuring ongoing professional development and mentoring of staff and by encouraging critical evaluation of standards of care.
- Use existing palliative care providers to train other health professionals (doctors, nurses, clinical officers, medical and nursing students) locally, to increase awareness of palliative care and to forge links with other care providers in the community.

REFERENCES

1 UNAIDS/WHO. *AIDS Epidemic Update.* Geneva: UNAIDS/WHO; Dec 2006.
2 Uganda Bureau of Statistics. *Uganda Demographic and Health Survey.* Kampala; 2006
3 UNAIDS/WHO. *2007 Sub-Saharan Africa: AIDS Epidemic Update Regional Summary.* Geneva: UNAIDS; 2008.
4 Uganda AIDS Commission/Uganda HIV/AIDS Partnership. *UNGASS Country Progress Report Uganda.* Kampala: Government of Uganda; 2007.
5 WHO (2007) *Model List of Essential Medicines.* Available at: www.who.int/medicines/publications/essentialmedicines/en/ (accessed June 2008).
6 Elston S. (2004) *Integrated Multi-agency Care Pathways for Children with Life-threatening and Life-limiting Conditions.* ACT: Bristol. Available at: www.act.org.uk/ (accessed 17 February 2010).
7 EAPC (European Association of Palliative Care) Taskforce. IMPaCCT: Standards for paediatric palliative care in Europe. *Eur J Palliative Care.* 2007; **14**: 109–14.
8 Elkateb, N. National Cancer Institute, Cairo, Egypt. Preventative approach to burnout among healthcare professionals. *J Paediatric Haematology & Oncology.* 2008; **30**: 105–6. (Workshop on the Stresses & Burnout of Working with Cancer Patients, a Collection of Abstracts, Cyprus, June 2007).
9 Niebuhr's Serenity Prayer – see Appendix 3.
10 United Nations General Assembly. *Follow-up to the Outcome of the Millennium Summit:*

Road map towards implementation of the United Nations Millennium Declaration. Report of the Secretary General. Geneva: United Nations; 2001.

11 United Nations Factsheet. *World Summit: High-Level Plenary Meeting.* New York: United Nations Department of Public Information; 2005.

12 United Nations General Assembly. *Resolution Adopted by the General Assembly: Political Declaration on HIV/AIDS.* New York: United Nations; 2006.

13 Steinbrook, R. The AIDS epidemic in 2004. *NEJM.* 2004; **351**(2): 115–17.

14 UNGASS. United Nations General Assembly Special Session. *Review of the Problem of Human Immunodeficiency Virus/Acquired Immunodeficiency Syndrome in all its Aspects: Special session of the General Assembly on HIV/AIDS.* Report of the Secretary-General, United Nations. 2001. Available at: www.un.org/ga/aids (accessed June 2008).

15 WHO *Child and Adolescent Development: The Role of the Health Sector in Strengthening Systems to Support Children's Healthy Development in Communities Affected by HIV/AIDS.* Geneva: World Health Organization; 2006.

16 Bedri A, Kebbede SK, Negassa H. Sociodemographic profile of children affected by AIDS in Addis Ababa. *Ethiop Med J.* 1995; **33**: 227–34.

17 UNICEF. *Children's Rights and Responsibilities: Summary of the United Nations Convention on the Rights of a Child.* London: UNICEF; 2001.

18 Nyambedha EO, Wandibba S, Aagaard-Hansen J. Policy implications of the inadequate support systems for orphans in western Kenya. *Health Policy.* 2001; **58**: 83–96.

19 UNICEF/UNAIDS. *The Framework for the Protection, Care and Support of Orphans and Vulnerable Children Living in a World with HIV and AIDS.* New York: UNICEF; 2006.

20 UNICEF and International Social Service, *Improving Protection for Children without Parental Care: A call for international standards: A joint working paper.* Available at: www.iss.org.au/documents/ACALLFORINTLSTANDARDS.pdf (accessed June 2008).

21 NEPAD, UNESCO & UNICEF. *The Young Face of NEPAD: Children and young people in the new partnership for Africa's development.* New York: United Nations Children's Fund; 2004.

22 Millennium Development Goals African Steering Group. *Achieving The Millennium Development Goals in Africa.* MDG Africa. International Herald Tribune. World Health Priorities. 2008. Available at: www.iht.com/articles/2008/06/09/opinion/edlet.php (accessed June 2008).

23 UNICEF *Enhanced Protection for Children Affected by AIDS: A companion paper to the framework for the protection, care and support of orphans and vulnerable children living in a world with HIV and AIDS.* New York: UNICEF; 2007.

24 Simbayi L, Jooste S, Managa A. Orphans and vulnerable children in distress. *HSRC Review* 2005; **3**(3). Available at: www.hsrc.ac.za/about/HSRCReview/Vol3No3/children.html (accessed 17 February 2010).

25 Goldman A, Hain R, Liben S. *The Oxford Textbook of Palliative Care for Children.* Oxford: Oxford University Press; 2006.

26 Norval D, O'Hare B, Matusa R. HIV and AIDS. In: Goldman A, Hain R, Liben S, editors. *The Oxford Textbook of Palliative Care for Children.* Oxford: Oxford University Press; 2006.

27 WHO and Global Health Workforce Alliance. *The Kampala Declaration and Agenda for Global Action.* Geneva: World Health Organization; 2008.

28 World Health Organization. *Child and Adolescent Health and Development Progress Report 2006–2007.* Geneva: World Health Organization; 2008.

29 International AIDS Society. *Conference Policy Report: XVI International AIDS Conference,* 2006 Aug 13–18; Toronto, ON: International AIDS Society.

30 Shetty AK, Powell G. Children orphaned by AIDS: A global perspective. *Semin Pediatr Infect Dis.* 2003; **14**: 25–31.

31 Bobat R, Moodley D, Coutsoudis A, *et al.* The early natural history of vertically transmitted HIV-1 infection in African children from Durban, South Africa. *Ann of Trop Paediatr.* 1998; **18**: 187–96.

32 UNAIDS/UNICEF/USAID. *Children on the Brink 2004: A joint report of new orphan estimates and a framework for action.* New York: United Nations Children's Fund; 2004.

33 ANECCA (African Network for the Care of Children Affected by AIDS). *Handbook on Paediatric AIDS in Africa*; Blanche, S. Natural history of HIV infection in children. In: Mok JYQ, Newell M-L, editors. *HIV Infection in Children: a guide to practical management.* Cambridge: Cambridge University Press; 1995.

34 Blanche S, Newell M-L, Mayaux M, *et al.* Morbidity and mortality in European children vertically infected by HIV: the French pediatric HIV infection study group and European collaborative study. *J Acquir Immune Defic Syndr Hum Retrovirol.* 1997; **14**: 442–50.

6

Organisation of care in South Africa

Joan Marston

There can be no better measure of a nation's soul than the way it treats its children.

Nelson Mandela

Children make up 43% of the total population of South Africa, a country that has been hardest hit by the HIV and AIDS pandemic in sub-Saharan Africa with an estimated 5.5–6 million people infected with HIV, including 300 000 children under 15 years of age, and 1.2 million children orphaned by AIDS. Tuberculosis (TB) co-infection is increasing with multi-drug resistant TB and extra multi-drug resistant TB increasing in incidence, especially in the rural areas.[1]

Statistics for children with other life-limiting and life-threatening conditions are more difficult to find, although the Cancer Association of South Africa estimates between 800–1600 children are diagnosed with cancer every year. Sadly, many are diagnosed very late, with over 80% presenting at stage 3 or 4.[2]

At present there are no up-to-date statistics for children with other conditions, or severe disabilities.

Although South Africa now has access to highly active anti-retroviral therapy (HAART), with excellent policies on prevention of mother-to-child transmission (PMTCT) and treatment guidelines, only 33% of children who need HAART are actually accessing clinics and many of these children have pre-existing morbidities such as heart or respiratory failure.[3]

Whilst palliative care has been provided in South Africa for the past 25 years, mainly through the hospice movement, and whilst both Cotlands in Johannesburg and St Nicholas Children's Hospice (now Sunflower Children's Hospice) in Bloemfontein have provided palliative care specifically for children for the past 12 years, in general, palliative care for children has only recently received focused attention due mainly to the Hospice Palliative Care Association (HPCA) of South Africa developing a national Paediatric Palliative Care Portfolio, managed by a national manager, regional officers and a sub-committee with representatives from hospices in each province, and a national development strategy.[4] This has seen children's palliative care programmes develop from 7 in 2007 to 46 in 2009 (*see* Figure 6.1).

Most children receiving palliative care are within general hospice programmes that

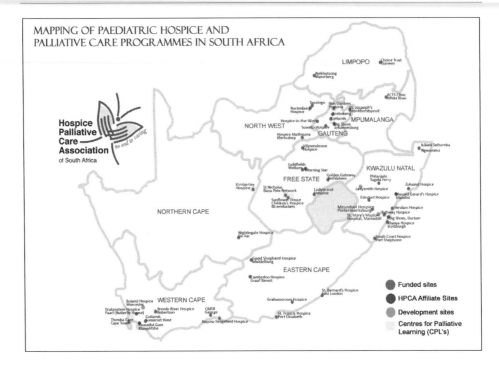

FIGURE 6.1 Mapping of paediatric hospice and palliative care programmes in South Africa

are predominantly adult-focused, with only six organisations specifically for children. A major challenge has been persuading these adult-orientated palliative care practitioners that children are different, have different needs and require services tailored to these differences.

South Africa does not have a national palliative care strategy at present although the HPCA of South Africa has recently written a draft strategy for the government that includes a comprehensive section on paediatric palliative care.[4] The National Strategic Plan for HIV, AIDS, TB and STIs 2007–11 has included palliative care as part of a comprehensive programme of home care within the plan. The National Cancer Control Guidelines also include frequent references to palliative care.

Within South Africa the combined problems of poverty, HIV and orphanhood, with children left to be cared for by elderly relatives, older siblings or caring neighbours, has led to complex social problems. Whilst South Africa has excellent legislation designed to protect children, and is a signatory of the UN Convention on the Rights of the Child, lack of social workers and community vulnerability has left many children with life-limiting conditions without social protection.[5]

STEMBILE'S STORY

Stembile was diagnosed with HIV when only three years old, after the death of both his parents from AIDS. He weighed only 9 kg and was unable to walk or talk. His 22-year-old uncle who was HIV negative cared for Stembile as well as his own disabled sister in a very neat shack in a township area. When Stembile was diagnosed with TB, he was admitted to a district hospital, where a further diagnosis of cardiac failure was made, and once on TB treatment he was referred to a local children's hospice in the grounds of the hospital. This enabled close continuity of care as the medical team from the hospital also consulted at the hospice. His clinical treatment included HAART, TB treatment and drugs to treat his heart failure. As his uncle had employment, the hospice staff met with the uncle and together they decided to keep Stembile in the hospice for long-term palliative care until his condition stabilised, and to provide intensive speech and physiotherapy for his other disabilities.

Stembile never learned to walk but did learn to say a few words, relying on his very expressive use of eyes, head and arms to convey his wishes. He enjoyed music, participated in day-care activities as far as possible, and gained weight steadily with a nutritious diet. He developed a wonderful relationship with the Hospice Chaplain, and with an older patient, and appeared to have a premonition of his own death, getting the staff to take him to his favourite places, and call all his favourite people in the two days before he died of heart failure aged four years.

Stembile was hospitalised for a short period to monitor his heart medication, and when he developed pneumonia, but the interdisciplinary team and the hospital medical team decided together that he was happiest in the children's hospice.

His uncle had very understanding and supportive employers who allowed him time off to be with Stembile at the end and also paid for the child's funeral.

Home-care staff followed up the uncle to provide bereavement support for him and his sister.

CARING FOR STEMBILE USING THE ACT CARE PATHWAY

This pathway (Elston 2004)[6] was not in use in South Africa at the time and has only recently been implemented in some areas. However a plan for continuity of care with steps very similar to the ACT Care Pathway, was developed for Stembile,[4] together with his uncle who was his legal guardian and his other healthcare providers. His uncle was informed of Stembile's prognosis and was kept informed of his status when he came on regular visits to his nephew. Stembile was cared for at home, in the hospital and in the children's hospice by the hospice team in collaboration with the hospital, ensuring continuity of palliative care and good communication regarding the little patient.

The uncle understood the implications of Stembile's HIV status and TB and went voluntarily for an HIV test and TB screening.

The uncle developed a good relationship with the staff and was provided with counselling as well as information on what would be needed to provide care at home, including training on the use of an oxygen machine. In preparation for his discharge he would take Stembile home with him for weekends and received training in giving anti-retroviral therapy and TB treatment at home. To ensure adequate income for food and other necessities for Stembile, the social worker assisted him to obtain a child support grant from the State as well as a disability grant for his sister. Whilst the uncle was dependent on township taxis for transport, the hospice also agreed to assist with transport for any clinic or hospital appointments. When, or if, Stembile was discharged he would be referred to the home-based care team, consisting of a professional nurse, a social worker and trained community caregivers who each have their own area and walk to each patient.

Despite all this, when Stembile was nearing the end of life, and required oxygen, the multidisciplinary team and the uncle together decided that the best place for Stembile to be would be in the hospice and when Stembile was asked whether this was accept-able for him he smiled and nodded.

Near the end of his life, his symptoms were managed with increased heart medica-tion, diuretics, oral morphine and oxygen therapy. His emotional distress was relieved through regular sessions of simple play, music and regular visits from the chaplain, his uncle and two favourite volunteers (*see* Figure 6.2).

Stembile's condition falls into Group 3 of the ACT categories, of progressive condi-tions without curative treatment options, where treatment is exclusively palliative and may commonly extend over many years.[7,8]

Stembile's uncle had been informed of his nephew's condition at diagnosis and was kept informed of his progress. Whilst the staff were adequately educated about HIV and AIDS, and TB, they required further education on cardiac failure and Stembile's specific disabilities. This was provided as in-service training.

The staff also had to receive bereavement counselling and support after Stembile's death as he had been with the hospice for a long period of time and was held in great affection by staff and volunteers.

PALLIATIVE CARE FOR CHILDREN LIKE STEMBILE

Implementation of the Care[8] Pathways can be used in further education on children's palliative care and to advocate for this to be included in government policy and guidelines.

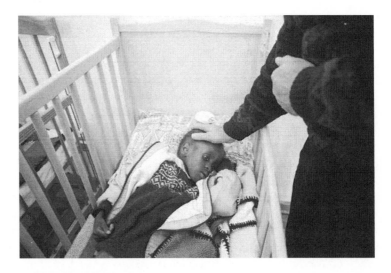

FIGURE 6.2 Stembile and pastor

Information and evidence on palliative care relevant to Africa is very rare. HPCA has developed a Toolkit[3] for Developing Children's Palliative care in Africa that organisations can use as a guide; and together with other practitioners in Africa, a textbook on Children's Palliative Care in Africa has been published by Oxford University Press.[10]

At present the only education for children's palliative care is that developed by HPCA and the Bigshoes Foundation collaboratively and includes an Introduction to Palliative Care for Children and short courses on issues such as pain management; psycho-social care; memory work; bereavement in children.

Training is carried out through 10 HPCA Centres of Palliative Learning, the University of Cape Town, and the Bigshoes Foundation in Johannesburg and Durban.

A new, more advanced, curriculum has been developed for implementation in 2009 and will also be included at university level as part of a multidisciplinary diploma with a paediatric elective.

The Diana Princess of Wales Memorial Fund is funding three Children's Palliative Care Training and Resource Centres in Africa, and a Virtual Children's Palliative Care Resource Centre in South Africa.

DEVELOPING A NATIONAL STRATEGY

In South Africa the development of palliative care has been carried out by hospices in the charity sector, and only in recent years has it received any government support to certain hospices.

The government Department of Health at national level and in the provinces, the Department of Correctional Services, the Cancer Association of South Africa and the Anglican Church of the Province of Southern Africa are in the process of signing Memoranda of Understanding with HPCA to integrate palliative care into their services.

In Johannesburg the Wits Palliative Care Centre of Excellence has been set up in partnership with the University of the Witwatersrand and has a department of paediatric palliative care that serves major hospitals in the Gauteng province.

There is a draft national strategy that still needs further development and approval by government; and palliative care is included in two major national plans – for cancer and for HIV, AIDS, TB and STIs. However, the majority of palliative care is provided by the HPCA of South Africa member hospices, many of whom work closely with primary healthcare clinics and hospitals.

BARRIERS TO PALLIATIVE CARE FOR CHILDREN AND YOUNG PEOPLE

Staff often have lack of knowledge of palliative care and limited formal education. Palliative care is still often seen as only end-of-life care and many doctors believe that palliative care will act as a barrier to people accessing HAART. Some adult-focused palliative care practitioners see palliative care for children as unnecessary use of resources. Until 2008 the government minister responsible for health promoted unorthodox methods to treat AIDS and supported AIDS 'denialists'.

This leads to direct consequences: Children requiring palliative care are seldom identified early[10] in the course of the disease due to a lack of knowledge and skills to assess children. Professional staff are often not aware of the WHO or ACT definitions on palliative care for children, nor of the four ACT categories. Pain in children is frequently under-diagnosed and pain assessment tools for children not always culturally sensitive. Dr Rene Albertyn at the Red Cross Children's Hospital has developed a Pain and Comfort Assessment tool that is suited to the South African situation. A major challenge is in involving children and often sick, young or elderly primary caregivers in decisions regarding their care. Early diagnosis of Stembile's HIV status with regular follow-up visits to the primary healthcare clinic where opportunistic infections would have been be treated and where he would have had early access to HAART would probably have prevented the cardiac failure. On HAART, if compliant, Stembile could have lived for many years. Cared for by sick parents and then a young uncle, his development was severely delayed and his health not monitored until after his parents' deaths.

Improved access to voluntary counselling and testing, to prevention of mother-to-child transmission, early and regular follow-up of all children born to HIV positive mothers and mothers living in poverty would increase early diagnosis and treatment access for these children.

There is a lack of continuity of care between formal healthcare services such as hospitals and community-based organisations. Whilst the HPCA is working to improve this in certain areas of the country, and has established strong ties with a number of primary healthcare clinics, where most South Africans receive their healthcare, this is not in place over all the country.

BANA PELE (CHILDREN FIRST)

St Nicholas Children's Hospice in Bloemfontein has established a new pilot project, the St Nicholas Bana Pele Network, to develop a network of services to children that includes hospitals, clinics, HAART sites, non-government and faith-based organisations, and comprehensive training, so that children requiring palliative care are kept within a safety net of services and receive continuity of care, but this is still in the early stage of the pilot.

In South Africa, the magnitude of the HIV and AIDS problem tends to overshadow all other illnesses which means children with other life-limiting conditions are not identified and may be dying without palliative care or, at times and in deep rural areas, any sort of medical or supportive care.

THE BENEFITS OF CARE PATHWAYS

The development of care pathways[4,6,12] for children would facilitate continuity of care and reduce the number of children leaving one service and being lost to further interventions, as well as enhancing communication between the different service providers.

Within the South African context, palliative care practitioners are aware of the complex social and emotional problems faced by vulnerable primary caregivers of children, and Stembile's uncle, a young man himself who had watched his sister and brother-in-law die of AIDS, and was also caring for his disabled sister with few material resources, was assessed from the beginning on his ability to cope. The uncle did not appear to have any family support but was fortunate in having understanding employers who also visited Stembile in the hospice and allowed the uncle to spend time with him when he was very ill. The uncle and Stembile loved each other dearly and Stembile's face shone when his uncle walked into the hospice. The hospice staff were sensitive to the fact that his uncle would have liked to continue to provide care at home but had no-one suitable to look after Stembile when he went to work. All avenues were explored with him, to try and get Stembile to spend more time at home, with suitable supervision and daily visits by the community caregiver supported by the professional nurse, but his deteriorating condition and increasing dependence on oxygen made this difficult as the shack had no electricity, and they shared a common tap and a toilet with 30 other shacks in their community.

A major challenge in South Africa is obtaining accurate statistics on the number of children requiring palliative care. Whilst statistics on children infected with HIV are collected and reported on annually, and we have some estimations on the number of children newly diagnosed with cancer, other life-limiting conditions are poorly documented.

The present St Nicholas Bana Pele Network model could be used as an advocacy tool to inform a national strategy on care pathways for children, along with existing effective hospice programmes that collaborate closely with other systems to provide continuity of care.

In the case of Stembile, leadership of his care management was taken by the hospice manager, who worked very closely with the hospital medical team and Stembile's uncle to ensure quality of care was maintained in the hospital, at home and in the hospice.

The hospice manager at that time was a professional nurse and she took responsibility for the care planning for Stembile, working closely with his medical team.

➤ The interdisciplinary team assessed Stembile and his social situation, taking into account the youth of his uncle, and the further financial and social needs of the whole family unit.

➤ Assistance was given for the family to obtain the social grants available in South Africa.

➤ The Chaplain became the leader of the team when Stembile was dying, at a time when both Stembile and his uncle required spiritual support.

➤ The chaplain's support continued to the uncle, to the other children in the hospice who had known Stembile, and to the staff, with regular visits and a special religious service where everyone had a chance to say their goodbyes.

However, this type of care management is not the norm in South Africa where a national and provincial policy on care pathways would benefit both adults and children, and facilitate continuity of care. Care is mainly delivered in 'silos' with a child entering and leaving one healthcare facility without any attempt to refer the child to another organisation for further care.

THE PRESENT SITUATION IN SOUTH AFRICA

Within the HPCA there is a plan to improve knowledge of care pathways through workshops and materials that document a culturally sensitive and relevant model. As HPCA is the major provider of palliative care in South Africa as well as the driver behind a national policy, and has networks in most regions of the country, HPCA would be the vehicle for implementing policies for care pathways in the country.

The main barriers to implementing the ACT Care Pathways include the lack of knowledge of both the care pathway model as well as of palliative care for children; few skilled practitioners in paediatric palliative care; under-staffed services both in government and non-government organisations; focus on providing immediate care without consideration of future planning; services working in isolation; competition for funding instead of collaboration; and poor identification of children with life-limiting conditions other than HIV means these children would not be identified to benefit from a care pathway.

Hospice, hospital and clinic personnel are overwhelmed with patient numbers, and lack of staff, due to lack of funding, makes implementing any new process daunting. In areas where the services are not used to collaborating a system for collaboration which takes up valuable time, may be difficult to develop. Support from provincial government departments of health is essential for new systems to be implemented.

Within the hospice movement, care pathways[3] will enhance present services and help staff to understand the concept of maintaining quality of care along a continuum for the benefit of the child. This is part of the ethos of palliative care but not necessarily of other healthcare providers. Inclusion of care pathways within the palliative care Standards of Care will encourage this integration.

HPCA has a strong advocacy department working closely with government and national non-government organisations. Within the hospice movement there is a paediatric palliative care portfolio that communicates and educates hospices and collaborating partners through centres of palliative learning and regional education forums. New process take time to implement as there is often resistance to change.

PALLIATIVE CARE FOR CHILDREN IN SOUTH AFRICA – WHAT IS NEEDED NOW

1 To develop a national policy regarding care pathways for children within the HPCA so that this will be reflected in the Standards of Palliative Care and included in education on palliative care for children. This will then disseminate to networking partners including government partners such as hospitals and clinics.
2 To improve advocacy on the benefit of care pathways to government at national and provincial level through developing documents relevant to South Africa, and inclusion of this in the national policy document.
3 To advocate for care pathways to be included in undergraduate training of all healthcare professionals through working with educational bodies such as universities and nursing colleges and national educational accreditation agencies.
4 To develop materials on the ACT Care Pathway relevant to the South African context.

5   To hold regional workshops to disseminate knowledge – and that include hospices, other non-government and faith-based organisations, and government agencies.

6   To assess the St Nicholas Bana Pele model once this has been fully-established as to the effectiveness of an integrated Care Pathway for children.

7   To implement the EMMA process in the development of care pathways – i.e. Education, Mentorship, Modelling, Advocacy.

The challenge in South Africa is maintaining quality of care whilst increasing access to palliative care for children. Through the implementation of care pathways linked to education, mentorship, modelling the process and effective advocacy this could be achieved.

N.I.C.E. analysis

Needs

- Better understanding of palliative care for children.
- Education on children's palliative care.
- Professional staff with skills in assessment and care.
- National policies to guide provincial and local policies.
- More children's palliative care units.
- Improved access to palliative care drugs at primary healthcare level.

Interests

- There is a growing interest in palliative care and palliative care for children in South Africa.
- There is increased donor support for children's palliative care and the development of a Children's Palliative Care Virtual Resource Centre for South Africa and other African countries.
- Increasing access to palliative care for children with the development of new sites each year.

Concerns

- Children with conditions other than HIV are not being identified.
- The main focus is on adult needs as their numbers are larger.
- There is fear of working with children due to emotional distress at children dying.
- Physicians working in the field of HAART believe palliative care will no longer be necessary.

Expectations

- Increasing acknowledgement of the need for children's palliative care.
- Improved collaboration through better communication.
- Advocacy for the care pathways to be accepted by service providers, led by the hospice movement.
- Increasing body of healthcare providers trained in palliative care for children.
- Care pathways to be included in undergraduate training of all healthcare professionals.

Reflection on the above analysis:

- Within the HPCA there is a plan to improve knowledge of care pathways through workshops and materials that document a culturally sensitive and relevant model. As HPCA is the major provider of palliative care in South Africa as well as the driver behind a national policy, and has networks in most regions of the country, HPCA would be the vehicle for implementing policies for care pathways in the country.
- The main barriers to implementing the ACT Care Pathways[6,12] would include lack of knowledge of both the Care Pathway model as well as of palliative care for children; few skilled practitioners in paediatric palliative care; under-staffed services both in government and non-government organisations; focus on providing immediate care without consideration of future planning; services working in isolation; competition for funding instead of collaboration; poor identification of children with life-limiting conditions other than HIV means these children would not be identified to benefit from a care pathway.
- Hospice, hospital and clinic personnel are overwhelmed with patient numbers and lack of staff, due to lack of funding, makes implementing any new process daunting. In areas where the services are not used to collaborating a system for collaboration which takes up valuable time, may be difficult to develop. Support from provincial government departments of health is essential for new systems to be implemented.
- Within the hospice movement, care pathways will enhance present services and staff understand the concept of maintaining quality of care along a continuum for the benefit of the child. This is part of the ethos of palliative care but not necessarily of other healthcare providers. Inclusion of care pathways within the palliative care Standards of Care will encourage this integration.
- HPCA has a strong advocacy department working closely with government and national non-government organisations. Within the hospice movement there is a paediatric palliative care portfolio that communicates and educates hospices and collaborating partners through centres of palliative learning and regional education forums. New process take time to implement as there is often resistance to change.

Action plan: next steps

- To develop a national policy regarding care pathways for children within the HPCA so that this will be reflected in the Standards of Palliative Care and included in education on palliative care for children. This will then disseminate to networking partners including government partners such as hospitals and clinics.
- Improve advocacy on the benefit of care pathways to government at national and provincial level through developing documents relevant to South Africa, and inclusion of this in the national policy document.
- Advocate for care pathways to be included in undergraduate training of all healthcare professionals through working with educational bodies such as universities and nursing colleges; and national educational accreditation agencies.

- Development of materials on the ACT Care Pathway relevant to the South African context.
- Regional workshops to disseminate knowledge and that include hospices, other non-government and faith-based organisations, and government agencies.
- Assessment of the St Nicholas Bana Pele model once this has been fully-established as to the effectiveness of an integrated care pathway for children.

REFERENCES

1 National Department of Health South Africa. *Guidelines for Management of HIV-infected Children*. Pinetown, NC: Jacana Media, Pinetown Printers; 2005

2 www.cansa.org

3 Lubega S, Zirenbuzi GW, Lwabi P. Heart disease in children with HIV/AIDS attending the paediatric infectious disease clinic at Mulago hospital. *Afr Health Sci.* 2005; 5(3): 219–26.

4 Boucher S, Marston J, Robbertze M. *A Toolkit for Children's Palliative Care Programmes in Africa*. Cape Town: HPCA; 2008.

5 UNICEF. *State of the World's Children 2009*. Available at: www.unicef.org/publications/files/The_State_of_the_Worlds_Children_2009_Exec_Summ.pdf (accessed 17 February 2010).

6 Elston S. *Integrated Multi-agency Care Pathways for Children with Life-threatening and Life-limiting Conditions*. Bristol: ACT; 2004. Available at: www.act.org.uk/ (accessed 17 February 2010).

7 Association for Children with Life-Threatening or Terminal Conditions and their Families and the Royal College of Paediatrics and Child Health (2003). *A Guide to the Development of Children's Palliative Care Services*. Bristol: ACT; 2007. p. 6.

8 UK Department of Health. *Better Care: Better Lives*. 2008. Available at: www.dh.gov.uk/en/Publicationsandstatistics/Publications/PublicationsPolicyAndGuidance/DH_083106 (accessed 17 February 2010).

9 Pfund R. *Palliative Care Nursing of Children and Young People*. Oxford: Radcliffe Publishing; 2007.

10 Amery J. *Children's Palliative Care in Africa*. Oxford: Oxford University Press; 2009.

11 Harding R, Brits H, Penfold S. Paediatric anti-retroviral therapy outcomes under HIV hospice care in South Africa. *Int J Palliat Nurs.* 2009; 15: 142–7.

12 Association for Children's Palliative Care. *The Transition Care Pathway*. Bristol: ACT; 2007. Available at: www.act.org.uk/ (accessed 17 February 2010).

SECTION 2

Focusing on families: hearing the evidence

Susan Fowler-Kerry

Section 2 of the text opens a door for readers to enter a very privileged place and for a moment they will have a brief glimpse into the lived experience of paediatric palliative care from the perspectives of those who are living it, parents, families, siblings and of course the children. You will become aware of triumphs and miracles, obstacles that were scaled and challenged throughout these narrative accounts. Also, you will gain a deeper appreciation and insight into the day-to-day struggles endured by these families just to live. Sadly some of the resistance and barriers these families face are a result of systems that were developed to ease their burdens but now are adding to their life challenges.

Every story is riveting and is not a simple retelling of details, but rather, you, as the reader will come to understand that they have been continually constructed and may be reconstructed by storyteller depending on the context. Personal stories are embedded in the larger stories and structures that permeate society.

The rationale for the inclusion of this section was to provide a platform for these powerful stories to be heard, a frequently untapped data source that clearly demonstrates how interlinked we are as global citizens and how our basic needs are the same everywhere. Unfortunately, there is no impartial global arbitrator to determine how privilege and oppression, fortune and misfortune are distributed within and across different sectors of the population, nor is there any fairness about which families will have a child with a life-limiting or life-threatening diagnosis.

The question for you to ask yourself is, should the state become involved in trying to leverage a more even playing field? That is not to say that the state would ever be in a position to change the reality of a child's diagnosis, but should all the devastating consequences from such a diagnosis be a foregone conclusion? Certainly from a social justice perspective the harm resulting from such a diagnosis could certainly be lessened through policies and practices that direct the provision and access of paediatric palliative care services to all those who require it.

Be mindful that every one of us is variously dependent, and that, at any given moment, any one of us or those we love may become life-limited, disadvantaged or disabled. Becoming so should never place an individual or family in a position of having no choice and no alternative, and of being forced to become reliant on unresponsive services or demeaning charity that renders them marginalised, dependent and voiceless.

7

A research perspective: narrative research

Sheila Greatrex-White

The 'self who writes' has no more direct and unproblematic access to the 'self who was' than does the reader; and anyway 'the autobiographical past' is actually peopled by a succession of selves as the writer grows, develops and changes.

Stanley 1992, p. 61[1]

Within nursing, health and social care research, one compelling reason often given for carrying out qualitative research is that it offers a means of exploring the ways in which people interpret the world, and their place within it.[2,3] Such interpretations are often extremely complex and nuanced, and would be difficult to access through other means. It has also been said that wherever you find humans you will also find narratives or stories.[4,5] This chapter considers one way in which such interpretation can be conceptualised within the context of Paediatric Palliative Care (PPC). It deals with the narrative dimensions of people's accounts, that is, the ways people make sense of the world, and themselves in it, by creating self-stories and using already circulating stories (including meta-narratives or public narratives) to interpret the world. Narrative is more than just another research method; it is a methodological imperative that enables us to ask critical questions of the significant and seemingly inconsequential moments of our own histories and the ways those histories inform and inflect our individual and collective understandings.[6]

Narrative, as used here, is not meant in the sense of a story that simply carries a set of facts or truths. I see narratives as social products produced by people within the context of specific social, historical and cultural spaces. Narratives are related to the experience that people have of their lives, but they are not transparent carriers of that experience. They are interpretive devices, through which people represent themselves, both to themselves and to others. In addition, narratives do not originate with the individual but rather circulate culturally to provide a repertoire from which people can produce their own stories:[7,8,9,10] this is the case within, and outside of, the research setting. According to Walker,[6] 'Our lives and experiences are not merely reflected in stories; they are instead actually created by and through them.'

Hence Taylor[11] speaks of 'intersubjective meanings'.

Narrative has been described as a natural human impulse, that is, a recollection of what happened, what was done, and what was of interest, in a temporal sequence. For example, Denzin[12] describes narrative as a story that tells a sequence of events that are significant for the narrator and her or his audience: he suggests it has an internal logic that makes sense to the narrator and relates events in a temporal, causal sequence. Thus, narratives are a central means with which people connect together past and present, self and other. They do so within the context of public narratives or meta-narratives which delimit what can be said, what stories can be told, what will count as meaningful, and what will seem to be nonsensical: herein lie the concepts of structure and agency.[13] Meta-narratives are those culturally dominant narratives that are regarded as the appropriate ways to experience and behave in the world by society at large. All narratives are from a particular point of view, in a context and to a particular audience.

Whilst narrative has gained respectability in nursing research, as evidenced by the burgeoning literature on carrying out narrative research, the term is often used interchangeably and uncritically with storytelling.[8,14] For example, Bingley *et al.*[15] define narrative as simply 'a form of expression recognizable as a story'. Similarly, Hinchman and Hinchman[16] state that, 'Narratives (stories) in the human sciences should be defined provisionally as discourses with a clear sequential order that connects events in a meaningful way for a definite audience and thus offer insights about the world and/or people's experiences of it.' What is helpful about this latter definition according to Elliott[17] is it stresses three key features of narrative: chronology, meaningfulness and that they are social. A useful distinction between storytelling and narrative has been offered by Wiltshire,[8] which suggests that, 'A narrative is conceptually more sophisticated and structured than a story.' He goes on to state that, 'Stories and tales are casual, informal, contingent. Narratives are pre-meditated, organised, more formal and have a structure that is their own.' Importantly, Wiltshire[8] warns that if narrative and story are to become a genuine focus for nursing inquiry, the meaning of each of these concepts will need to be adequately defined and delimited. According to Ricoeur[7] narratives have certain properties that must be present in order to speak of a narrative as such. First, a narrative describes not a single event or idea but a sequence over time; second, it has a plot; and third, narrative entails a timeline: the possibility of drawing a configuration out of a series of events as they are placed in relation to each other. All of these aspects draw attention towards the narrative as complete, unified and with an extension over time. The core argument of narrative theory is that narratives are 'the primary schema by means of which human existence is rendered meaningful' (p. 11).[4]

Although narratives are most closely associated with life history research, narrative can be an extremely useful way of conceptualising the kinds of accounts people (children, professionals, parents) produce in qualitative PPC research. To understand PPC it is not enough simply to watch: we need to ask what different events mean to people and why they are happening. Narratives, whether personal or public, neither begin nor end in the research setting: they are part of the fabric of the social world. Nevertheless, the PPC research setting is one arena within which narratives can be elicited and explored. These narratives may be fragmentary, incomplete, even unfair, but can nevertheless tell us a great deal about PPC, the person and the social world she or he inhabits. The process of narrative re-telling, in interviews for example, involves the narrator convincing the researcher, who was probably not present when events happened, that these happenings had credence for the narrator. A particular narrative self is constituted through the narrative, occasioned by the presence of a listener who brings their own set of historically, culturally and theoretically framed questions and comments to the encounter. Thus, research narratives can be understood as a form of reflection upon an event. [7,14] Research which explores the narratives people produce will necessarily be interpretivist in nature: it will work from the basic premise that individuals and groups interpret the social world and their place within it.

Narrative research is the study of stories[18] and can be seen as a means of confounding the false dichotomy by which a research participant's account is conceptualised either as an unproblematic transparent, accurate reflection of lived experience or as 'a distorting screen that always projects experience out of its own categories'.[19] It is not so much that 'the facts do not matter', nor is it the case that 'only the facts matter': rather, facts (or experience) and the interpretation of those facts (or that experience) are envisaged as necessarily entwined. Similarly, narrative knowledge involves more than simply the transmission of 'the facts' from one who knows to one who does not: a narrative also carries an implicit message about the culture and society in which it is being told. Narrative research as an alternative 'culture of research' recognises the whole, the unity or coherence of a life-story in which the experience of, for example, living with a life-threatening illness, is nested. Working with multiplicity, it is about new ways researchers and participants can engage with each other. Such relational forms of inquiry have the potential to advance PPC beyond the boundaries established by methodologies that claim to know 'an-other' on the basis of brief or detached encounters and which may unduly restrict the revelations of research participants.

The study of narrative has been associated with literary texts that largely centred on the technical components of the narratives themselves.[20] However, more recently social-scientific work has drawn attention to the significance of narratives for a study of the social world. This recent work is drawing on a relatively long tradition in social science, from the nineteenth-century philosopher Wilhelm Dilthey,[21] through the ethnographic work of the Chicago School (which elicited individual biographical accounts) and life history work, to contemporary qualitative research, for example Frank,[22] Lather and Smithies[23] and Thomas.[24] Narrative has become a meeting ground and a battle ground of the disciplines and is fast becoming a discipline in its own right.[25] Such work, although different in many ways, has been in marked contrast to positivism. Positivists would hold that the only social phenomena worth consideration are those phenomena which are directly observable and (in some sense) measurable. For some scientists if something cannot be measured, then it is either illusion or impossible to conceive: not true and/or not real. Arising out of a 'methodological fundamentalism' that returns to a much discredited model of empirical inquiry in which 'only randomized experiments produce truth',[26] it has been argued that current over reliance on measuring leaves large areas of inquiry either poorly researched with inappropriate methods, or ignored.

From the perspective of narrative research, what can be seen, observed and measured is not all there is to say: a much more interesting issue is that of interpretation involving how people interpret the social world, and their place within it.[2] For example, Ricoeur[27] recalls that, '. . . the same gesture of raising one's arm can, depending on context, be understood as a way of saying hello, of hailing a taxi, or of voting'. As McNay[28] argues, 'Meaning is not inherent to action but is the product of interpretative strategies amongst which narrative is central'. Thus, narrative has numerous advantages, not least of which is that it provides a sophisticated response to some of the philosophical and methodological problems raised by postmodernists.[29]

In the health and social sciences, narrative research searches out, analyses and works with stories that relate significantly to people's lives (Elliot[17]), and narratives related to illness, dying and bereavement have become a significant sub-genre of these (see for example Bailey and Tilley;[30] Brown and Addington-Hall[31]). Frank[32] argues, whether ill people (and I would add ill children) want to or not, becoming seriously ill calls for stories. He suggests that these stories repair the damage that illness has done to the ill person's life trajectory, and these are stories that have to be told to many people (family and friends, employers and healthcare professionals). Frank is one of a growing number of writers who attest to a therapeutic influence from the use of narrative. Some even consider narrative research to be unique in that it is at one and the same time a research method and a therapeutic intervention.[33,34] Mattingly[35] points out, 'We make as well as tell stories of our lives and this is of fundamental importance to the clinical world.'

Narratives have conventionally been treated merely as (more or less transparent) carriers of a set of facts: they have not in themselves been seen as social products.[24] Somers and Gibson,[36] however, suggest that contemporary researchers and theorists have adopted a position which postulates that

> social life is itself storied and that narrative is an ontological condition of social life. Their research is showing us that stories guide action; that people construct identities (however multiple and changing) by locating themselves or being located within a repertoire of emplotted stories; that "experience" is constituted through narratives; that people make sense of what has happened and is happening to them by attempting to assemble or in some way to integrate these happenings within one or more narratives; and that people are guided to act in certain ways, and not others, on the basis of the projections, expectations, and memories derived from a multiplicity but ultimately linked repertoire of available social, public and cultural narratives.

However, not all view narrative research this way: over the last few decades, many have problematised the so-called 'narrative turn' and many remain sceptical of its use as a research methodology. Atkinson and Silverman,[37] in their attack of the narrative turn in social science, refer to narrative research as 'a blind alley', a 'preoccupation with the revelation of personal experience through confession and therapeutic discourse', and as 'misleading', 'sentimental', 'exaggerated' and a 'romantic construction of the self'. The narratives that they object to are the personal, autobiographical, and illness narratives, particularly when these are unanalysed, not treated as social facts, or are presented without recourse to methodological scepticism. They condemn both the form of these narratives and the methodology of face-to-face 'empathic' interviews that often is used to produce them. In doing so Atkinson and Silverman express a manifestly scientific (or positivist) viewpoint; personal narratives cannot be trusted and must be subjected to methodological scepticism (see Bochner[38]). It is perhaps this kind of argumentation that has led healthcare narrative researchers to try to make their methods consistent with the positivist methodologies of the majority of healthcare research.[3] Interestingly, the practical, ethical and moral focus of narrative inquiry, which Atkinson[39] regards as a prominent threat to recognising the significance of narratives, is precisely what writers such as Frank,[22,40,32] Polkinghorne[18] and Mishler[41] believe gives narrative research its importance. For these latter writers, how we use narratives does not come down to a choice between morality and methodology. Frank,[22] for example, observes that one of the main challenges of illness is to construct a story that can turn mere existence and stigmatisation into a meaningful social and moral life that is self-validating.

The issue of bias or trust in narrative research is important: is the narrator misremembering, misrepresenting or simply lying about earlier events? How do we know that the narratives, stories, interpretations are the right ones, what alternatives might be available? The debate draws on issues regarding what is truth in narrative text and involves the so called 'crisis of representation'. But as Riessman,[42] has noted whilst this is a 'thorny problem in narrative research' (p. 21), this focus misses the point: there is no unbiased access to the past. She argues that 'a personal narrative is not meant to be read as an exact record of what happened nor is it a mirror of the world out there concluding that this is the case precisely because narratives are always located in discourses (e.g. scientific, feminist, and therapeutic)'[42] (p. 64). Indeed, the past is constantly worked and re-worked to provide a coherent sense of the subject's identity. We all live in narrative; we tell stories about our lives, both to ourselves and to others and it is through such stories that we make sense of the world, of our relationship to that world, and of the relationship between ourselves and other selves. Narratives then are a means by which people make sense of, understand, and live their lives. Moore[43] follows White[44] and Ricoeur,[27] arguing that, '. . . narrative is a strategy for placing us within a historically constituted world, and thus our very concept of history is dependent on narrative. If narrative makes the world intelligible, it also makes ourselves intelligible.' The 'truths' people produce through such narratives are not 'truths' as conventionally understood in positivist health and social science: nevertheless, they do speak certain 'truths' about people's (socially located) lives and identities.[2]

People constantly produce and reproduce narratives on the basis of past experiences or memories; interpreting the past through the lens of social information, and using this information to formulate present and future life stories. Narrative provides a means of conceptualising people in the context of history: if the past is always interpreted through the present, then equally, this interpreted past informs the present. If we look at the chapters within this book, it is clear that the writers are producing their own narrative, not from the past, but out of the present. They are interpreting their earlier life experience in the light of what they now know. Indeed, earlier events gain significance only through events that come later. Despite expressions of change, the movement of the plot leads to them becoming what they are. To a certain extent, the connections drawn in these narratives can be seen as a search for a PPC plot that may keep the events of a story together as a clear, unified and understandable story: a way of keeping PPC in a constant state of becoming. This presupposes an audience, narratives are told to make a point, and they touch the other person by offering a different perspective and by that challenge both our self-understanding and perception of others.[45,46] It is in this sense, as Plummer[47] points out, that narrative research might be seen as 'joint actions'.

The task of researchers using narratives is multilayered. First, they must set in place the conditions in which people (including children) are likely to produce narratives. Researchers ask a 'trigger or stimulus question' of personal significance to the participant which, according to Holloway and Freshwater,[10] (p. 708) limits the use of irrelevant questions, and as such researchers are less able to misuse/abuse their power in the often unequal research situation. The researcher to some extent empowers the participant to set the agenda, helping to prevent the fragmentation of the narrative. Therefore, structured questionnaires and straightforward observation are unlikely to produce narratives. As Chase[46] explains, researchers are more likely to elicit narratives when simple questions are asked that clearly relate to the participants' life experiences. This might be seen as one of the positive aspects in narrative research especially when carried out with children in the context of PPC. Narratives however, come in many forms, including oral narratives, written narratives (including autobiographies, letters, journals, personal web pages and diaries), visual narratives, and performative narratives (e.g. those transformed to stage, poetry and fiction).[48,17,49] Narratives do not have to be lengthy or full accounts of a life: they simply have to incorporate the processes of 'emplotment'[7] (pp. 21–2).

Second, researchers have to analyse those accounts in terms of narrative. Elliott[17] points out that 'there is no single narrative method, but rather a multitude of different ways in which researchers can engage with the narrative properties of their data.' Usefully, Bingley et al.[15] distinguish between qualitative analysis applied to narratives and narrative analysis as method. 'In the former, general methods of qualitative analysis such as thematic, discourse and conversational analysis may be applied to the interpretation of narratives as well as other sources of data, while in the latter, specific analytic techniques have been developed devoted to narratives alone.'[50]

Third, researchers need to consider the kinds of public narratives or meta-narratives on which both researchers and research participants draw, and which operate as constraints on the kinds of narrative they can produce. Finally, they have to consider the relationship between these public or meta-narratives and the personal narratives produced. This relationship need not be harmonious or smooth: the process of constructing a personal narrative is creative work (even if it is not self-consciously so) and people may well use public or meta-narratives only to oppose them. Further, people frequently combine fairly contradictory forms of narrative in producing their personal narratives. So, for example, people may postulate a self that is the product of genetic inheritance at the same time as postulating a self that is the product of socialisation processes or social engineering. In this, they are drawing on competing narratives, yet combining them in a new narrative form. Above all, the researcher must consider the processes of interpretation going on, both personally and publicly.[9,51]

There are, however, at least two other levels of interpretation going on in narrative research; that of the researcher and that of the reader.[17] It is important to reiterate here that narratives are not produced solely in the research setting nor are they simply imported more or less wholesale into the research setting. If narratives are constantly worked and re-worked outside of the research setting, then they are also being re-worked within and throughout the research processes. In this sense, they are co-produced between the researcher and the research participant.[52,53,54] The kinds of questions asked, the whole direction of the research processes, will to some extent influence the kinds of narrative participants produce in the research itself, as will the location and ontological positioning of the researchers themselves.[55] By interpreting and editing the narratives, the researcher essentially creates a 'hybrid story' to re-present what the experience collectively means.[51] The issue here is not one of bias or distortion, but one of the inevitability of interpretation and reinterpretation. Additionally, narrative research might position readers of narratives as responders and thinkers in the sense that 'the audience teaches you something' and that 'we need other people to help us think' and not only as readers, but also as enhancers and messengers of the stories.[56] As Rolfe[2] points out, a narrative without listeners is a pointless exercise because it is in the act of being read that status is bestowed on the narrator, so the listener is just as important in the act of narration as is the narrator. Narrative research in PPC might help in securing a place in history for childrens' and parents' voices and stories. This means getting the stories told and out.[54]

NARRATIVES IN PPC

A growing number of researchers from a variety of disciplines have either taken or are in the process of moving towards the narrative turn.[8,14,2] Narrative has long been used to convey nurse's knowledge of individuals to each other and has always been part of how we explore the shared work of patients and clients. Street[57] argues that nursing is a narrative culture. PPC nurses will have many examples of these narratives. Some will be stories about self: the personal events that may have triggered interest in nursing, leading to the bedside of children nearing their end of life, or what it is like to do this work (*see* Chapters 3, 4 and 5). Other stories will be told about patients, through case studies, to colleagues on courses, or written in personal or reflexive diaries (*see* Chapter 3). Many will reflect and remember the particular child to whom you continue to refer when the occasion arises to do so; stories about colleagues (perhaps of their thoughtful support of a child reaching their last hours), or towards families (bewildered, angry, heartbroken), or towards you (as you struggled with meeting the needs of patients and families after a long and tiring shift). Added to these are the childrens' and families' stories that will have been told to you, of how illness was discovered, diagnosed, and treated; how they or their family were treated; how they have tried to live with illness, disability, disfigurement and the fear of death. These personal narratives may be subjective legitimisation of personal concepts and beliefs that are in conflict with other, often dominant, meta-narratives or public narratives such as those of health experts. Such personal narratives might serve to help the PPC nurse to develop new understandings of the children they care for, give direct access to key dimensions of the nursing context, be an essential tool in the understanding of suffering as a human experience: a way of transcending the often limited perspectives and insight into illness.

According to Bamberg and McCabe[58] narratives have many purposes: they are created to remember, argue, convince, engage or entertain their audience. Crucially, they help make sense of experience, ordering events into a more coherent structure that helps create meaning; an especially important and challenging dimension in the context of PPC where patients, parents and healthcare professionals ask questions about the meaning of disease, the meaning of the life that has been led, and, indeed, the meaning of life itself. Though narratives have been shown to have a therapeutic value of their own, both for the narrator and for the listener,[22,40,32] many still question the value of narrative research as a form of research to PPC nursing: How does such research help beyond the daily practice of listening to, and telling stories?

Speraw's[59] moving research, which illuminated life-long experiences of suffering, healing and the quest to be human as perceived by a 16-year-old girl disfigured by multiple cancer treatments, stands as an exemplar. She states it 'has relevance for health care education and practice in that it challenges professionals to examine their views on personhood and self-care agency, and the ways those views impact the care they provide.'[59] Having read the case study I have to agree; Kelly's voice raises a number of questions that all healthcare professionals should think upon if we are to be true to our ethical promises. Woodgate's[60,61] and Woodgate and Degner's[62] research, which describes the experiences of childhood cancer and its symptom course by children and their families not only uncovers the participant's battle for life, but also their battle for dignity and support, and it is this dimension that offers a compelling insight into an often hidden aspect of patient/parent experience. Adolescents in Woodgate's[61] study valued the support they received from healthcare team members, friends and especially family. 'Being there' was identified as more than merely a physical presence; rather it also involved a psychosocial – emotional presence within a supportive relationship that was also sometimes a source of stress. This gives PPC nurses insight into how they might focus more attention on how significant relationships in adolescents can be strengthened, considering that 'being there' was seen as a way to maintain connections with their families, friends and others. In one of the few studies to use children's narratives of their cancer experience, Bearison[63] found that the narratives the children produced during the research provided each narrator with an outlet to construct and understand the self: the narratives reflected their struggle with cancer and their attempt to resolve it. Importantly, Bearison showed that not only were all the children in his study able to tell their stories through interviews, but they also wanted others to hear their stories. He concludes that this gives healthcare professionals a means to understand children's experiences of cancer from the children's perspective.

Woodgate and Degner's[62] description of the family's experience of the child's cancer path as 'getting through all the rough spots' by trying to 'keep the spirit alive' has a similar impact. Bjork *et al.*[64] in their study of families experiences of having a child diagnosed with cancer reported that the parents involved in the study suggested that in-depth narratives, used to collect data, should be part of the general care afforded parents and not merely a research approach. It is reported that parents in the study felt that relating their experiences to someone was both comforting and satisfying. This supports the notion that narrative research can be therapeutic. In a recent review of qualitative research on the childhood cancer experience from the perspective of siblings, Wilkins and Woodgate[65] conclude that such research is still in its infancy, but what few studies have been carried out should be encouraged, as accessing children's personal accounts provides us with the opportunity to hear their voices. Such accounts provide us with valuable insights into the changes siblings encounter, the intensity of their feelings and the resources they find helpful. All these studies make a number of suggestions for future research from which PPC healthcare professionals might take up the mantle.

Perhaps of equal importance are healthcare professionals' narratives, which have a great deal to teach us about the many, often invisible, aspects of PPC work, including the conflicts and challenges of working in this setting. In a study of nurses' narratives of unforgettable patient care events, Gunter and Thomas[66] report that nurses appear to use narrative to make meaning of incomprehensible events and to cope with their distress by identifying how lessons learned from these events changed their practice. Macpherson,[67] in her study of peer-supported storytelling for grieving paediatric oncology nurses, suggests that the opportunity to tell their stories to peers who could understand such stories was highly valued, concluding that storytelling may be therapeutic for nurses in PPC.

Supporting children and their families is a key element of the role of nurses working within PPC and is currently high on the healthcare agenda.[68] As Brett[69] points out, the provision of support is particularly important as a means of mediating stress faced by children with complex health needs and this support is vital from diagnosis, throughout the illness trajectory, and during and after the death of a child. Evidence suggests that the use of narrative and stories in PPC education may deepen practitioners' understanding of children's and parents' experiences in this context and enable them to provide the much needed support in a sensitive and meaningful way. Patient and parent stories have been used within palliative education programmes. In a study by Read and Spall,[70] students reported that reading such material encouraged them to explore personal perspectives on palliative care, deepened their understanding of emotions that are often not disclosed, and highlighted the gap between personal and professional perspectives.

Despite the many advantages of narrative research[71,10,59] and an increase in qualitative research publications generally,[72,73] narrative research in PPC (especially in the UK) is rare. More pointedly, studies involving children's and young peoples' voices in PPC is virtually non-existent.[74,75,76] This is an unacceptable position because as Savage and Callery[77] point out, the proxy accounts of parents cannot be accepted as representative of young peoples' views because their objectives of care can differ from those of their parents. The same might be said of proxy healthcare professionals' accounts. The young people narratives that are available are mostly written in books (*see*, for example, Chapters 6 and 10), magazines, on the Internet (personal home pages, ACT),[78] television or in film and radio drama.[15] This seems ironic in an age where research for/with children who are receiving palliative or end-of-life care has been identified as a priority within PPC.[79] What the dearth of research does show is the value of narrative as a vehicle to improve practice, patient care, education and training; as a means to explore the experience of illness and the interaction between professionals; and the potential therapeutic nature of narrative.[10] In this capacity, narrative could make a significant contribution to the practice of PPC healthcare professionals.

PPC healthcare professionals and researchers have the opportunity to draw and build upon a wide range of narrative research methods with the potential to inform and improve healthcare policy, medical and health sciences education and practice. Perhaps more importantly, narrative might hold the potential for caring for each other by greater eliciting and listening to the stories being told and those circulating in society.

NARRATIVE RESEARCH IN PPC: SOME OF THE CHALLENGES

Narrative research in any context is not an easy option, in PPC this is even more so. Whilst there is an identified need for increased narrative research in PPC,[80] recruitment to studies is particularly challenging. Narratives are grounded in personal lives; they invoke feelings, thoughts and emotions and can be profoundly introspective. Thus, narrative research can generate fears, doubts and emotional pain; there is vulnerability in revealing personal experiences, in not being able to take back what might have been shared in an interview or in having no control in how readers (including researchers) interpret the narrative.[14] In a recent review of the literature, Tomlinson *et al.*[81] found that the challenges to participating in PPC research, commonly reported in published papers between 1966 and 2006, were methodological issues relating to the sensitivity of what might be seen as a vulnerable population and especially gaining entry to participants (getting past the gatekeepers including parents/guardians and ethics committees). Concerns included: the potential vulnerability of the research participants and the threat of coercion, the burden of participation, the potential that the child is unaware of their diagnosis or that they are terminally ill and the possibility parents have not come to terms with the inevitability of their child's condition. Vulnerability can be variously defined as 'the incapacity to protect one's own interests' and/or 'capable of being physically or emotionally wounded or hurt'.

Children and adolescents may be vulnerable, depending on the context within which their consent to participation in research is obtained. Positions of dependence and vulnerability can be experienced in any controlled setting, but if a child is in a crisis, his or her ability to give consent may be particularly diminished.[82] However, the belief that children are highly vulnerable and easily influenced has been challenged and is not necessarily supported by empirical evidence.[83] According to Savage and McCarron[80] young people have traditionally had little research opportunity to make their voice heard. Indeed most of the research I located and read during the writing of this chapter relied on parental reports. For many this is unacceptable.

The ethics of narrative research involves being in relationship with human beings, which requires accountability and responsibility. The principles of ethical practice are significant in terms of what is right to do, of achieving what is good, and of exemplifying the qualities of character necessary to live well. From these emerge goodness criteria for the researcher, such as considering participants first; safeguarding participants' rights, interests and sensitivities; communicating research aims; protecting the privacy of participants; not exploiting participants; and making written material available to participants.[84,85] In order to carry out narrative research ethically it is critical for researchers to understand how tenuous and in need of negotiation their relationships with participants are. By honouring research participants in a continually negotiated relationship throughout, the researcher is in a better position to know when and how to explain oneself to them whilst simultaneously trusting in their ability to shape what is of concern to them. With regard to the recruitment of parents, Tomlinson *et al.*[81] recommend researchers include strategies that will eliminate the potential unnecessary emotional burden by specifically eliciting opinions on study design from experienced families. They also briefly discuss the concern of ensuring the inclusion of the child's views, pointing out this is a sensitive topic which raises many ethical issues and requires greater debate and discussion. There is, however, conflict in the literature regarding whether or not children should be involved in any type of research and although there is considerable discussion about children's rights, these rights may not be realised if they can be overridden by adult decisions, including those of the ethics committee. Those who are competent, yet have their decisions overridden by others, can suffer substantial injury to their self respect.[86] With regard to narrative research in the PPC context, it is possible that children might also be missing an opportunity of the simple therapeutic value of telling their story and more importantly of having it heard.[40] Using only universal principles of ethics to make decisions about child participation in research may not help researchers to decide about individual cases.

According to the United Nations Convention on the Rights of the Child, children should be encouraged and enabled to make their views known on issues that affect them.[87] This has led to growing awareness and acknowledgement that children have the right to have their voice heard and to participate in research. Thus health-related research involving children is shifting from seeking information on or about children to seeking information directly from them.[88,89] Although what the nurse, doctor or parent perceive to be the child's experiences, fears, wishes, concerns, etc. are important, children must have the opportunity to express their own thoughts and experiences. If we are serious about respecting the rights of children then we must explore ways in which their voices can be heard.

There are a number of reasons why people wish to tell their stories and how they use them. Holloway and Freshwater[10] have suggested the following: as a device for individuals to come to terms with their experiences, as a way of sharing their emotional experiences, to dramatise their experience for maximum effect and to be heard perhaps by those in more powerful positions, to attribute responsibility, blame or praise to specific individuals or by way of taking control and to subsequently feel empowered. Common to all these is the idea that it enables the narrator to distance themselves and gain a different perspective on the experience; in other words, it can be a useful coping strategy.[10] If this is the case, should children not also be afforded such opportunity?

Many writers have defined narrative in terms of being a representation of a personal reality. In sharing the stories contained within this book we continue to construct our lives, and in doing so, our role within PPC. In this we hope that something will resonate with you the reader and that we make some kind of connection. When narratives are withheld we are deprived from gaining direct and intimate knowledge of collective experiences. When narratives are shared, it creates a sense of belonging and community which is a powerful way of enabling us to transform self and practice.[14] In terms of this book, the question is what happens after the narrative? Readers might reflect on their own experience, surfacing yet different interpretations, new meanings, and shifting thoughts while taking a parallel journey through each of the chapters. Thus, we hope to keep PPC and narrative research in a state of constant becoming.

N.I.C.E. analysis

Please reflect on the issues raised in this chapter in relation to your own practice.

Needs
- Young people need to be visible and have their voices heard and listened to.
- Palliative care professionals need to hear their narratives.
- There is a need for an increase of narrative research, both from a user and carer, but also professional perspective.

Interests
- There is considerable drive to have user and carer input within healthcare and healthcare education.
- Narrative research can serve to integrate this input.

Concerns
- There is very little narrative research currently available.
- Narrative research is often seen as unscientific.
- It is often difficult for researchers to engage patients and families with palliative care needs in research.

Expectations
- Narrative research needs to become more accessible and to be given more credibility.
- More qualitative researchers to sit on approval boards for research committees.

From the above analysis please reflect on:
- How might you engage in narrative research with children, young people and their families?
- What are the barriers for young people to have their voice heard? And listened to?
- How can you and your area of practice be truly reflected in research in paediatric palliative care?

Action plan: next steps
- To get involved to engage paediatric palliative care in narrative research.
- To raise the profile of narrative paediatric palliative care research by engaging with/utilising the findings.

REFERENCES

1 Stanley L. *The Auto/biographical I*. Manchester: Manchester University Press; 1992.

2 Rolfe G. *Research Truth and Authority: postmodern perspectives on nursing*. London: MacMillan Press; 2000.

3 Ezzy D. Are qualitative methods misunderstood? *Aus and NZ J Public Health*. 2001; **25**(4): 294–7.

4 Polkinghorne DE. *Narrative Knowing and the Human Sciences*. Albany: State University of New York Press; 1988.

5 Cobley P. *Narrative*. Routledge: London; 2001.

6 Walker K. Nursing, narrativity and research: towards a poetics and politics of orality. In: Rolfe G, editor. *Research, Truth and Authority: postmodern perspectives on nursing*. London: MacMillan; 2000.

7 Ricoeur P. *Time and Narrative*. Chicago: Chicago University Press; 1986.

8 Wiltshire J. Telling a story, writing a narrative: terminology in health care. *Nurs Inq*. 1995; **2**: 75–82.

9 Lawler S. *Mothering the Self: mothers, daughters, subjects*. London: Routledge; 2000.

10 Holloway I, Freshwater D. Vulnerable story telling: narrative research in nursing. *J Res Nurs*. 2007; **12**(6): 703–11.

11 Taylor C. *Sources of Self*. Cambridge, MA: Harvard University Press; 1989. pp. 57–8.

12 Denzin NK. *Interpretive Interactionism*. London: Sage Publications; 1989.

13 Hollis M. *The Philosophy of Social Science: an introduction*. Cambridge: Cambridge University Press; 1999.

14 Freshwater D. *Therapeutic Nursing: improving patient care through self-awareness and reflection*. London: Sage; 2002.

15 Bingley AF, Thomas C, Brown J, *et al*. Developing narrative research in supportive and palliative care: the focus on illness narratives. *Palliat Med*. 2008; **22**: 653–8.

16 Hinchman LP, Hinchman SK. *Memory, Identity, Community: the idea of narrative in the human sciences*. New York: New York State University Press; 1997. p. xvi.

17 Elliott J. *Narrative in Social Research: qualitative and quantitative approaches*. London: Sage; 2005. p. 4.

18 Polkinghorne DE. Validity issues in narrative research. *Qual Inq*. 2007; **13**(4): 471–86.

19 Ezzy D. *Qualitative Analysis. Practice and innovation*. London: Routledge; 2002.

20 Hevern VW. *Narrative Psychology: internet and resource guide*. 1997 (last updated July 2008). Available at: web.lemoyne.edu/~hevern/narpsych/narpsych.html (accessed 17 February 2010).

21 Dilthey W. *Selected Writings*. Cambridge: Cambridge University Press; 1976.

22 Frank A. *The Wounded Storyteller: body, illness and ethics*. Chicago: University of Chicago Press; 1995.

23 Lather P, Smithies C. *Troubling with Angels: women living with HIV/AIDS*. Boulder, CO: Westview Harper Collins; 1997.

24 Thomas C. Cancer narratives and methodological uncertainties. *Qual Res*. 2008; **8**(3): 423–33.

25 Carr D. Discussion: Ricoeur on narrative. In: Wood D, editor. *On Paul Ricoeur: narrative and interpretation*. London: Routledge; 1991. p. 160.

26 House ER. Methodological fundamentalism and the quest for control(s). In: Denzin NK, Giardina MD, editors. *Qualitative Inquiry and the Conservative Challenge: confronting methodological fundamentalism*. Walnut Creek CA: Left Coast Press; 2006. pp. 100–1.

27 Ricoeur P. Life in quest of narrative. In: Wood D, editor. *On Paul Ricoeur: narrative and interpretation.* London: Routledge; 1991.

28 McNay L. *Gender and Agency: reconfiguring the subject in feminist and social theory.* Cambridge: Polity; 2000. p. 95.

29 Ezzy D. Lived experience and interpretation in narrative theory: experiences of living with HIV/AIDS. *Qual Sociol.* 1998; **21**: 169–80.

30 Bailey PH, Tilley S. Storytelling and the interpretation of meaning in qualitative research. *J Adv Nurs.* 2002; **38**(6): 574–83.

31 Brown J, Addington-Hall J. How people with motor neurone disease talk about living with their illness: a narrative study. *J Adv Nurs.* 2008; **62**(2): 200–8.

32 Frank A. What is dialogical research, and why should we do it? *Qual Health Res.* 2005; **15**(7): 964–74.

33 McKenzie R. Vulnerable story telling: narrative research in nursing. *J Res Nurs.* 2007; **12**(6): 713–14.

34 Pennebaker JW. Telling stories: the health benefits of narrative. *Lit Med.* 2000; **19**(1): 3–18.

35 Mattingly C. The concept of therapeutic 'emplotment'. *Soc Sci and Med.* 1994; **38**(6): 811–22.

36 Somers MR, Gibson GD. Reclaiming the Epistemological 'other': narrative and the social constitution of identity. In: Calhoun C, editor. *Social Theory and the Politics of Identity.* Cambridge, MA: Blackwell; 1994. pp. 38–9.

37 Atkinson P, Silverman D. Kundera's immortality: the interview society and the invention of the self. *Qual Inq.* 1997; **3**: 304–25.

38 Bochner AP. Narrative's virtues. *Qual Inq.* 2001; **7**(1): 131–57.

39 Atkinson P. Narrative turn or blind alley? *Qual Health Res.* 1997; **7**: 325–44.

40 Frank A. The standpoint of storyteller. *Qual Health Res.* 2000; **10**(28): 354–65.

41 Mishler EG. *Research Interviewing: context and narrative.* Cambridge, MA: Harvard University Press; 1986.

42 Reissman CK. *Narrative Analysis.* London: Sage; 1993.

43 Moore H. *A Passion for Difference: essays in anthropology and gender.* Cambridge: Polity; 1994. p. 119.

44 White H. Desire in narrative In: De Lauretis T, editor. *Alice Doesn't: feminism, semiotics, cinema.* Bloomington, IN: Indiana Press; 1984. pp. 129–72.

45 Taylor C. Understanding the other: a Gadermarian view on conceptual schemes. In: Malpass J, editor. *Gadamer's Century: essays in honor of Hans Georg Gadamer.* Cambridge: MIT Press; 2002. pp. 279–97.

46 Chase S. *Ambiguous Empowerment: the work narratives of women school superintendents.* Amherst, MA: University of Massachusetts Press; 1995.

47 Plummer K. *Telling Sexual Stories: power, change and social worlds.* London: Routledge; 1995.

48 Chase S. Narrative inquiry: multiple lenses, approaches, voices. In: Denzin N, Lincoln Y, editors. *The Sage Handbook of Qualitiative Research.* Thousand Oaks, CA: Sage; 2005.

49 Suzuki LK, Beale IL. Personal web home pages of adolescents with cancer: self-presentation, information, dissemination, and interpersonal connection. *J Pediatr Oncol Nurs.* 2006; **23**(3): 152–61.

50 Squire C. Reading narratives. *Group Anal.* 2005; **38**(1): 91–107.

51 Reissman CK. Exporting ethics: a narrative about narrative research in South India. *Health: An Interdisciplinary Journal for the Social Study of Health, Illness and Medicine.* 2005; **9**(4): 473–90.

52 Frank A. *At the Will of the Body: reflections on illness.* Boston: Houghton Mifflin; 1991.

53 Mason J. *Qualitative Researching*. London: Sage; 1996.

54 Lather P. *Getting Lost: feminist efforts toward a double(d) science*. Albany, NY: State University of New York Press; 2007.

55 Greatrex-White S. Thinking about the nature of research findings: a hermeneutic phenomenological perspective. *Int J Nurs Stud* 2008; **45**(12): 1842–9.

56 Lather P. To appear other to itself anew: response data. *Cultural Studies <=> Critical Methodologies*. 2008; **8**(3): 369–71.

57 Street A. *Inside Nursing: a critical ethnography of nursing*. New York: State University of New York Press; 1992.

58 Bamberg MGW, McCabe A. Editorial. *Narrative Inquiry*. 1998; **8**(1): iii–v.

59 Speraw S. Talk to me – I'm human: the story of a girl, her personhood, and the failures of health care. *Qual Health Res*. **19**(6): 732–43.

60 Woodgate RL. *Symptom Experiences in the Illness Trajectory of Children with Cancer and their Families*. Unpublished Dissertation. Winnipeg, MB: University of Manitoba.

61 Woodgate RL. The importance of being there: perspectives of social support by adolescents with cancer. *J Pediatr Oncol Nurs*. 2006; **23**(3): 122–34.

62 Woodgate RL, Degner L. A substantive theory of keeping the spirit alive: the spirit within children with cancer and their families. *J Pediatr Oncol Nurs*. 2003; **20**(3): 103–19.

63 Bearison D. *They Never Want to Tell You: children talk about cancer*. Cambridge, MA: Harvard University Press; 1991.

64 Björk M, Wiebe T, Hallström I. Striving to survive: families' lived experiences when a child is diagnosed with cancer. *J Pediatr Oncol Nurs*. 2005; **22**(5): 265–75.

65 Wilkins KL, Woodgate RL. A review of qualitative research on the childhood cancer experience from the perspectives of siblings: a need to give them a voice. *J Pediatr Oncol Nurs*. 2005; **22**(6): 305–19.

66 Gunter M, Thomas SP. (2006) Nurses narratives of unforgettable patient care events. *J Nurs Scholarship*. 2006; **38**: 370–7.

67 Macpherson CF. Peer-supported storytelling for grieving pediatric oncology nurses. *J Pediatr Oncol Nurs*. 2008; **25**(3): 148–63.

68 Craft A, Killen S. *Palliative Care Services for Children and Young People in England: an independent review for the Secretary of State for Health*. London: Department of Health; 2007.

69 Brett J. The journey to accepting support: how parents of profoundly disabled children experience support in their lives. *Paediatr Nurs*. 2004; **16**(8): 14–18.

70 Read S, Spall B. Reflecting on patient and carer biographies in palliative care education. *Nurse Educ Prac*. 2005; **5**(3): 136–43.

71 Frid I, Ohlen J, Bergbom I. On the use of narratives in nursing research. *J Adv Nurs*. 2001; **32**: 695–703.

72 Borreani C, Miccinesi G, Brunelli C, *et al*. An increasing number of qualitative research papers in oncology and palliative care: does it mean a thorough development of the methodology of research? *Health Qual of Life Outcome*. 2004; **2**: 7. Available at: www.hqlo.com/content/2/1/7 (accessed 17 February 2010).

73 McKibbon KA, Gadd CS. A quantitative analysis of qualitative studies in clinical journals for the 2000 publishing year. *BMC Med Informat Decis Making*. 2004; **4**: 11. Available at: www.ncbi.nlm.nih.gov/pmc/articles/PMC503397/?tool=pubmed (accessed 20 February 2010).

74 Woodgate RL. Part I: An introduction to conducting qualitative research in children with cancer. *J Pediatr Oncol Nurs*. 2000; **17**(4): 192–206.

75 Woodgate RL. Part II: A critical review of qualitative research related to children's experiences with cancer. *J Pediatr Oncol Nurs.* **17**(4): 207–28.

76 Callaghan EE. Achieving balance: a case study examination of an adolescent coping with life-limiting cancer. *J Pediatr Oncol Nurs.* 2007; **24**(6): 334–49.

77 Savage E, Callery P. Weight and energy: parents' and children's perspectives on managing cystic fibrosis diet. *Arch Dis Child.* 2005; **90**(3): 249–52.

78 www.act.org.uk/

79 Hinds PS, Pritchard M, Harper J. End-of-life research as a priority for pediatric oncology. *J Pediatr Oncol Nurs.* **21**: 175–9.

80 Savage E, McCarron S. Research access to adolescents and young adults. *Appl Nurs Res.* 2009; **22**: 63–7.

81 Tomlinson D, Bartels U, Hendershot E, *et al.* Challenges to participation in paediatric palliative care research: a review of the literature. *Palliat Med.* 2007; **21**: 435–40.

82 Pieranunzi VR, Freitas LG. Informed consent with children and adolescents. *J Child Adolesc Psychiatr Nurs.* 1992; **5**(2): 21–7.

83 Broome ME, Stieglitz KA. The consent process and children. *Res Nurs Health.* 1992; **15**: 147–52.

84 MacIntyre A. *After Virtue.* Notre Dame, IN: University of Notre Dame Press; 1981.

85 Newton AZ. *Narrative Ethics.* Cambridge, MA: Harvard University Press; 1995.

86 Bishop A, Scudder J. *Nursing Ethics: holistic caring practice.* 2nd ed. Sudbury, MA: Jones and Bartlett; 2001.

87 Bellamy C. *The State of the World's Children.* New York: UNICEF; 2003.

88 Carter B. Chronic pain in childhood and the medical encounter: professional ventriloquism and hidden voices. *Qual Health Res.* 2002; **12**(1): 28–41.

89 McPherson A, Forster D, Galzebrook C, *et al.* The asthma files: evaluation of a multimedia package for children's asthma education. *Paediatr Nurs.* 2002; **14**(2): 32–5.

8

Part 1: 'Where's my sitcom?' The young adult's voice

Greg Wilford

For my family, with love.

Did anyone ever see 'All About Me' or 'I'm With Stupid'? No? Ah, just me then, oh well. What's the significance? Well, these two names I've seemingly drawn out of the hat were sitcoms commissioned by the BBC that feature prominent wheelchair-bound characters. The former programme was (according to the 'ever so reliable' Wikipedia) a situational comedy about a multi-cultural British family (tick one box) living in the Midlands (tick another box) with the youngest child of the family being confined to a wheelchair through cerebral palsy (a demographic hat-trick). Refreshingly, the actor portraying the wheelchair user is for once actually . . . disabled.

It wasn't very good. It wasn't bad, it just wasn't very good. To be fair I only caught a few episodes so am probably not in the best position to be casting a fair critical review.

Same can be said for 'Stupid'. It features a lead protagonist in a wheelchair, played by an actor who incidentally has cerebral palsy. Again, this good news – the same condition as the character he plays in the show. Cerebral palsy and paralysis, interestingly, seem to be the only two reasons for being in a wheelchair according to television.

The premise of the show centres on 'Paul's' adventures, in and around the 'home for the disabled' he resides in. As with 'All About Me' it's ok. It fulfils the objective of light-hearted entertainment expected from it, but that's all it does. To say these two programmes feature such disabled-focused characters, you would hope (or dread even) that the BBC may portray the themes associated with disability in a realistic and mature fashion. Alas, they don't. They never do – and to be fair to them, they aren't the only party guilty of this 'wimping out'. Is this through unintentional ignorance or deliberate avoidance? I don't know. I have a pretty good idea which; because the norm in television when presenting disabled people either falls under a series of undeveloped caricatures or melodramatic, morose depressives (as seen in any soaps). 'All About Me' was very well intentioned there's no doubt – the 'wheelchair' character (I forget his name) often conveyed his thoughts through articulate narration conveying that despite his 'fragile' exterior, he was one of the most perceptive and, at times, the most rational member of the cast; it's just a shame the makers of the programme chose not to expand on this. I think the same could unfortunately be said about 'Stupid'. The creators will have been well-meaning when wanting to make this show – of course they will have. They will have endeavoured to construct a refreshing portrayal. Yet they ended up confining the character and the rest of his 'disabled' fraternity to the interior of the 'home' rather than having them mix with the outside world. The important themes such as education, creating understanding and social integration with members of both the disabled and non-disabled communities are not discussed. Instead the programme turns to reliable, yet bromidic, devices or stereotypes that have been used time and time again. The programme was also located in the dated facility of an all-purpose 'residential home'. I was a bit disappointed that this was the situation of choice as now, thanks to sweeping changes in the field of 'Independent Living' projects, the concept of living in a 'home' is something that is reality for the minority for disabled people nowadays rather than the majority.

See, this rant – it'll be over soon, just bear with me – stems from a module I'm studying at the moment entitled *'Cultural Identity within British Television'* – again . . . please bear with me – a point is coming. Essentially within this course I study a variety of social groups that make up the length and breadth of twenty-first-century Britain today (e.g. gender, ethnicity, class, sexuality) paying particular attention to the way they have been represented on television since its inception. I was intrigued reading our topics for the semester, and surprised even, that 'disability' wasn't one of the sessions listed. Now usually I'm not one to pick on things like this, but this really did surprise me. After a period of thinking about programmes I'd seen over the years about 'disability' I came to this conclusion – that there are hardly any examples to draw upon; hence that's why it isn't on the list. As a lad 'who thinks he can write good' and an obsessive fan of film and good programming in general, this was a bit of a head scratcher. Over the years, I've come across some amazing individuals who have to live with some really tough conditions – conditions that make mine look pretty tame – with some even more amazing stories. Really I guess it would be just nice to see someone use these people as a basis to create a piece that is profound, different, but most importantly *true* to the issues it deals with. No mawkish, over-sentimental melodrama and at the same time no show about the kid who overcomes his chronic muscular dystrophy, triumphs in the face of adversity, and tops it all off by scoring the winning goal for Leeds United in the FA Cup Final – 'we can all but dream'. I mean, in my opinion I reckon you're hard pushed to find a better representation of disability on television than *South Park*'s 'Timmy'! A controversial choice I'm sure, and one that isn't to everyone's taste, but please let me elaborate. Timmy is portrayed as having a profound disability that is never disclosed during the show, though it seems to display characteristics of both cerebral palsy and autism. Timmy can only communicate through screaming his own name and other choice phrases; thus making communication with other characters potentially difficult. This often leads a series of misunderstandings of Timmy on the part of the adults, and demonstrates their belief that Timmy needs constant protection from the world around him due to his vulnerable condition. *South Park*'s main characters, a group of eight-year-olds, differ in this approach and choose to accept him as one of the group rather than isolate him like the adults try to do. It was a risky portrayal by the creators; prior to their first show featuring the character, there was an anxiety from the producers that the nature of his disability would be considered in poor taste and the audience would not respond well to it. In reality the opposite happened – Timmy went down a storm, and in subsequent appearances raised awareness for people with disability. I don't put this effect wholly down to the actual character itself, I believe that it was through observing the other characters interact and accept Timmy that this resonated through to its fan base.

I think because of the lurid material *South Park* features, it will always be looked at askance. So, really, it is unlikely that the general public will see past the surface and appreciate what a clever representation of disability it is. What I would like to see from a programme is a frank, fresh portrayal of disability that challenges and at the same time educates its audience rather than conform to an artificial stereotype. Until then at least we can rely on the 2-D Timmy and, at a push, the always-believable . . . erm . . . ugh . . . Ironside?

It's about 4.30 am; at least I think it is. I haven't got a clock on hand to correct me, though given that it's still dark outside it seems my guess would be a close one. Still, that doesn't escape the fact that it's 4.30 in the morning and I can't get to sleep. Why? I don't know. I've just been rolled onto my side – so it can't be that, the ventilator mask is all nice and secure. Not too tight so it puts pressure on my nose, but not too slack so excess air isn't blowing in my face every time I breathe, so it's not that either. I'm not dried up in my throat so I don't need a drink or anything. In fact, in the last 10 minutes I've gone through a litany of possible reasons for my insomnia yet none seem to offer any solution. So what could it be then? Why am I still awake?

I wouldn't mind, but I've got to be up early for a lecture tomorrow – too early in fact. I bet you I'll want to sleep when nine o'clock in the morning comes. Maybe my leg's rubbing on a crease from my pyjamas . . . nope that's not it either. Hang on. Perhaps, I'm looking at this the wrong way. Instead of trying to force myself to sleep by squeezing my eyes as tight as they will go till my eyelids just get fed up and submit, letting me have some much needed kip, which really isn't working, why don't I just – relax? So I try it and hey, you know what? It works, within five minutes I'm beginning to drift off to sleep . . . slowly . . . veerrrrryyyyy sloooowllllyyyyy . . .

Suddenly, I hear a faint scratching sound outside our communal door; the unmistakable racket of a pair of keys trying to be guided into its respective lock by a certain inebriated individual, who instead of hitting the target first time, continues to scrape the keys across the door due to a lethal combination of quaking nerves and blurry vision. Annoyingly, after what seems like 3000 attempts at getting the bloody key in the blasted lock, he's managed it. The door flies open and instead of walking down the corridor to his bedroom and his bed, this arrival decides to stagger in the opposite direction – slurring something incoherent in a thick Irish drawl as he does so; all the way to my bedroom door, where subtly, and intently with the knowledge that I have an early start in the morning, he announces his presence with a pounding series of knocks and a tender cry of, 'ARE YOU AWAKE [insert expletive here]!? I'M GOING TO MAKE US SOME CURRY . . .' This usually continues for another 10 minutes, waking up the poor PA, who wearily stumbles into my room and urbanely asks if I'd like to let my prat of a flatmate in. I say yes, so long as she'll lovingly throttle him for me. See I wouldn't mind – but I haven't woken him up at this time of night for at *least* three days . . .

That's where I am now, a sleep-deprived student (he's not that bad really) in my second year at university, but things weren't always that bad . . .

I was born in 1988, in a small Yorkshire town to my father, a structural engineer (he drew car parks and constantly tried to assure me it was more interesting than it actually sounded) and my mum, a nurse of some shape or form. I also had a younger sister, who as far as sisters go isn't too bad. In a nutshell, growing up was pretty wholesome for me and, well, I would say pretty unremarkable if you place it within the grand scheme and compare it to the things that have happened to me since. That's not to say I didn't have a happy childhood. On the contrary, I did, all things considering. I was fortunate enough to go on holiday to America, I learnt to ride a bike – I'll rephrase, I tried to learn how to ride a bike, I played football, I did what was done at that age.

I don't remember much about the time when I was finally diagnosed with Duchenne muscular dystrophy (DMD) nor the occasion when I finally went off my feet. It is surprising really when you think how monumental an event it was but . . . no I don't remember a thing.

What I do remember from that period of time though is when they were eliminating the possibilities as to what could be wrong with me; the physiotherapist was adamant that my unsteadiness when walking was caused by one leg being minutely longer than the other. This alleged extra length was so minute in fact, that it was cunningly invisible to the naked eye . . . and I would predict the microscopic eye at that. In fact it was so tiny that when measured against a tape measure it could be said it was almost non-existent. It's funny the things you remember isn't it?

I think I'm about 5 or 6 at this point; I'd definitely started primary school by then so, yeah, I must have been 6. See, I always remember my mum being very sceptical regarding this (mis)-diagnosis. She was always convinced there was something they were missing; that they were clutching at straws. I mean she couldn't talk; her 'scientific deduction' was based on the fact that I could never draw a perfect circle – my ends wouldn't join together – which doesn't really hold a lot of weight in the scientific community as a basis for diagnosis. My auntie tells me that when she used to bring the 'circle thing' up with friends, family, etc., everyone thought that she was worrying about me too much. 'It's just a phase,' they used to tell her, 'nothing to worry about.'

But in the end it turns out she was right.

Personally, I can't speak for my family on how they felt when they first heard the news about my disability; obviously they were shocked and gutted, but I couldn't say what their instinctual reaction was. I'd imagine when a parent hears news like that, they tend to go down one of two common trains of thought, either it'll be one of courageous 'well that's not going to stop us' or the fatalist 'well that's it then isn't it.'

I'm not a parent of a disabled child; to me it is one of the most unenviable positions for a person to be in, therefore I can't speak with any authority or judge those that are – not even my own – and the decisions they choose to or choose not to make. To be honest, it's not a subject that comes up in conversation that often, and that's not because it's impossible for us to sit down and talk about it. My mum and dad were always on hand to give me frank, honest answers to any question I had regarding my condition though looking back, my dad's answer to any questions I did ask regarding any subject usually consisted of some variation of the phrase, 'I don't know. Ask your mother!' The thing was, growing up, they never . . . umm . . . they never . . . I'm going to use the word 'deluded' here, yeah they never tried to create a pretence for my benefit on the nature of my condition; they never sugar-coated the details for me. Was that a good idea looking back? Personally – yeah, I think it was. I mean I need to be clear here, DMD is a hard pill to swallow I think we can all agree with that, especially at 16, when I truly understood the severity of the condition.

For those of you who aren't familiar with the condition, Duchenne Muscular Dystrophy is essentially a mutation in the dystrophin gene – a gene responsible for the creation of protein that creates a kind of membrane around the muscle. With no dystrophin, the muscle degenerates and is replaced with a combination of fat and fibrotic tissue – in layman's terms, this gives the muscles no substance. The effect of this really is the progressive weakening of every single muscle in the body; first causing difficulty in walking, which eventually leads to a dependence on a wheelchair; then curvatures of the spine that if not treated accordingly will lead to skeletal deformities, and to wrap things off the cardiac and respiratory muscles experience a 'wasting' effect, leading to respective difficulties in later life. Phew. I do worry myself sometimes with how easy it is for me to rattle the above description off without so much as a shudder, but hey that was the gist of what I was told and I think that upbringing is what made me so content with my situation. The approach for my parents, then, despite all that – and for me to this day – runs along the lines of 'well, let's see what happens'. To give you an example; I think one of the first things they did after I was diagnosed was sign me up for judo practice: can you believe?

I was never mobile enough to win a fight; in fact I was lucky if I could stay on my feet long enough between the start of the bout and the time it took for my opponent to walk over to me and toss me over their shoulder. Once I was on my back, I was like a bloody ladybird, I was stuck. But that didn't stop my *sensei* from dragging me back onto my feet and sending me back in the ring only to peel me off the floor again five minutes later – all this at my mum's insistence of course, and do you know what? I loved every minute of it and I think she knew that – I mean what sort of cruel parent takes pleasure from watching their child get systematically beaten by each and every one of his peers (yes, girls too – they were the better fighters) with no real chance of retaliation. Actually, now that you mention it . . .

As you can see, they weren't members of the 'cotton-wool wrapping' brigade, that's for sure. In essence, they wanted me do whatever I could do, be whatever I could be and enjoy whatever I could enjoy – within reason of course. It was that simple.

Their next big decision was to sack off any advice given to them by 'those in the know' who believed I'd be best suited in an establishment colloquially known as a 'special school' for my later years of compulsory education, and instead packed me off to the only mainstream school in the area that catered for the disabled at the time. Yes, it was undeniable that a 'special school' provides the facilities that would cater for my physical needs – I would be around staff and peers alike who would understand my limitations and compensate accordingly; but this would be at the expense of my academic pursuits and most importantly the social side – which is, as we can all agree, the best thing about school.

To the school's credit, my time there was great. I have no complaints. I was well supported through my education both by a fantastic team of teaching assistants – many of whom worked with me all the way through school – and a close group of friends. The faculty as a whole was very good to me, the teachers were inclusive and always encouraging me to do the best I could and that with the right mixture of equipment, support and my own input I could be as successful as the next student. I think it was thanks to them and a tiny bit of effort on my part that I managed to come away with a collection of grades that put me in good shape for whatever I wanted to do next in life. They even allowed time in the schedule for me to access the school pool for my PE; a definite benefit for me as it kept me as active as possible. The facilities provided by the pool included a designated disabled changing room all with hoist, bed and roll-in shower; and for the poolside, the school had purchased a hoist that could transfer someone straight from a bath chair into the water. Not only was this facility put in place for my benefit, but for the benefit of the community as well, though since I left I hear the only use it's had has been as a glorified storeroom. Bit of a shame really.

I have a couple of friends in wheelchairs whose parents opted to utilise the facilities a 'special school' offered. These guys are 20 . . . 21 and now attend a mixed residential college – mixed meaning both disabled and non-disabled students – which they love. It gives them everything they need from a higher education course. Though . . .

I go back to a conversation we had last year when we were comparing our respective experiences of education. I think in the nicest way these guys regret not having the opportunity to integrate with their peers, instead only having the company of 'other disabled people' – not that that's a bad thing; it's just nice to have a bit of variation I think, that's all. One lad in particular remarked that he felt much more confident round 'able-bodied' people his own age now he is constantly in an environment where they are present. To be honest with you the only difference I've noticed since he's become a student is his capacity to drink twice as much beer as he used to without being sick (two pints).

Another issue raised was how he felt being in a 'special school' had compromised his chances of getting decent grades by the time he left school. I don't know if this is dogma, but my friend tells me that he was only allowed to take two GCSEs and that A-levels were a 'pipe dream'. You could say that perhaps he didn't possess the ability to keep up with the work, but as I mentioned before, he's now in his final year of his first college course and relishes the challenge of doing another degree, so clearly his ability to complete the work is not an issue.

I asked him:

'So if you could go back and change things, would you want to go to a mainstream school then?'

'No. I don't think I would.'

'Why the hell not? I mean you've just been telling me how you didn't get to do the things you wanted to do as a kid because of being in "special school".' (I have to confess that was not the term I used at the time.)

And he replied with this; I SWEAR this was what he said:

'Yeah, but I might have been bullied.'

Let me dispel a myth for you if I may. I and several other people with an array of disabilities all attended a mainstream environment and I am pleased to say that I have heard very few stories about disabled people being victims of bullying. In my mind it is a rare occurrence. An unfortunate one, yes I agree, but there are so many opportunities and benefits from being in as relatively 'normal' an environment as possible that the ends will always justify the means.

I'll admit when I started in my first year there was a sense of feeling different from the rest of the group. Course there was. I mean crudely put, I had wheels and they didn't; and some kids picked on that difference through a combination of ignorance, misunderstanding and a case of kids just being kids. This was a minority and often not people that I knew. The students who I spent most of my time with gave me banter about being in a wheelchair, but also about being ginger, and I gave them cheek for being a bit tubby or the usual kind of insults lads give each other. In a strange way this constant stream of insults and gestures made me feel very much involved because it was what everyone else did. A different form of integration, but in my friendship group insults and offensive nicknames seem to be a kind of warped term of endearment for us.

Moving on: its 2003, I'm now 14 and I'm about to make one of the biggest decisions of my life. The muscles in my back are weaker, I'm beginning to lean over on to my left side; my scoliosis is pretty prominent now and pretty destructive in terms of my health. The curvature is causing pressure to be placed onto one of my lungs and heart – that's not good apparently – and this is something that's going to manifest into something much worse unless drastic measures are taken … But like I said, I'm 14, and all of this is going in one ear and straight out of the other. I mean I understood the complications perfectly. Crushed heart + crushed lung = BAD! Thing is, I just wish – I didn't understand the conditions perfectly. I was at the wrong age to be caring about trivial stuff such as 'respiratory failures' and 'skeletal deformities'; for me, 14 was the age where my priorities were girls and … and I'm pretty sure there was another interest back then, it's just not springing to mind right now, so I'll just say girls again for the time being. Reflecting on all this, there was certainly naiveté on the part of the doctors, the nurses and my parents when they left it up to me to decide whether I should have titanium, spinal rods screwed to my back to rectify the scoliosis. I was in no way ready enough to make an informed decision on that big a scale; but I still managed to bluff, and made the right choice. To be honest, they sold the operation to me when they said I'd have metal in my body; everything else was a bonus at that point. So I did the op, all 11 hours of it; I did the recovery, no problems there; and I corrected the warping of my spine – everything was sorted. Was I ever worried? Well no, to be honest, I was blissfully ignorant about the whole process – I was told what was going to happen – thing is it never clicked, which in itself was a blessing in disguise. If I knew step-by-step what the surgeon was going to do to me in the operating theatre; if I knew that invasive surgery was going to be executed on my spine where severe nerve damage could be caused; that because of my already then poor lung function there was a risk I wouldn't come round from the anaesthetic; that when bolting the metalwork to my bones there was a chance they could have broken my back, would I still have had the operation? Yes, course I would. Not because of the benefits I described earlier mind, I just think the scar kicks ass.

But I think we should lift the mood; operations can air on the side of depressing at times. Let's lighten the mood, let's make things a bit more cheery . . . hmm let's talk about near-death-experiences!

When I was 16, I had what some may call 'a life-altering experience'. I nearly died! Over a period of time I had begun to be accustomed to nocturnal ventilation. This was proving to be unsuccessful. I was finding the machine too invasive and was struggling to sleep with it. Funny thing was, I wasn't respiring at night as well as I should have been, hence a build-up of CO_2 began to occur. This reached such a level that one night my body shut down and I effectively stopped breathing. Not one of my better ideas!

I came to in an ICT unit and was surprised to find an enormous tracheotomy protruding from my throat and according to the medical staff it was to become a permanent fixture of Greg Wilford. Scary stuff indeed and for the first time in my life I was that. Scared! Shitless! I thought that was it for me; the end of any aspirations I would ever have and for the rest of my life I would be stuck at home – bored. I think this was what my family were thinking as well; I mean aside from my spinal operation, nothing like this had ever happened to me before. I always maintained a healthy lifestyle and I was hardly ever ill.

So what did I do? I did what anybody would do; I ignored whatever I was told and did my best to get that bloody thing out of my throat. It took me four months, but with help and encouragement I did it. That experience taught me a lot; first, however much I like to think so, I am not invulnerable and it is important to manage my condition with effective treatments and my own awareness – within reason. Second, I found that four months in hospital can offer you either a lot of chances to sleep or too much time to think. Within this period I considered every single avenue on what I was going to do once my life at school was over . . . or to be more precise what I *could* do. I wanted to leave home, that was a given. I wanted to go to university, that was also a given; I felt I worked hard enough, but what was I going to do – what course would help me discover a career that I could do as much *myself* as possible for the *longest* amount of time. No small feat.

I still hadn't made a choice when I got back to school, my mum and dad weren't much help; they just sat on the fence and said they would support me in whatever I chose to do or didn't do. I think credit needs to go to my head of year at the time, who one day sat me down and took me through every university course and job opportunity possible, bearing in mind my strict parameters. He then suggested that maybe I should consider writing as a possible career – I'd written things before and at the time of this discussion I was writing a play for my drama course so that's what led me to that. It would be a career that would be based on my creative skill and effort; with technology and computer aids I could potentially have it as a career for a number of years. I just have to find something mildly interesting to say first . . . I'm still working on it.

Don't get me wrong, I didn't just work all the time in my final years at school. Oh no! It was also the time when I was becoming more and more involved in going out, getting drunk and staying up till all hours of the night with my mates. Unfortunately my parents weren't as keen. Again I need to be clear; my folks were great at encouraging me to go out and socialise and were always there at the end of the night to nurse my drunken state when my friends remembered to return me home. Thing is, they were getting on a bit and when you're the age they are you need eight hours of sleep a day . . . and six hours at night – your son rolling in at three in the morning really isn't what you want . . . or need. That was my main reason for leaving home I think; not for university itself, but just to get away from home so I could live the life that I wanted – and so my family could live the life they wanted as well; to enjoy a parent–son relationship with them, rather than a parent/carer–son relationship; and since I've been away that's just what happened.

I'm 20 years old now – that awkward age when you're too old to be a teenager but too young to be classed as a man yet. I guess I'm at that age where one calls himself a 'lad'. On top of that I'm also a student, so any notion of responsibility really goes out the window. I say that, next year is my final one at university – providing I don't stay to do a masters – and I still have no idea what to do with myself. I do have ambitions though; it may be a fantasy, it may be a dream – I don't know. My main one is when I and a few mates decided we would take a large camper van, convert it as best we can in terms of disabled access and drive as far across Europe and beyond as possible. We are on a bit of a sticking point when it comes to the vehicle, mind . . .

So that's a brief insight. Do I have a point? I hope I have a point. Really the only advice I can give is none – I don't have any advice. If I break it down, if I really think about it, then I guess I just did my best with the resources I was given; I enjoyed myself the most I could with the resources I was given; I drank beer and slacked off as much as I could with the recourses I was given! It never occurred to me that DMD would stop me from doing whatever it is I strived to do. Obviously there are things that are beyond the realms of possibility for me – I've accepted that – but there are still a lot of *things* to do. There's nothing inspirational about that statement, nothing brave. Despite my circumstance I still have a life that needs to be lived; yeah things could be a little bit easier for me, a little less tough; but my situation's not going to change – and I've had a pretty good laugh so far.

Enough rambling; it's now 4.30 in the morning and know a certain Irishman who's going to have his door banged on.

Part 2: Commentary on the young adult's story

Mike Miller

What responsibility do we have as professionals to help families help young people to grow up and become independent? In his passage, Greg obviously had the inner drive to achieve in general and to achieve independence. There are strong clues in his writing that this came from his parents, although Greg might argue it came from him! When faced with a child who has a life-limiting illness it is important that, as for any child, no restrictions are blindly applied. Life is very much about taking risks and obstacles being there to be overcome.

There are tasks that a teenager has to undertake to become an adult. The fact that these were described as long ago as 1952 by Havighurst[1] doesn't mean to say they aren't relevant today.

They are:
- ➤ forming a clear identity
- ➤ accepting a new body image
- ➤ gaining freedom from parents
- ➤ developing a personal value system
- ➤ achieving financial and social independence
- ➤ developing relationships with both sexes
- ➤ developing cognitive skills and the ability to think abstractly
- ➤ developing the ability to control one's behaviour according to socially acceptable norms
- ➤ taking responsibility for one's own behaviour.

It is easy to argue that these are true for any young person, independent of their physical and mental abilities. Those young people with severe cognitive difficulties who are unable to complete these tasks will need continuing support.

It is notable that Greg's parents never deluded him about his physical difficulties. This made it possible for him to contemplate the future. How could Greg complete the tasks above without clear knowledge and understanding of his physical condition? One's physical state is a very important part of one's identity. Once accepted it is then possible to develop the care system to compensate for any deficiencies, to work with and direct other carers and begin to take responsibility for oneself.

In the 'Talk about Change' video by the KOSH company,[2] one young man says that teachers and parents should have been more explicit about the future. At school he was given the impression that he could have done anything. This may lead to not preparing yourself for what you might do. It has become apparent from such open discussion and unselfconscious essays that these young people consider themselves as people first, people who have a disability (possibly a significant disability) second and no more life-limited than anyone else! They want and deserve all realistic opportunities, to be listened to and to be heard. In the same video it becomes clear that these young people who have a life-limiting disease do not see themselves as dying (certainly no more than we are all life-limited to some degree) but have accepted they have limitations from their various conditions. At the same time the limitations are there to be overcome.

So how are we to help? We should encourage families to talk about the future of the condition with realism and hope. Not all possibilities are open. The young person should be gently encouraged to learn about his condition and take responsibilities for it. They should manage their own condition and know when appointments are and what medication they are taking and why. They may need to understand any genetic implications. They should be allowed to take the same risks as their peers and be allowed to experiment.

The passage on to adult services then becomes much easier, although it is up to the professionals to ensure that adult services are educated about the condition and taught any special techniques (accessing porta-caths, use of overnight ventilation) so that there is no reduction in quality of support.

I would suggest the following tasks that children's services have to accomplish before the child can be passed on.
1 The child understands their condition as far as possible.
2 Any genetic implications are fully understood.
3 The young person knows who to call for emergencies – and that person is known to them.
4 Adult services are aware of the young person and trained to manage their needs.

As in all things paediatric, this is a development process and needs to start very early so that during that confusing time the young person can become an adult at 16 years (for inpatient services), at 18 years for social services and at 19 years for education and many outpatient services.

How does the introduction of the Mental Capacity Act[3] help in these thoughts? I have heard this Act described as not being a threat but simply codifying existing good practice. If life is about taking risks, it is also about making choices and everyone should be empowered to make those choices that they can. I remember one young man who doesn't seem to register my presence yet can clearly choose which CD he wishes to listen to on journeys when shown two CD cases. He can make those choices for which he is competent and should be allowed to make them even if they are not to our taste. The Mental Capacity Act, though, has clearly determined that parental rights do not continue after the age of 18 years. Whilst the parents will often be the main carers and be in a position of knowing the young person best, they are some of the people to be consulted, not the only people to be consulted, when choices have to be made outside the competence of the young person. This age is also a transition for parents as well the child and understandably creates many concerns.

The Act should be a stimulus to allowing young people as much independence as possible. They are given various protections that help to balance any loss of protection that they may seem to have lost from their parents and in strict legal terms, never had. These protections aim to ensure the young person is viewed objectively and by all those who are involved in their care. Parents may have to accept (as do all parents) that choices are made that they themselves would rather were not.

In this way, one of the tenets of palliative care, that of making the most of the present, remains important throughout transition.

N.I.C.E. analysis

Please reflect on the issues raised in this chapter in relation to your own practice.

Needs

- Staff working with young people need to be able to communicate at a level appropriate to the young person and be able to understand that needs and aspirations differ based on the age.

Interests

- I have found that many staff have an interest in working with young people, and there is a lot of good practice. It really will help if this is shared, so that staff working with young people become more confident and can assist young people more effectively in the future.

Concerns

- Young people might miss out on social and academic opportunities presented by a mainstream environment due to the feeling that the comfort and securities offered by more specialised centres would be more beneficial for them.
- That they're young people and their families who struggle to access vital support from due to not being aware of what provisions they are entitled to. The reason for this is often through poor communication from the relevant authorities.

Expectations

- There are many young people making transitions between children's and adult services, and for many at the moment this experience is not good and needs to improve significantly.

Action plan: next steps

- Overall, there is a vast number of opportunities for young people that weren't available 10 years ago. It is important that this progression continues as medical advancements increase the life expectancy of young people with chronic diseases meaning that issues such as independent housing and work will need to be examined.

REFERENCES

1 Havighurst RJ. *Developmental Tasks and Education*. New York: David McKay; 1952. Also see www.childdevelopmentinfo.com/development/teens_stages.shtml

2 www.thekosh.com/projects.htm

3 www.publicguardian.gov.uk/mca/mca.htm

9

Part 1: The parent's voice

Anna Gill

I am writing this as the parent of a young man who has a supposed mitochondrial cytopathy and who has managed to defy all expectations, all medical 'best guesses' and has survived into young adulthood against the odds.

This really is cause for celebration and delight, but sadly the reality is far harsher, because whilst we as a family can adapt and change over the years we have found that palliative care services for children have not kept pace. With all the many advances in interventions and care there are ever increasing numbers of young people surviving as young adults, most of whom would not have done so even a few years ago.[1]

Ours has been a very long and challenging journey that has been, we are told, the typical rollercoaster ride faced by families with children diagnosed with degenerative metabolic conditions. For professionals in the field this is a relatively common experience; but it must always be borne in mind that for the families it is always without doubt a frightening journey into the unknown; a process where the outcomes are utterly dependent on the care and support a child and the family receive.

I am only too aware that I am writing from a personal perspective, from one small area of the UK and about a rare condition. I realise I can never relay the feelings and experiences of families facing the very different journey faced with a diagnosis of cancer; but I do know that as the parent of a severely disabled and life-limited child my experiences are replicated all over the UK.

THE EARLY YEARS

Our son Jamie was born in 1991, after a normal, uneventful pregnancy. He was slow to respond and needed suction, oxygen and considerable stimulation to take his first breaths. I am a nurse and was only too aware at the time that his start was less than ideal, but after a couple of days in a special care baby unit (SCBU) with poor feeding, he finally came home and we had one month of having a 'normal' baby – what turned out to be the only month in his whole life.

At one month old he was suddenly ill with a urinary tract infection and was rushed into hospital in respiratory distress. He recovered quickly, but even with hindsight I did not anticipate that this unusual incident was the start of the multiplicity of medical challenges and emergencies that were to follow.

By six weeks old it had become every obvious that Jamie was totally blind and unable to respond to any visual stimulus. We were seen very quickly by a consultant ophthalmologist, who gave me the first indication of how advice and support given sensitively and positively can make such an enormous difference to parents of a sick or disabled child. This was our first foray into the world of disability and by being a very constructive and supportive experience set the tone for all future contact with the team. The consultant concerned explained that he was quite sure that the lack of vision was from a neurological source – that Jamie's brain had not developed sufficiently yet to programme the visual stimuli. He quickly referred us to the visual impairment team at a time when every day of waiting was so painful. As a parent in this situation you need prompt and timely support, which for me was immediately! By giving us guidelines and exercises to promote and help develop early emerging vision we were given a crucial opportunity to do something for our son rather than to just sit by, to 'wait and see', which for many of us is sometimes the only feasible option offered.

The level of Jamie's neurological deficit became more and more obvious as his very poor tone became apparent; his lack of head control and his general floppiness was causing increasing concern. His eyesight gradually started to emerge, and by four months he was responding to light, and by six months he was tracking and responding to faces. However, this improvement was tempered by the realisation that he was severely delayed in every other area of development.

In these early stages we were referred to the Child Development Unit at our local hospital and started to embark on the regular round of therapists and investigations. All results were totally inconclusive and so started the long and arduous search for a definitive diagnosis; a journey that 17 years later we still have not completed. This need for a label will be recognised by many medical staff, but I cannot over emphasise its personal importance. I needed to know what I was up against, I needed to know what to expect and I really needed to know if this was something that was inherited and, if so, what the chances were of nature repeating itself.

By nine months it was quite apparent that the outlook for Jamie was very uncertain and I had a difficult and memorable discussion with his consultant to outline what outcomes we might expect. In retrospect it was very early on to be asking such questions as, will he walk, read and write, etc., but at the time I needed to know what I was going to have to face. It's a very hard decision, I appreciate, for any doctor to face but for many parents it's actually the fear of the unknown and our imagination of things to come that can be far worse than the reality. Honesty is very much appreciated and respected by families, and the first venture into this 'new world' can have far reaching ramifications if it is a poor experience for families.

What helped me so much in these early days apart from the very strong relationships with the various therapists were the chances to meet other parents of disabled children, to discover a whole world out there that until now had never even occurred to me. For many parents of children in the palliative care categories 3 and 4[2] it is the prospect of having a disabled child that is the very first hurdle that has to be overcome before the prospect of a limited life span is broached or even considered.

EMERGING CONCERNS

Up until the age of 2½ Jamie merely had a label of 'delayed development', a euphemism for 'we don't know what's wrong or what's going to happen'. This is a very difficult and challenging diagnosis for parents to accept as 'delayed' strongly implies something that will arrive, albeit late.

Matters changed suddenly and irrevocably when just before his third birthday Jamie developed diabetes and epilepsy within months of each other and the multi-systemic nature of his illness was becoming apparent. He coped well with these changes and, luckily for us, due to his learning disabilities he was not frightened of the implications of this diagnosis and has accepted with equanimity his daily round of five to six insulin injections.

He was presenting with a wide range of alarming conditions, from severe ataxia, protracted diarrhoea, difficulty with speech and swallowing, severe heat intolerance and wildly swinging blood sugars that never responded to all attempts to control them. We were referred to Addenbrookes Hospital and then, after exhaustive investigations, to Great Ormond Street Hospital, as it was becoming apparent that Jamie had something rare and possibly life-threatening.

The metabolic specialist from London who had been informed that I came from a medical background contacted us. We discussed what investigations and conditions she was considering, which for me, was a bonus that I really appreciated. I fully support the need to identify just how much information and involvement parents can sustain, but I for one, like many of my parent colleagues, had become really quite knowledgeable about my son's supposed condition of mitochondrial disease. This level of prior information is not everyone's choice, but for me it meant I had prepared all my questions, and made very good use of the valuable time spent in this tertiary centre. I am an enthusiastic ambassador of partnership working with parents (and later with young people themselves), and this was a very good example of the efficacy of this approach.

We returned to Great Ormond Street Hospital to receive our result – an occasion that will live with me forever. Again it was all handled so well and followed perfectly the guidelines in the ACT Care Pathway.[3] We were seen without my son, as I had requested not to take him; it was a long and potentially stressful car journey and I needed to be able to take in as much as I could from this consultation.

We were seen in a private room with the specialist nurse there too. We were given plenty of time and told the appointment was as an hour long which gave me confidence to take my time to digest the news, collect my thoughts and ask all the inevitable questions. In essence we were told that Jamie 'almost certainly' had mitochondrial disease, and that young people who do well with this condition can live to maturity. However, neither I nor my father who accompanied me actually asked what 'maturity' meant; it emerged we had very different images of this prognosis. I thought probably aged 21, but in actuality what was meant were early teenage years or puberty. It was a salutary lesson in enforcing the need to make sure that all parties are speaking the same 'language' and have the same understanding of what's been said.

We returned home and it became incumbent upon me to tell my husband and family what had been confirmed – that Jamie had a short life-expectancy and that our lives were to change forever.

It should be noted here that at this time we had approximately 32 different practitioners and medical staff working with us and no key worker. I had to tell all these people about the news we had just received – letters from tertiary centres take weeks to reach the local hospital, then further days to reach community staff, by which time the family themselves have had to repeatedly tell their story, reinforcing the devastating news over and over again.

In many ways, life then settled down again. I finally had a direction, some understanding of what we were facing and the endless search for a diagnosis seemed over. We found the different reactions of people quite surprising in many ways. Some were overwhelmed by the news and expected Jamie to go into a rapid decline and die, whilst others could not accept the devastating diagnosis because he did not look ill, and also, of course, it was not proven, not definitive.

This uncertainty has always haunted me and now, so many years on, it still does. How can you plan for something that no one can quantify, qualify or even adequately explain? In the end I think to some degree I put my life on hold and completely immersed myself in caring for Jamie and in being involved in his 'special needs' world. I was a committee member and, later, trustee, of a local, parent-led charity that ran music groups for disabled children; I was the Portage Parent Rep and became a governor at his special school, all within a very short while. For many parents with time and confidence this is the way they cope – there is nothing you can do for your child but you can work hard to change their world and the circumstances that families find themselves in.

Much of my early support came from other parents, from being able to be open, quite frank and honestly angry and frustrated in the company of those who know exactly what you are facing. I have always been involved with parent groups and believe one can never over-value the therapeutic effect of finding you are not alone in these very hard and often harrowing times.

Jamie himself was very happy and blissfully unaware of his limitations, taking endless massive swings in his blood sugar with amazing stoicism. He was, however, very strong-willed and stubborn and many was the time in the ensuing years that he ended up in hospital on an IV to correct his severe keto-acidosis because he had starved himself into a dangerous state. Trying to rationalise and cajole a child with his level of learning disability proved a thankless task!

Any childhood illness rendered him either semi-conscious, dehydrated and severely hypoglycaemic or, just for fun it seemed sometimes, in an acidotic, vomiting hyperglycaemic state! The consultants, both in our local hospital and at Great Ormond Street Hospital, had never seen anything quite like it. He has the ability, though no one ever knows why, to actually go seriously 'hypo' when actually on a dextrose infusion with very limited insulin. On one occasion he was given a large 50% IV dextrose bolus by our GP in order to get him conscious enough to be transported by ambulance to the hospital. Within half an hour he again had a blood sugar of less than 2 mmol.

Many times in these early years comment was passed that it was very 'lucky' that I was a nurse and so could cope with all these events. It may well have helped to manage him clinically, but trying to use any level of professional detachment in an emergency involving your own child is of course nigh on impossible. Also, of course, I knew only too well what all these catastrophic events were doing to his brain cells, his overall chances of survival and certainly to the frayed nerves of our entire family. My daughter went through stages of coming home as an 8- to 10-year-old, never knowing if we would be there or yet again hanging on for dear life in the hospital. This strain takes an enormous toll on a family and perhaps knowing what might be still to come is no comfort whatsoever.

THE MIDDLE YEARS

Jamie's life so far has almost been divided into neat sections, the early years, the middle section where we settled down and just 'got on' with life, and then his teenage years and the journey into the wonderful world of 'transition'!

So, in many ways these middle years were a time of stability, acceptance and many fond memories. It's a stage that many families are lucky enough to experience, though sadly many others go straight from diagnosis, lurch through crisis followed by crisis until they find themselves in an end-of-life phase.

He was very settled in his special school, had friends with a wide variety of levels of ability and learnt to successfully manage an electric wheelchair, to develop a love of singing (very badly!) and a wicked sense of humour that has stood him in good stead over many years. He attended specialist respite play-schemes with other children and spent many happy days and nights at our local children's hospice – where, he says, he would now live full-time given the opportunity.

We would not have managed all this long without the hospice; the understanding, support and regular respite care that has been the crutch for our lives over the last 14 years. It is a typical and ironic fact that children as complex and 'demanding' as Jamie have very few choices in life as their care is deemed just 'too difficult' to manage. Such are his care needs (*see* Part B) that mainstream services just are not geared up to make daily clinical decisions. It is a constant source of amazement to me that following all the recent years of technology-dependent children and complex health children that although parents are constantly taking on new and much extended roles, the services that look after our children are so far behind in their own development.

The need for highly specialised care for such children has been discussed at national level for many years and I have been party to many of these reviews and conversations, but we still have children too ill or just too complex to manage. My plea here is that it's *not* our children who are too complex, it is instead, the systems, the processes and hoops that we have to negotiate, that are far, far too complex and slow to act. Joined-up, holistic, integrated, child-centred care is something I have been working to promote for several years now, whilst my own son is an example of just the very children and young people that we are unable to support outside the very specialist world of children's palliative care teams or children's hospices.

When Jamie was about eight years old we had a pivotal meeting with the neurologist who cared for him, to discuss future plans. We had become increasingly concerned about the uncertainly surrounding Jamie by this stage as he had obviously 'plateaued' for some time but was now showing signs of further changes, such as the slowing, and sometimes slurring, of his speech and an increasing tiredness and intermittent lack of strength. We decided to have this meeting whilst he was still in reasonable health and I am eternally glad that we did this at a time when we could plan and reflect on what we wanted for him, not at a time of crisis or under any sense of pressure. We discussed a range of interventions that we did or did not want to happen and also for the first time what might be the most likely events that could lead up to his death. Obviously this would not be every parent's choice, but for me, it was just what I needed. I had been worrying about all sorts of things that were put to rest. For example, I had been fretting considerably about whether we would be pushed into Jamie having a gastrostomy, or his being resuscitated at all costs, and also too about the possibility of a post mortem (PM). I had feared that as he was essentially still undiagnosed that he would routinely need a PM and this really worried me as I did not want him to have to go through this procedure on top of all he had faced when alive.

I am now so glad that I had the confidence to ask for this meeting and that my request was met so promptly and with such sensitivity as obviously many of my fears were unfounded. (I had been worrying quietly for quite some time.) I am now a fervent supporter of encouraging families to look at discussing 'End-of-Life Care' plans, to help them realise they do have a very important role to play in discussing their child's death, just as they do in caring for them when alive.

ACT produced a Family Companion to its Care Pathway[4] in May 2009 and this is a really useful resource to guide parents through the maze of services and to help them to plan in advance for their child's care including the end-of-life phase.

Jamie continued in his own inimitable way: his general health improved in that having grown out of childhood illnesses meant that he was less prone to endless admissions and as the level of care in the community increased then our reliance on the acute services lessened. Our close links with the team that cares for him did not lessen and I have always been grateful for an open door policy and for very regular appointments to keep on top of the myriad challenges we had to face.

Whilst it became slowly obvious to all around him, that Jamie was slowing down both physically and intellectually, he maintained a very happy outlook on life and has never ever questioned his lot in life, for which we are eternally grateful. This has helped us all immeasurably and I have been only too aware over the years of discussions that other friends have had to endure with their children, about their illness, disability and worst of all, their prognosis. The escape from this harsh reality has been a blessing that we are only too aware of.

Whilst becoming very obviously much slower and often very tired, Jamie still continues at his special school nearly full-time. He has been able to benefit from regular, but not frequent, respite visits to the hospice and, when necessary, 'rest days from school', where he would miss school or go in late. But this is only made possible by the fact that my husband and I are self-employed and can often make ourselves available to be home with him. It is a testament to the skills of the school staff that he has never been aware that he is at best, standing still academically whilst his peers are forever moving on – albeit at a very slow pace. I am a great believer in making the very most of life and feel that a special school where there are many life-limited or life-threatened pupils is exactly what has made his life as 'normal' as possible. He has lost over eight peers that he has known well during his school life but has gained immeasurably by being in a community for whom this is, sadly, a regular occurrence. The ethos and atmosphere is one of celebration and achievement. Personally, I know how he would never have managed in mainstream provision being the only youngster facing such a catalogue of challenges.

THE TEENAGE YEARS

In many ways we have faced the universal challenges of parents of teenagers everywhere. Its really gratifying to see that even a very disabled youngster will fight the idea of getting up for school, will develop a passion for television soaps that are on after bedtime and decide his parents are boring, bossy and embarrassing! Those reading this with disabled children will understand how much we parents celebrate the normal, the everyday and love to see any spark of challenge or resistance from our youngsters as that is what we have always expected from their siblings. Sad, quiet, passive compliance is far harder to endure.

Jamie put on huge amounts of weight as a young teenager; he had slowed down to the point that it took all his energy to try to pull himself up onto a low sofa and he had stopped crawling or attempting anything too physical. This, coupled with his appallingly wild diabetic control, meant that his weight ballooned and he looked very Cushingoid for a couple of years. He went through a very sad patch of seeming to be quite depressed and angry. He was probably beginning to gain an awareness of this tiredness and general deterioration; however, it was so insidious that it was often hard to measure but was always there at the back of my mind. At this stage he seemed most upset about his inability to read and write like his close friends – many of his best friends at school had muscular dystrophy, so although they shared many experiences and great trips to the hospice together he was gradually getting left behind intellectually and was probably aware of this, in his own way.

The school responded very proactively with the arrival of a new head teacher and the year group was split into two groups: one following the national curriculum, and the other, Jamie's group, which concentrated on a much more holistic, independence-based curriculum. I mention this because this decision had far-reaching, very positive outcomes for several of the young people in the class. I believe that this demonstrates very well that we must not forget that even the most profoundly disabled young people can be aware of their changing health and whilst not understanding the implications they too can suffer the same lack of confidence as that experienced by other teenagers.

Matters started to become more unsettled, and much more worrying, when Jamie was about 14. Alongside his slow deterioration there were several other things going on that were to cause concern amongst the medical professionals involved in his care.

It was noticed that he had an enlarged optic disc on one side and some neurological examinations were providing cause for concern. The most dramatic and frightening, though, was a seemingly sudden weight loss that went on for months and which at its peak meant that Jamie was losing up to 4 kilos per week. He was seen by the dieticians but a detailed food diary proved his intake was quite sufficient. He started to show obvious muscle loss when seen undressed.

It was this change that really has proved one of the hardest things to cope with. When dressed in typical baggy teenage sweat shirts, etc., he still looked himself and so many people tried to tell me at first that it was 'just a growth spurt' or 'it's a teenage thing, they change now you know'. What I was actually seeking was someone who could see what I saw and could validate my concerns. It took really quite some time to get others to see what I thought was so obvious. You know all the contours of your own child's body when you have washed and dressed it every day for 14 years and actually it was not false reassurance that I needed. In the end it was care staff at school and the outreach respite nurses who were the ones to pluck up courage to talk to me about this – everyone seemed to want to allay my fears, but sometimes that is just not what a parent needs.

In time Jamie was obviously showing signs of gross muscle wasting and I was told he would have an 'urgent' MRI scan. Thereby hangs a tale. As a professional you will know what an urgent scan means, but to a worried parent 'urgent' means very, very soon. When I am training practitioners who work with disabled children I always ask them, now how long do they think this would take, then to think again as a parent — are the times the same?

I did not go out for a couple of days whilst waiting for the phone call to come, then I rushed out and rushed back for a week to check the phone and post every day. In the end I was so worried that I called the diabetic outreach nurse. She got back to me straight away. Urgent was, of course, in about for to six weeks at best as he needed an anaesthetic, it was an 'emergency' scan that was the really fast one. Even as an ex-nurse, so supposedly able to speak the jargon, I still did not understand when it was my own child who was ill.

The scan proved that Jamie's cerebellum had become very atrophied since his first scan at age three. Worrying – but in reality no further forward.

He continued to actually just waste away and was beginning to look drawn and very tired, but was still his old self regardless of what worry he was causing us all. I then asked his consultant at this time what we could expect. We had had so many years expecting Jamie to leave us, and then had settled down to just enjoying his life and now once again everything was looking very stark.

We agreed that there was no way he could keep losing weight at this rate and that it would be a matter of wait and see, but obviously unless he settled again he would not be likely to survive more than a year at best. We then discussed what plans we wanted to make and I really knew that I needed everything all sorted now, and that I was in no fit state to just wait and see. I also had huge concerns about losing Jamie before we ever had a diagnosis to help us know what the future held for any possible grandchildren and I really needed to feel some sense of control over all this.

We had a very good meeting, if there ever can be such a thing, to discuss an end-of-life plan. This meeting was everything such an event should be – the people involved were the ones I wanted, the venue and timings, etc. were all agreed with me and my respite coordinator took on the role of key worker – never in my life have I needed one more. Everything was planned out including responses and actions expected from the ambulance trust, etc., and everyone we could think of has a copy. It was so much better to go through this when Jamie was not in crisis and when we had time to slowly absorb so many emotions.

Needless to say, in true Jamie spirit he decided to defy us all! His weight loss stopped a few months after this meeting and he is still happily plodding on nearly two and half years later! He certainly does have many, many problems including severe and quickly increasing scoliosis, but his quality of life is great and he is very happy being a typical teenager!

There is only one problem – we have had no real transition plan in place. He just was not expected to make it this far and there is nowhere within the whole county that could care for him to the same level of nursing that he has been used to at home and at the hospice all these years. And as a family we feel that, after 18 challenging and restrictive years, we deserve the opportunity to have something of the normal life enjoyed by others.

He wants to leave school as soon as he turns 18, he also wants to leave home and live at the hospice. They have a huge TV, a jacuzzi bath, he does not have to attend school and they give him breakfast in bed – what more can you want!

We have managed after a long, protracted and admittedly fraught time to finally secure his continuing care funding into adult services, but he is forging a new path here and it has become very obvious that the system is just not ready for the challenges that young people like Jamie have to offer. There is no one in post yet to co-ordinate this transition and he seems to be just too complicated and too expensive for 'mainstream' disability services to cope with.

We are going to manage, and indeed flourish, given time, because of the special and hugely appreciated efforts of one or two local champions. However, I know we are very lucky with the team we have supporting us – so many families are left high and dry at this crucial time.

This may seem a harsh indictment of the system that has helped us so much over so long, but it is the hard, inarguable reality. However, I now have an active part in trying to change things for the better because, as a Parent Trustee of ACT, I am a member of the national group that has oversight of the first ever and much-awaited Children's Palliative Care Strategy.

Until provision matches the newly extended life spans of many of 'our' young people, what exactly are they going to transition to? We have found the perfect place for Jamie in a neighbouring county, but it's a much needed, heavily over-subscribed, very expensive specialist service, and is only for three years, so what then . . .?

REFERENCES

1 www.ucl.ac.uk/neuromuscular/publications/rahmanpublications
2 www.act.org.uk
3 Elston S. *Integrated Multi-agency Care Pathways for Children with Life-threatening and Life-limiting Conditions*. Bristol: ACT; 2004. Available at: www.act.org.uk/ (accessed 17 February 2010).
4 ACT. *A Family Companion to the ACT Care Pathway for Children with Life-limiting and Life-threatening Conditions*. Bristol: ACT; 2009.

Part 2: Jamie's continuing care domains

Anna Gill

CHALLENGING BEHAVIOUR

Jamie does not exhibit any manifestations of challenging behaviour outside the family home. At home he is becoming increasingly resistant to parental control and is very aware of his inability to control any aspect of his life – his dependence on adults is of a level that ensures he is physically totally dependent and becoming increasingly aware of his limitations, failing strength and lack of control, i.e. bedtimes/getting up/bathing, etc. He is happier and much more compliant with care staff that he knows.

He was exhibiting signs of depression in 2004 when his deteriorating health and resultant skill loss at school was very evident against his peers. The introduction of a new curriculum and effective peer grouping has increased his self-confidence.

COMMUNICATION

Jamie has indistinct speech that is difficult to understand and uses symbols at school to aid his understanding. He is unable to read or write but will persist with his verbal requests if encouraged with sensitivity. He becomes very frustrated if carers do not understand, and if they make assumptions or ignore what he is trying to say. He lacks confidence in making strangers understand him so is very reluctant to alert carers to any medical needs unless staff are well known to him or he associates them with being able to help him, such as the school nurse, who he knows well. For example, if in pain or feeling hypoglycaemic, he does not speak out and thereby places himself at considerable risk in unknown situations.

MOBILITY

Jamie is totally dependent on carers for all his physical needs. He can, when well, move himself on a sheepskin and lie against a beanbag, but has severe ataxia, especially when not well-supported. He is unable to weight bear and no longer has sufficient strength in his upper body to assist in transfers from chair to bed, etc. He needs hoisting with a sling and two staff members for all transfers. He has considerable loss of feeling in his extremities and is totally unaware of keeping himself from inappropriate positioning. He needs assistance and encouragement to change position, which he finds difficult due to extensive muscle loss and wasting. He has regular pain in his shoulder girdle, neck and spine due to crush fractures as a result of osteopenia and resultant osteoporosis. His scoliosis (spinal curvature) is severe and is increasing, which is compromising his sitting position, posture, and more recently his chest capacity.

NUTRITION, FOOD AND DRINK

Jamie is able to finger feed appropriate food but needs feeding at all other times as he is unable to sustain sufficient energy whilst feeding himself to take in sufficient nutrition. He lost approximately 25% of his body weight and mass in the last few years but has continued to grow. He is considerably taller but his body weight remains the same as two years ago. The paediatric dietician reviews his diet and his intake is deemed sufficient although he is showing signs of compromised absorption, with severe intractable diarrhoea if not treated daily. He has had intermittent and increasing episodes of dysphagia and has his feeding regime carefully monitored. He requires a straw to enable him to control liquid intake and has to have his diet carefully monitored to reduce choking. He suffers from reflux and on occasions this causes some erosion and damage to his oesophagus and trachea, causing further dysphagia and associated pain with coughing and swallowing. This is treated palliatively with losec and he sleeps in an electric bed with the head end raised to reduce bile reflux. He is totally unaware of the need to avoid sweet food and has no understanding of the dietary implications of his diabetes. The possible future need for a gastrostomy has been discussed, but we are keen to enable Jamie to continue eating as long as possible as it's one of his main pleasures and central to his social life.

CONTINENCE AND ELIMINATION

Jamie is doubly incontinent and wears pads. He has consistently high sugar levels in his urine and as a result suffers from very frequent perineal candidiasis (thrush) that needs oral and local treatment. His stools are very loose and he needs daily varying doses of imodium to try and control this; if unsuccessful his perineal skin breaks down very easily. Care needs to be taken not to induce bowel obstruction, however, as the treatment has very variable responses due to his poor absorption control. He cannot therefore be on a standing order for dosage; it needs to be calibrated on a daily basis.

SKIN AND TISSUE VIABILITY

Jamie has had profound and prolonged muscle wasting and almost total loss of body fat. He has extensive deformities in both his feet, which result in the anklebones being particularly vulnerable. He has some paraesthesia (loss of feeling) in all extremities but these are difficult to measure due to his learning difficulties. All his bony protuberances are vulnerable to reddening and pressure after a very short time. For example, his spine becomes very red and stays so for some while after only five minutes of lying on the floor when changing, if not suitably padded. He needs considerable careful monitoring of his feet due to the deformities, lack of sensation and his poorly controlled diabetes. Once any small wound does appear, on any extremity, Jamie has a slow healing time and becomes very distressed by any injury he can see, however small. For example, he went swimming recently and because of dragging his feet on the bottom of the pool he ended up with 2 cm long friction burns on each foot that caused blisters and skin loss, but he was totally unaware of the injuries till he saw them and until the blisters became raw. It is only due to very diligent monitoring and care that he has not suffered pressure sores on a regular basis. He sleeps on a low-air-loss mattress on an electric bed.

BREATHING

Currently Jamie has no difficulty with breathing. He gets regular coughs and some occasional chest infections but they do not threaten his health at present.

DRUG THERAPY AND MEDICINES

Jamie has many different medications. However, the main challenges and concerns all centre on his uncontrolled diabetes and its interaction with his epilepsy. He has had this since age 3 but it has never been controllable to 'normal' standards. He needs his blood tested five to six times a day and during the night. All his doses of insulin are then calibrated against his blood sugar, food intake and general health. It is not possible to have rigid standing orders as his health is too varied, the absorption of food uncontrollable and the effects of the insulin doses are not standard but vary daily. He frequenting becomes ketotic and this is usually after fasting overnight or if ill. He has separate care plans as for hypoglycaemia and hyperglycaemia, for keto-acidosis and for in the event of a hypo and resultant epileptic fit.

If Jamie is ketotic and nauseated he will refuse any food, so his morning insulin has to be omitted until his food intake is sufficient to sustain the insulin dose without causing loss of consciousness. If he is nauseated in this fashion then IV fluids may be needed to combat keto-acidosis. When unwell Jamie is reluctant to eat, so Hypo-Stop gel or IM glucagon may be needed. If vomiting for any reason he needs immediate IV fluids to maintain stability. If he becomes hypo and his blood sugar does not respond to food, Hypo-Stop or IM glucagon he may continue to have a prolonged hypo attack during which he usually loses consciousness and then tends to vomit and fit at the same time. Airway integrity is compromised and he needs immediate experienced medical intervention. This has happened twice in recent years, both times treated by his mother who is a trained nurse.

All nursing staff who care for Jamie have open access to the Assessment Unit at the local hospital and have access to a consultant paediatrician for advice re treatment and drug doses, etc. Jamie has a detailed care plan for emergency and end-of-life care and this is shared with the school, hospice, community team, acute teams and the ambulance service. There are clear directions for non-resuscitation signed by the family and paediatrician.

Jamie is prescribed drugs to control his epilepsy and any previous attempts to wean him off have been unsuccessful. If he is ill and not taking oral medications then care needs to be taken to ensure he does not have a seizure.

Jamie is unaware of his epilepsy, is compliant taking his medications including his injections but is totally unable to take them himself, understand their implications or take any responsibility for them. He is aware at times of being ill, but his condition usually deteriorates so quickly he is losing consciousness before he becomes aware or afraid of what is happening. He does not usually recognise his fluctuating blood sugars and can be at considerable risk of harm if not carefully monitored at all times by someone able to assess, interpret his rapidly changing condition and its ramifications, and intervene appropriately and promptly. To date this has always been carried out by a qualified nurse in all settings, including at home.

PSYCHOLOGICAL AND EMOTIONAL

Jamie, as mentioned above, has low self-esteem and has little confidence in his ability to communicate. He often has to miss time at school due to his deteriorating health and has an absence rate of approximately 25–30%. He is happy being cared for by a range of carers but becomes stressed with too many changes at any one time. He is very friendly and outgoing and is now frequently expressing an interest in leaving home, although the only place he identifies for this is the hospice at Quidenham. He would like to live there, but we have not discussed the topic of leaving home with him yet. He becomes obsessed and frets about changes, choices and above all, the unknown. He has no understanding of his illness or prognosis and this has *not* been discussed with him, in agreement with the hospice and all involved in his care.

SEIZURES

Jamie has petit mal seizures on a daily basis but only usually has grand mal and loss of consciousness with severe hypoglycaemias, as described above. He has a separate care plan for this.

OTHER CARE NEEDS

A consultant ophthalmologist has monitored Jamie annually as he was blind until approximately four months old and has been exhibiting further eye changes that are currently being investigated. He also now requires glasses but his compliance will be questionable.

His continuing neurodevelopmental regression means that he is not able to maintain the same academic levels at school, but with considerable careful planning Jamie is less aware of this. He is though, gradually becoming much weaker and is often tired and frustrated by this.

He has trismus (uncontrollable grating of the teeth) after drinking and after brushing. Due to the reflux he has considerable loss of enamel on his lower molars and has regular specialist dental care for this, and uses Difflam spray for pain when required.

Jamie is under investigation at Great Ormond Street/Queen's Square for his assumed mitochondrial cytopathy and for possible current or future cardiac involvement.

ACT
*Young life
matters*

ACT Integrated Palliative Care Pathways Standards: Parent Service Assessment Tool

This assessment tool is based on the ACT: *Integrated Multi-agency Care Pathways* and aims to identify the aspects of best practice within a local area.
The stages of the assessment are:

- Stage One – Using this tool, assess service provision against whether the standards & goals were achieved;
- Stage Two – Local areas to review the findings and produce and implement an action plan aimed at achieving best practice;
- Stage Three – Local areas to review achievement towards best practice;
- Stage Four – Local areas to disseminate improvements and or review action plan.

This assessment tool provides local areas with a process of considering the experiences of families in relation to current practice and services received and will enable the identification of good practice and areas of practice which need further development.

As a parent you may find services mentioned have not been offered, but would be helpful. In this case please ask your local service provider for a contact person to discuss this with.

The Goals and Standards listed below correlate to those in ACT's *Integrated Multi-Agency Care Pathway*.
For more information contact ACT on 0117 922 1566 or visit the ACT website at www.act.org.uk

Goal	Goal & Standards	Were these goals & standards achieved?				
		Yes	No	Not applicable	Don't know	Comments
• **Breaking News**	*Every family should receive the disclosure of their child's prognosis in a face-to-face discussion in privacy & should be treated with respect, honesty & sensitivity. Information should be provided both for the child & family in language that they can understand*					
A1	Was your child's diagnosis shared with you during face to face discussion?	x				Have had several points of diagnosis but
A2	Was the news shared with you in a private setting?	x				always well handled and
A3	Was the news given to you with a relative/friend to support?	x				support given
A4	Was useful written material provided to you?		x			
A5	Was an interpreter offered, if you needed one?			x		
A6	Was appropriate information available for your child/ren?			x		

FIGURE 9.1 ACT integrated palliative care pathways standards: parent service assessment tool

Goal	Goal & Standards	Were these goals & standards achieved?				
		Yes	No	Not applicable	Don't know	Comments
• Discharge home	*Every child & family diagnosed in the hospital setting, should have an agreed transfer plan involving the hospital, community services & the family, & should be provided with the resources they require before leaving hospital.*					
B1	Did/Do you have a key worker?		x			Needed a key worker many times especially in early years
B2	Was your GP informed?	x				
B3	Were community services informed e.g. health visitor; community nurse?	x				
B4	Was a community children's nursing service available.	x				
B6	Were you involved in your child's discharge plan?			x		
B6	Was your child's discharge planned early?			x		
B7	Were home visits arranged pre discharge?			x		
B8	Was shared medical care between the lead centre and your local service planned?	x				
B9	Did you receive the equipment you needed to care for your child?	x				
B10	Were your transport needs addressed?		x			
B11	Were you/carers trained before transfer?			x		
B12	Were clear communication lines agreed with you?	x				
B13	Were you provided with a 24 hr contact number?		x			
B14	Was a Keyworker identified before discharge home?		x			
• Assessment	*Every family should receive a multi-agency assessment of their needs ASAP after diagnosis or recognition, and should have their needs reviewed at appropriate intervals*	Yes	No	Not applicable	Don't know	Comments
C1	Were your child & family's needs assessed ASAP following diagnosis?	x				
C2	Were assessments coordinated across services?	x				
C3	Were you fully involved in assessments?	x				
C4	Was your Child kept central to and included in the process?	x				
C5	Did the assessment include all of your family?	x				
C6	Did the assessment recognise and respect your child's individuality?	x				
C7	Were your transport needs considered?		x			
C8	Was information gathered and recorded systematically?	x				
C9	Was non-jargon language used?	x				
C10	Did the process address confidentiality and consent?	x				
C11	Were you given a copy of the assessment information?	x				
C12	Was the key worker's role clear to you?			x		Never offered a key worker

FIGURE 9.1 ACT integrated palliative care pathways standards: parent service assessment tool (continued)

Goal	Goal & Standards	Were these goals & standards achieved?				
		Yes	No	Not applicable	Don't know	Comments
• Care Plan	*Every child & family should have a multi-agency care plan agreed with them for the delivery of co-ordinated care & support to meet their individual needs. A keyworker to assist with this should be identified and agreed with the family.*					
D1	Was a Keyworker identified?		x			
D2	Was the Care Plan available to you and you child?	x				
D3	Does the Care Plans include the whole family?	x				
D4	Was Symptom Management, Nursing Care & Personal Care planned for?	x				
D5	Was psychological care available for your whole family?	x				
D6	Was benefits advice/financial information given to you?	x				
D7	Were flexible short breaks available for your child?	x				
D8	Was social care and support available?	x				As he was not expected to survive
D9	Were there opportunities for play/social activities?	x				
D10	Was your child's education fully supported?	x				
D11	Did the Care Plan address your health issues?	x				
D12	Was a Community Children's Nurse been allocated to your child?	x				Transition was not really
D13	Were aids/equipment available for home and school?	x				addressed till
D14	Did the Care Plan address transition to adult services?		x			very late on but
D15	Were there regular updated reviews?	x				this was a
D16	Were you able to request reviews?	x				mutual decision
• End of Life	*Every child & family should be helped to decide on an end of life plan and should be provided with care & support to achieve this as closely as possible*	Yes	No	Not applicable	Don't know	Comments
E1	Do you have an End of Life Plan?	x				
E2	Are your professionals open & honest in discussing the end of life?	x				Really good
E3	Are resuscitation plans agreed, written up & communicated appropriately?	x				support in end of life care
E4	Do you have access to 24hr symptom control?	x				planning and on

FIGURE 9.1 ACT integrated palliative care pathways standards: parent service assessment tool (continued)

						going support
E5	Are symptom control staff suitably qualified & experienced?				x	
E6	Is emotional/spiritual support available?				x	
E7	Are your choices able to be supported with resources?				x	
E8	Have you and your child & family given a choice in the place of care?				x	

Thank you for completing the assessment this far. The questions on the next page relate to goals and standards for bereaved families and will not be applicable to all.

The following questions relate to care and services provided for bereaved families and will therefore not be applicable to all. If you have experienced the death of your child, and feel able to complete this section, we would be very grateful for your comments. However, we understand that it may be too painful to comment on your experience and you may prefer to leave this section blank.

Goal	Standards	Were these goals & standards achieved?				
		Yes	No	Not applicable	Don't know	Comments
• After Death						
F1	Were you and your family given time & privacy with your child after death?					
F2	Were you in control & supported in making choices?					
F3	Was practical advice & written information available?					
F4	Were the needs of your other children & grandparents considered?					
F5	Was fully informed consent given for post mortem examinations?					
F6	Were professional contacts informed about the death of your child?					
F7	Was bereavement support available for as long as needed?					
F8	Were your other children's bereavement needs supported?					

Your Name:
Anna Gill

Thank you.

ACT is the only organisation working across the UK to achieve a better quality of life and care for every life-limited child and their family.
ACT, Orchard House, Orchard Lane, Bristol BS1 5DT. Telephone: 0117 922 1556 Fax: 0117 930 4707 Email: info@act.org.uk
Registered Charity No: 1075541 Company Registration No 3734710
ACT Integrated Palliative Care Pathways Standards: Parent Service assessment Tool, © ACT (Association for Children's Palliative Care), August 2007.

FIGURE 9.1 ACT integrated palliative care pathways standards: parent service assessment tool (continued)

Part 3: Commentary on the parent's story: the key to integrating services

Peter Limbrick

There are certainly medical experts who can talk with authority about their specialism and offer expert advice about treatment. There are no experts when it comes to supporting families in their life with a disabled child because children and their families are unique, and Jamie's life is a path that will only ever be trodden by one person – Jamie. What I can do, as a non-expert, is make some comment on this chapter in terms of my experience of other children and families and of the services in the UK that support them or fail them.

My own path, as a worker in the disability field, began in the 1960s when there were far fewer children needing multiple interventions – either because they did not survive birth or because they were decanted into institutions as infants. Families, nurseries and schools simply did not have to meet the challenges they would have brought. Jamie's mother comments that '. . . the services that look after our children are so far behind in their development'. This is my experience too. Of course there are some exemplary services in the UK, but they exist as bits of colour in a grey patchwork and too often their valued support comes to an end at one of the major transitions; hospital discharge, into school, between schools or into adult services. What Jamie and other children should be able to expect is a seamless service that begins as soon as concerns are raised, is child- and family-centred, is a well coordinated collective effort between all agencies involved, is led by actual needs, and continues into adulthood. This is my vision but we are a million miles short of it.

Jamie's mother makes the profound observation that 'it's not our children who are too complex, it is the systems . . . we have to negotiate that are far, far too complex . . .' Though a child can have a range of conditions leading to a multiplicity of needs, a baby is just a baby and a child is just a child for all that – and baby and child should be welcomed and celebrated.

So where does the problematic complexity come from? In Jamie's case one level of complexity came directly from his evolving medical conditions and the treatments for them. I have known babies of a few months go home from the neonatal intensive care ward or special care baby unit (SCBU) with a list of medications as long as your arm – and with the requirement on the parent to follow intricate regimes, to observe the baby very carefully for unusual responses and to exercise fine judgements about when to vary a particular dose, offer some emergency procedure or call for help. I do not see any prospect of simplifying complicated treatments but I do see a need to offer parents ongoing support in this extremely demanding and potentially stressful role – both as a regular routine and as a rapid response to problems as they arise.

The other level of problematic complexity has, in my view, a historic cause and is remediable – in part if not in full. Children like Jamie, and their families, will be looking for support from very many practitioners from many separate services and agencies. The big ones in the UK are health services, education services and social services, and each of these has its own departments and sections. For the vast majority of children it is acceptable for each practitioner to do what they do more or less separately from the others, and services have largely been designed with these children in mind. But when Jamie or even 'Jenny' comes along with a growing number of other children who have a whole bunch of needs spanning all the agencies, then practitioners are severely challenged to start working together, to see themselves as part of a whole support system and to see Jamie as a whole child inside a whole family. Separate practitioners focusing on separate bits of Jamie or Jenny are almost certain to fail. Jamie invites us to learn the humbling lesson of collective competence; not one of us can go it alone with a child who has sensory needs, physical needs, learning needs, etc. We learn the art of collaborative teamwork or we risk being ineffectual.

But because of how our public services have evolved we find ourselves stuck with separate agencies with staff who speak separate professional languages, are trained separately and enjoy vastly differing working conditions and pay structures. Very, very few practitioners have any training in teamwork or in how to work with others and when they are in post they are hampered in joint working by outdated management systems and even incompatible software. Agency boundaries can be as meaningless to families as are national boundaries to migrating birds. The task then is to create structures for joining these agencies together around children like Jamie while acknowledging that they are likely to persist as separate organisations.

What would have helped Jamie and his family? His mother has given us the answer in her description of the meeting to discuss an end-of-life plan. This came in response to her need and gave her some sense of control. It was attended by the people she wanted, it happened at a time and in a place to suit the family and one of her practitioners, the respite coordinator, took the role of key worker. A joined-up plan was made for an agreed anticipated future. This is an example of support that is child- and family-centred, that is a well coordinated collective effort between all agencies involved, and that is led by actual needs. What a pity that this well organised joint working was so late in coming. The approach of giving the family a key worker within a collective system that creates successive multi-agency plans is the ideal and in my experience families need it from the very beginning.

Jamie's mother tells us that in the early days, when Jamie was three years old, there were 32 different practitioners and medical staff working with them but without the benefit of a key worker. So what do we know about key working and about what a key worker does? A UK charity called One Hundred Hours[1] provided a large part of the answer in its pioneering work in the 1990s in which it provided key worker-based child- and family support to new families who had neurologically impaired babies. The role of the key workers evolved in response to the needs of families and can be summarised as:

1 offering a listening ear and emotional support to parents
2 helping parents get information about their child's condition, strengths and needs
3 helping the parents get timely and relevant information about all available services that can help the child and the family
4 helping the family get relevant services
5 helping to join everything together which can be at two levels:
   ➤ coordinating appointments, meetings, assessments, etc. to reduce time wastage, travelling and stress on child and family
   ➤ helping to integrate separate discipline-specific programmes into a whole-child programme that recognises that vulnerable, young children do not come in separate bits
6 helping the parent to operate as an equal partner with practitioners.

Jamie's mother valued partnership working with the metabolic specialist in which she (the specialist) shared all the information she had. Professor Hilton Davis[2] tells us more about working in partnership and suggests that all practitioners from all the agencies should be trained to work in this way with families and older children. The approach is characterised by empathy, honesty, trust and respect, and should be an integral part of the seamless service, not just a rare treat for a family happening to meet a particular enlightened practitioner.

Let us assume, in our ideal service, that families like Jamie's or Jenny's have key workers and that those key workers are trained in partnership working. If the services offering support to the child and family are all choosing to work separately from each other (and perhaps even offering contradictory advice and interventions) then the key worker will be just as disempowered by the chaos as is the family. The constructive environment for key worker support is a local integrated pathway which must be created by senior managers in the separate agencies working together with Jamie and Jenny in mind. The integrated multi-agency pathway has been described by the author[3] and will take the child and family through the stages of:

1 meeting the new child and family – the meeting phase
2 learning about the child and family – the learning phase
3 planning how to support the child and family – the planning phase
4 supporting the child and family – the support phase
5 reviewing the support for the child and family – the review phase.

Despite being a collective effort by separate agencies, the integrated pathway appears seamless to the family. In the pathway, support is reviewed as often as necessary and a new plan is made. In this way Stage 5 continually loops back to Stage 3.

These multi-agency plans, which are typed and given to all involved, are a key part of the process. With an agreed plan everyone knows what is happening and what is expected of them. Ideally, for children who are born with some disability or possible disability, the first multi-agency plan will be written on discharge from the neonatal intensive care ward or SCBU. There will then be successive plans in early support leading up to a transition-into-school plan. Around the age of 14, school staff, parent and young person will work with practitioners in adult services to create a transition-out-of-school plan. For some children and young people the sequence will be interrupted by a multi-agency end-of-life plan as we saw with Jamie. (Although Jamie had other ideas!)

At whatever stage in the child's life, both the family and the key worker are supported by multi-agency plans, which carry agreement about what the needs are and about what interventions are going to be provided. It can be a large part of the key worker's role to chase people up to make sure everyone is doing what they should be doing at the time they should be doing it.[4] At the risk of stating the obvious, and with the plan for Jamie's transition out of school firmly in mind, if some of the main elements of needed support are of poor quality or entirely missing, then no amount of joint working and no efforts of even the most committed key worker are going to put it right. Multi-agency planning has no magic formula for turning sows' ears into silk purses!

Being a parent of a child who needs ongoing multiple interventions can be exhausting and stressful with, of course, times of joy and celebration. Jamie's mother is not alone in feeling she had to put her own life on hold. No one can take this tremendous challenge from a family and any practitioner who tries risks burning herself out very quickly and depriving the family of its opportunity to respond and grow. But the key worker can take some of the load at particular times, can show the parent they are not alone in their struggle, and can help the family gather the resources they need to face the future.

In my work in all parts of the UK, I have encountered many exemplary services offering wonderful support to particular children at particular stages in their lives. We have all the good models we need. We know what helps children like Jamie and their families and we know full well how to do it. What we have not yet done is join it all together so that effective support is available to every child like Jamie in all parts of the country, so that it continues from the very beginning for as long as necessary.

N.I.C.E. analysis

Needs
- A key worker for all families who need and want one.
- Recognition and acknowledgement at all levels that many young people (YP) with life-limiting conditions are surviving much longer.
- Development of a workforce able and confident to deal with such YP in all settings, not just specialised ones.
- A rapid and imaginative response to provide such YP with places to live, work if able and fully participate in society with their peers.

Interests
- There is an increasing awareness of the need for key workers beyond just the Early Years settings.
- Interest in transition challenges for all YP with disabilities is increasing and finally becoming a political issue.
- Parents and YP themselves are now more than ever at the forefront of emerging Policy and Practise.
- Emerging knowledge about metabolic diseases such as mitochondrial disease.

Concerns

- Key workers are deemed too costly, too difficult to provide.
- Multi-agency true 'Partnership Working' is deemed too challenging or too demanding.
- YP with such complex care needs are deemed just too difficult, too expensive to provide holistic services for and are not being allowed a fulfilling experience of adult life – however short that life might prove to be.
- There is too much 'drift' in this area. There has been much talk about YP living longer but services are not keeping pace.

Expectations

- All YP should have a multi-agency team working with them and their family to provide an integrated pathway that reflects their needs, not based on what services have to offer.
- A seamless service is not too much to expect – survival into transition should not be a burden.
- Families should be able to feel fully involved in their child's care, in all aspects of planning and should be treated by all as true partners.
- With recent England-wide initiatives families should be able to expect an improvement in children's palliative care services.

From the above analysis please reflect on:

- How can your service/your work ensure that a longer life remains a meaningful life?
- What barriers do young people with a life-limiting or life-threatening illness face over and above their peers, and what can you do to overcome those barriers?
- How does your service/your work truly reflect the opinions of the child or young person and their family?

Action plan: next steps

Highly supported, independent living should be a reality not a dream – that is what we should all be planning for our young people who have palliative care needs and who have survived into young adulthood. Just keeping our children alive is *not* enough.

REFERENCES AND FURTHER READING

1 Limbrick-Spencer G. *The Keyworker: a practical guide.* Birmingham: Handsel Trust with WordWorks; 2001.
2 Davis H, Day C, Bidmead C. *Working in Partnership with Parents: the parent adviser model.* London: Harcourt Assessment; 2002.
3 Limbrick P. *An Integrated Pathway for Assessment and Support – for children with complex needs and their families.* Worcester: Interconnections; 2003.
4 Limbrick P. *Early Support for Children with Complex Needs and their Families: team around the child and the multi-agency keyworker.* Worcester: Interconnections; 2004.

10

Part 1: A child's life path

Gordon Martell

STANDING IN THE CENTRE OF THE PATH: A CULTURE OF AMBIVALENCE AND POLICY ABSENCE

'Standing in the centre of the path' evokes competing images. One may perceive the act as pondering beauty or a pleasant pause. Standing in the centre of the path could just as easily be perceived to be exhaustion or pondering how to overcome an obstacle. The only way to discern which perception is accurate is to listen to the traveller's story. The story of my pause in the path considers not only the path and my journey as a father of a child living with a life-limiting condition, but also the societal and policy context. The journey will be familiar to many who struggle each day with the miracle of a child that has survived against insurmountable odds only to gain entry into a unique membership that has as its privilege a continued struggle for basic supports that most enjoy as the spoils of a democratic victory.

I can describe the context of the pause but you have to understand the lens of my worldview to fully appreciate that context. I am an Indigenous Canadian from the Waterhen Lake First Nation in the Western Canadian province of Saskatchewan. My Indigenous community is a Cree community that was established in the early 1900s as a federal government invention to compartmentalise Indigenous peoples and gain access to the land. I identify with the international Indigenous experiences of colonisation and marginalisation. My identity is continually reinforced by the ever present struggle over the definition of Indigenous rights played out in Canada. The Canadian Constitution recognises Indigenous and Treaty Rights. This fact has resulted in many Canadian Court decisions favourable to Indigenous rights. Unfortunately, most interpretation unfolds in the much less glamorous arena of daily interactions of Indigenous peoples with paternalistic government policies and negative public opinion. There exists a most troubling paradox of government maintaining control over Indigenous peoples while shirking responsibilities for Indigenous peoples as described in the Canadian Constitution and the terms of Treaty.

Public social policy, such as that which influences paediatric palliative care, is complicated by the clash of interpretations of Indigenous peoples and governments. The struggle associated with the control versus responsibility paradox casts interpretation in conflict. I cannot yield my Cree community worldview. My story is characterised by my status as an Indigenous person in Canada. My worldview contributes to my perspective that we are all autonomous beings influenced by the will of the Creator. The essence of my worldview is my belief in a sacred circle of life in which I participate but that I don't control. My journey, then, looks for a path through life that I can trust rather than one I feel compelled to exercise dominion over.

I struggle as Sarah's father with a society that values dominion over life through science as an appropriate response to health challenges. This is the antithesis of my belief in the beauty of life in its varied forms and my responsibility to honour that diversity. The dual challenges of being an Indigenous person in Canada are both the fight to maintain Indigenous and Treaty rights and the struggle to negotiate a contemporary Indigenous worldview amidst a society imbued with western interpretations. So the story begins.

'*Creator, I understand if you call my daughter home but if it is not to be, please give me the strength to care for her.*' This was the prayer that ran through my mind; my head pounding from lack of sleep. Leaving the neonatal intensive care unit in the middle of the night for a few precious hours of fitful sleep, I prayed that my daughter's path would be made easy, in whichever direction it proceeded. Ten years later I am now aware of the role of the potential in a continuum of care under the auspices of paediatric palliative policy and I wonder how these supports could have influenced the struggle to live a life-affirming experience amidst a context that sees only illness and cure.

SARAH'S STORY

There are two ways to introduce my daughter. One follows a pathological approach that attempts to deconstruct the child into neat piles of disease, deficit and genetic anomaly that represent an affront to the human ideal. I employ this metaphor for the Canadian response to children with life-limiting conditions. The second introduction looks at the whole child. This matter of introduction concentrates on the human being, which fosters recognition of the fullest humanity of the child. This is the holistic approach that, when used as a metaphor of care, provides a response that honours the humanity of the individual.

PATHOLOGY

The following pathological description of Sarah is filtered and softened by my interpretation as a parent and layperson. Still, the description rolls easily as I have either heard or recited the litany in medical and educational settings for 10 years.

Sarah was born at term with myelomeningocele (spina bifida) which was discovered via ultrasound four days prior to delivery. The ultrasound also identified a single kidney and hydrocephalus resulting from the myelomeningocele. Shortly after birth by caesarian section, it was discovered that Sarah had low haemoglobin and she received a blood transfusion. Two days later, Sarah was again transfused because of continued low haemoglobin. A vigilant neonatal unit nurse discovered that Sarah had colobomas in both eyes which render her legally blind. Sarah's heart has a malformed valve causing aortic backflow.

The anaemia became chronic and Sarah underwent a bone marrow aspiration. This revealed an anaemia suspected to be Diamond Blackfan. This is an aplastic anaemia that does not support the generation of red blood cells. Sarah survives on monthly transfusions and, as a result, she is chelated with desferrioxamine to avoid iron overload in her organs. Iron was typically measured annually with a liver biopsy but is now measured through MRI technology. The difficulty of undergoing testing with the presence of transfused blood has not resulted in a definitive diagnosis. Diamond Blackfan patients sometimes respond to steroid therapies. Sarah has been unresponsive to prednisone and other steroid treatments.

Prognosis ranges widely based on the range of complications associated with Diamond Blackfan. Patients typically succumb to complications related to iron overload or blood-borne infections resulting from intravenous chelation. It was determined that Sarah is not a good candidate for a bone marrow transplant with an estimated 5% chance of survival. Remission is possible but not likely.

HUMANITY

This description of Sarah is generated by a loving parent but it is more than commentary that accompanies a beaming tour through a family photo album. The holistic introduction of Sarah holds vital information that could influence both the perception of Sarah and the manner in which societal supports are actualised. This description is what we hope to sustain and we require supports to achieve this goal.

Sarah is characterised by a remarkable tenacity that allows her to mobilise her skills and abilities not only to meet daily needs but also to excel in certain areas such as art, singing and reading; and she has an acute sense of humour and an outstanding ability to foster human relationships. Sarah is highly adaptable and easily navigates able-bodied environments with minimal support. She has an innocence which manifests as an absolute trust in those with whom she interacts. She also has a deep sense of gratitude that characterises her response to family and caregivers. Physical limitations never render Sarah helpless. As she accepts her mobility as her normal, so, too, do those around her. Sarah builds bridges and exemplifies acceptance. These qualities draw care and support to her and join those around her closer together and closer, ultimately, to Sarah.

I often carve out my role as Sarah's father as mediating these dichotomous descriptions. Mediation is necessary because without it the experience of a child with a life-limiting condition is bound to unfold in the clinic rather than the home. I am thankful each day that the Creator's will sustained Sarah's presence in our family. I never considered, though, that my prayer for the ability to take care of her needed to consider the social and policy environment to the extent that it does.

The phenomenon that renders a child with a life-limiting condition less worthy of the social benefit than others is dismaying as it is out of step with the democratic and socially just Canadian experience. Where the introduction of mainstreaming in schools and the dismantling of an institutional response to varying levels of ability may have been forged in a social awakening, Canadians have drifted back to sleep and while not openly embracing a marginalising system, have rather, fallen into it. When the obviousness of systemic limitations is exposed, the effect of Canadian ideals should fill the void and extend into paediatric palliative care.

My role as Sarah's father is like any loving and concerned parent. I help her where I can, advocate for her where I must and worry for her a lot. As an Indigenous person, I have come to realise that I will usually experience an added layer of complexity. The shade of my lens on the world sees wholeness rather than fragmentation, it aims to work within a natural order rather than controlling the natural world and it recognises value in all that *form the circle* rather than valuing those who *sit atop the pyramid of success.* Add to my father's role and my Indigenous lens recognition that, considering paediatric palliative care, the Canadian policy cards are stacked against those in the most need of society's support, and being Sarah's dad comes with complex considerations.

A VIEW OF WELLNESS

I consider the international paediatric palliative care movement that has worked to entrench support for children living with a life-limiting condition into the continuum of wellness supports an issue of a *standard of care.* Consideration for a common standard of care for marginalised sectors of society is able to overcome the pitfalls that accompany difference, based on subtleties such as ability, ethnicity or income. The pursuit of a standard of care that purports to accompany each individual loses momentum in the translation from a universal standard to an adjusted standard commensurate with our collective vision of wellness.

Where the victory of a scientific–medical response is seen as the pinnacle of success in care for the unwell, those who live with jeopardised wellness are forced to participate in a cycle of pathology and cure. Simply, accepting illness as a normalised characteristic of a child is an affront to a society that values the act of overcoming illness. Where equitable access to resources for people of different races is obvious, few are willing to accept that the sick can be called normal next to the healthy.

Without possibility of cure, what is wellness? Achieving life characterised by dignity is perceived by some to be a fantastic pursuit. In a society characterised by almost hedonistic pursuits, survival is the best that can be afforded children living with life-limiting conditions. As a parent I am not angry at the lack of a cure, but I am confused by the lack of a response that extends a dignified life experience to all. I continually feel that expressing my concern in this manner sounds like complacency. The paediatric palliative care community resists that characterisation as it pursues the dignity aspect of the continuum of care.

An Indigenous perspective on wellness is characterised by the concept of the circle where each individual must be balanced in the mental, physical, spiritual and emotional part of their being. The community as a whole is also healthy in balance achieved through respect for the diversity of humanity. The value of one is the value of all. Failure to affirm the value of the unwell fails to affirm the value of society.

IMPEDIMENTS

The difficulty in overcoming the marginalisation of children living with life-limiting conditions is a result of a suppressed voice of children living with life-limiting conditions, the replication of marginalising contexts familiar to society and the perception of the need to maintain stratification in society. The victory that can be achieved through the achievement of a supportive context and common standard of care is a victory for the children and a victory for all. In undoing one of the last remaining vestiges of stratification, society can embrace its fullness. That is not to say that improvements in the context of paediatric palliative care is a magic fix for an otherwise utopian society, but that marginalised children are all of our children and their continued marginalisation defies what we collectively desire. Unintentional marginalisation sustains our least desirable qualities, while reducing this anomaly clearly celebrates who we aspire to be.

VOICE

The fact that becomes all too clear for a parent of a child living with a life-limiting illness is that prior to the arrival of our child, one's whole experience may have been within a context of privilege. What makes my perspective unique is that I have experienced the marginalisation of Indigenous peoples in Canada. When I interact with parents of children living with life-threatening illnesses, I find many parallels between the effects of marginalisation of Indigenous peoples and marginalisation of the children and families living with life-limiting conditions. The pursuit of a common standard of care for children living with a life-limiting condition should have been achieved through accomplishments for basic human rights. Children with a life-limiting condition often emerge from a context of privilege. There is often no history of marginalisation which means that there is also no *liberating* history. The voice of advocacy falls to associations of parents and healthcare providers. Communities of support are fragile voices for the voiceless as the need for advocacy is most often at times when advocates are least able to advocate because of new challenges and often grief. As a parent and an Indigenous person I identify an opportunity to offer insight from the perspective of my liberating history in hope that it contributes to enhancing voice for the voiceless.

MARGINALISATION SUSTAINED

Canada, like most societies born of colonial intrusion upon Indigenous territories, generates and maintains divisions. The replication of familiar subordinating contexts is a mode easily adopted. Like the root of many dominant-subordinate relationships, the experience of children living with a life-limiting condition is seen to consume an inordinate amount of resources. We know that slipping into a familiar reaction that resists unique considerations for some is an affront to our vision of equity but old habits of division are not easily purged. The pursuit of a common standard of care for children with life-limiting conditions, through advocacy for paediatric palliative care, needs to be pressed to the point that a routine is established. This victory would demonstrate the potential for all in a victory for marginalised children.

MAINTAINING STRATIFICATION

Societies built on stratification have a hard time overcoming that orientation. The antithesis of a modern, capitalist, outcomes-oriented society is an Indigenous worldview. Indigenous worldview values individuals that depart from the norm. Unique individuals exemplify diversity and illuminate other parts of the circle that makes us whole. A society that values survival of the fittest has a harder time adopting a paradigm of acceptance even when those disadvantaged in this view are our neighbours, relatives or even our own children. Where the life experience of people with unique needs is subordinate to the life experiences of most, the difference must be the subject of critical dialogue. Referencing stratification against the values and goals of society fosters opportunity for resolution. South Africa's Truth and Reconciliation Commission or Canada's Royal Commission on Aboriginal Peoples are examples of healthy resolutions.

ANALYSIS

Obstacles in my path include an absence of authentic dialogue, jurisdictional confusion and a vision of childhood and life that does little to meet the real needs of children living with life-limiting conditions. The Canadian conversation regarding paediatric palliative care is situated in advocacy. Families of children with life-limiting conditions and their supporters from the fields associated with wellness and palliative care keep the dialogue current. The national policy referring to paediatric palliative care is an advocacy policy that has yet to be adopted by government in Canada. Absent voice allows absent leadership. Championing the cause for ill children is more apt to be a charitable response that offers extraordinary experiences when the end of life is inevitable rather than easing the journey when the end is uncertain but the journey is just as tumultuous.

LOST IN DIVERSITY

Canada's strength in universal healthcare also presents challenges. The autonomy of the provinces results in a lack of consistent national policy. While it may be argued that services across provinces are not dramatically different, it is more difficult for local policy victories to be applied nationally. The vastness of the country and the concentration of services within population density means that my daughter receives paediatric haematology services from the Hospital for Sick Children in Toronto, Ontario; over 3000 km from our home in Saskatoon, Saskatchewan. The complexity is compounded because Sarah is an Indigenous person and under the Constitution of Canada, a responsibility of the federal government. Referral to an out-of-province hospital is determined by our provincial government while funding is approved by the federal government. An appropriate standard of care is hard to find in a system with such a complex jurisdictional roadmap.

An example of the jurisdictional complexity is that if Sarah was not an Indigenous person, the provincial government would pay for the installation of a wheelchair lift in our home. The federal government does not recognise this benefit for Indigenous children. We paid for Sarah's lift to avoid carrying Sarah, and her wheelchair in two separate trips, up the stairs and into our house. Systems that talk to each other may expose and overcome these jurisdictional wranglings and achieve a standard of care that protects children and their families from frustrating confusion of policy and practice. Moreover, if the ultimate goal is the care of the individual, jurisdictional wrangling becomes subordinate to that goal.

As an Indigenous parent I feel compelled to hold the government to account for its responsibilities under the auspices of the Treaty between government and Indigenous peoples. I also feel compelled to hold the government accountable to its responsibility to ease the journey of children with life-limiting illnesses. My frequent calls to government officials at various levels are the least that a parent can be expected to do, but I am troubled when systemic limitations based on an antiquated view of human diversity and dignity means that my advocacy won't be taken up because of a lack of desire to fully actualise the breadth and depth of our democracy.

AN ELUSIVE NORMAL

The most disturbing aspect of raising a child with a life-limiting condition is the pursuit of the elusive arrival at normal. The continuum of care for children resides in the medical-technical fields. It is complex and demoralising to translate the highly technical information into a format usable to children and families. For example, the experience of being told, following Sarah's assessment for a bone marrow transplant, that she was not a good candidate with an estimated 5% survival rate was a relief to us as parents. It was not, however, without an incredible sense of guilt for being happy with the news that meant that a long and painful chapter of Sarah's story could be avoided. I do feel guilt associated with being happy with what, for others, might have been a bad news story. A view of life over cure might have come to the same conclusion, but a view to a dignified life would marshal resources for life without a bone marrow transplant just as it would have for a transplant. Life is the *consolation* rather than the *plan*.

NORMALISING DIALOGUE AND POLICY

Paediatric palliative care victories like England's 'Better Care: Better Lives' bridges from a family's challenge to a place of belonging in a community gathered around common issues and establishing a sense of normal for what are sometimes extraordinary considerations. In the Canadian context there are few places to attach to find the experience of contributing to and benefiting from the experiences of other families. Ironically, contributing this story gave me a glimpse of the Canadian paediatric palliative care support network. I add this on-line support network to my frequent tasks of looking for new leads on managing everyday challenges for Sarah.

The absence of a national framework and policy erodes universality in service and care. It is hard to evaluate universality when the measuring stick is so elusive. Standards of care for cancer patients, paraplegic children or children with a blood disorder are fragmented where the more pertinent gathering place is paediatric palliative care. Families gather and share stories and advice from a platform without a name. Paediatric palliative care may instil fear of loss in some but for parents walking the difficult journey, it is a place of refuge.

Our affluence and sense of entitlement to life marginalises the sick as the antithesis of dominance, progress and an authentic life. This orientation is replicated in schools where integration is too often a policy without the support to be actualised. In Sarah's case, moving from a supported pre-school to a publicly funded grade school began the end of a near appropriate level of care. The level of care at the preschool was described as barely adequate. A fraction of the care is present in grade school but the service purports to be adequate for the same child with the same challenges. Without a policy driver, the perennial cry of being underfunded is simply complacency. We always hear that supports through the schools are underfunded, but we don't see any significant efforts to increase that funding. Education authorities don't go out on a limb for someone else's sick child without a policy motivator.

MOVING FORWARD

Having identified the pathway impediments and offering a perspective on the root causes, the *where to from here* extends the pathway metaphor and offers solutions. Paediatric care must undergo a deprogramming similar to the decolonising project of Indigenous communities. This is manifest in the creation of a global dialogue about the effects of colonisation and how we, as Indigenous peoples, gather our strength to recover from colonisation with tools familiar to us. It is essentially a global Indigenous recovery. What Indigenous peoples have taught all of us is that it is easy to maintain oppression when we assume the role of the *oppressor* and oppress ourselves. The decolonising project is most effective when society recognises its colonised state and attempts to cease colonisation and its accompanying subordination. Paediatric palliative care not only must mobilise those currently walking the path but also it must hold a mirror up to society as a whole so that the limitations of the status quo can be identified and dismantled.

Mobilisation is tricky business when entry to the exclusive club of a child or family living with the effects of life-limiting conditions comes at an amazingly tumultuous time. Often it is the alumni of this club that are the best advocates. Good policy not only answers the pleas of these people but mobilises a context of support around them. Canada has a responsibility to assist the organisation and accomplishments of parents, families and caregivers.

The liberating effect of achieving a standard of care for paediatric palliative care ensures that Canada's ideals are achieved, but it does much more than that. Diversity is the norm in Canadian schools and communities as the image of a Canadian reflects Canada's increasing image as a globally influenced society. Achievements in paediatric palliative care model processes and standards for the myriad other challenges of diversity that emerge. Canadians need to let go of resisting change and diversity in favour of counting victories in achieving supportive policy and practice.

CONCLUSION

What this story says about my reason to pause is that I, by virtue of being an Indigenous person and Sarah's father, am sensitive to the dichotomies that characterise issues of rights and perspective. What this story says about the environment around the path is more complex. I liken it to a national that chooses to fight for a vision of her country even when that vision is not actualised. It's what we aspire to. We advance a position based on the best of who we are. Sarah is a great individual with great potential and some significant challenges. She need not convince society that she wants as others do and contributes also as they do. The circle is wide enough for all to occupy a space. Shoulder to shoulder, Canadians will look to the centre and discover, yet again, the beauty of the ideal that was once imagined. My role as Sarah's father is worth wading through the complexities and conceptualising solutions to problems most don't need to consider. It is worth it because there are children waiting for the re-discovery of the ideal of equity and inclusion. Sarah also waits.

Part 2: A philosophical perspective on a father's tale

Gosia Bryckzynska

A COMMENTARY ON A FATHER'S TALE

Philosophy is essentially about analysing matters in detail and about getting rid of preconceived notions. Moreover, it is not easy to analyse and comment on powerful personal narratives; but as Gareth Matthews[1] (p. 13) in his iconic monograph about children and their capacity to philosophise, notes, since '... much of philosophy involves giving up adult pretensions to know' perhaps this is not a bad sentiment to bear in mind as we listen to the father's story. The father's story stands on its own merits, as his personal testimony, concerning his child and the care that his child is receiving. It is certainly, therefore, not the intention of this commentary to restructure the tale into something else, an academic text for example. The story stands as it was told – neither a piece of literature nor a strictly clinical report; but a father's tale told with compassion, courage and political awareness. It is a tale told to anyone willing to listen to it and reflect upon what is being said. It is a tale told to further the '... development of insight [and] the development of compassion ...' among those who choose to listen to it.[2] It is his story that we will now be engaged in reflecting upon.

Why bother looking at this tale so closely? Why attempt to deconstruct this one-of-a-kind tale? And why attempt to look at this narrative primarily from a philosophical perspective, when one could also listen to it and analyse it from a political, sociological and/or spiritual perspective to just name a few possible approaches? What benefits can a philosophical perspective bring to the narrative that may be of value to members of the healthcare and social welfare professional communities? What part of the story is not being told to us, and why not? Are some aspects of the story too painful to be recounted? Or has the narrator taken certain aspects of the story for granted? What can be added to the father's unfolding and unfinished narrative and should such activities on our part, even be our aim? I will attempt to address some of these questions; others will be left to stimulate the philosophical imagination.

As the father comments: 'I can describe the context ... but you have to understand the lens of my worldview to fully appreciate that context.' Just as Socrates started his philosophical dialogues by commenting that he will be walking down a *path* to the sea port of Piraeus[3] so I will start by taking a closer look at the *path* which the father took. I will consider what moral philosophy may have to say about some of the issues which he raises. Lastly, I will address the question – of where is little Sarah's voice in her father's tale? True, we were asked to listen to the father's tale; a tale about *his* daughter; but part of me is aching to hear Sarah's own tale and to listen to what she herself has to say about her own life. Sarah's tale of course would be a tale told in a different voice and it would therefore represent a different perspective. It would be a tale told by a young girl who enjoys 'art, singing, reading . . . has a sense of humour and an outstanding ability to foster human relationships.' In this era of granting children their rights, the right for little Sarah to be heard directly and not through an advocate – however articulate and concerned that advocate might be – is increasingly growing in political if not social momentum (Article 12 and 13 UNCRC 1989).[4] Therefore, what has political philosophy to say about Sarah's right to be heard? As the philosopher Gareth Matthews[1] noted concerning children and their ability to express novel insights – 'One of the exciting things that children have to offer us is a new philosophical perspective' (p. 14).

The father starts his tale by stating that he is standing in the middle of a path and contemplating his unknown future. Now the concept of a *path* or *way* or *road* is heavily loaded with spiritual and developmental significance. On the one level we really do have a father telling us that he stopped to pray and reflect on a path outside a hospital somewhere in Canada; and on another level we have an ancient symbol of life's trajectory and spiritual growth. We are presented almost without warning with the father's encounter of a transcendental moment. The father's introduction of the concept of *way* in his narrative is therefore fascinating, but it is also frontloaded with foreboding. Like in ancient Greek dramas – we dread for him and with him in respect to what might come down that path and confront him – but we also know that that particular road, that specific path he has chosen, is significant for him and unique to him and his life. It is his path and he has to go down it. Indeed the North American poet Robert Frost[5] would say that he chooses consciously to go down that particular path –

> '. . . long I stood
> And looked down one as far as I could
> To where it bent in the undergrowth;
> Then took the other.'[5]

This notion of path is a common metaphor therefore and is much utilised in contemplative psychology and encountered daily in such existentialist expressions as spiritual journey, journeying, maintaining a journal, enlightened way, spiritual path and so on. Thus *paths* and *ways* are referred to as essential aspects of the pursuit of religious and spiritual development, notions well recognised by moral philosophers and moral theologians.[2] We also refer to *pathways* – meaning trajectories or directions of movement from an alpha to a beta position. This use of the term pathways is clearly reflected in this book as it is a term much utilised by health and social care clinical and managerial professionals. But the pathway this father is being made to undertake is a *path-way* through the forest of life – a route which he cannot predict or foretell where it will take him or where and when it will end. There are no maps to the ways he has to traverse; and yet the healthcare and social care systems under which he is living would as soon as not impose upon him a clearly defined *pathway of care* – a predictable trajectory for the delivery of care to his daughter although that trajectory (package of care) is along an uncharted and unknown route! As the father observes, 'where advanced considerations for paediatric palliative care can make the journey a life affirming experience, the absence of these supports render the journey a frustrating struggle.' Thus as Greenlaugh[6] commented '. . . stories embrace complexity and are embedded in other stories' (p. 49) – in this case the story of Sarah's existence is embedded in the story of the Canadian Healthcare System, which is also fast becoming part of the story of the father's life.

The distraught father has now taken a road less travelled even if he would have initially preferred not to take it – as he notes: 'I prayed that my daughter's path would be made easy, in whichever direction it proceeded.' Over time he started to notice things that hitherto had not given him concern, e.g. the marginalisation of certain children, the lack of resources surrounding the care of patients with particular conditions; various social inequalities and a general lack of justice. The road less travelled can be a hard road but one not automatically to be considered insurmountable or to be even avoided at all cost.

> Two roads diverged in a wood, and I –
> I took the one less traveled by,
> And that has made all the difference.[5]

Han de Wit[2] in his fascinating book on the pastoral role of contemplative psychology notes that one of the benefits of contemplative reflection is that it encourages the growth of a relationship between insight and an overall state of one's being. By pondering on certain realities and then becoming more aware (firstly to self and subsequently by being shared with others) this process can result in a gentleness and genuine caring for other people. De Wit goes on to note that '. . . the development of spirituality is thus based on the unity of view (insight) and action (compassion)'. This statement by de Wit that insight can lead to an increase in compassion (and spirituality) is certainly not unique to him. Any benefits from acquired insights however are contingent on the motivation of the person doing the reflection and their subsequent intentions and actions. This has been one of the leading axioms concerning virtue ethics since the writings of Aristotle. Moreover, compassion is one of the most important virtues to be cultivated and one commented upon quite extensively in the philosophical and existentialist literature.

Compassion, courage and a sense of justice (often accompanied by the feeling of righteous indignation) and many of the other social virtues are subject to being manifested in our lives by our unique psychological personalities and reflect to a larger or lesser degree how we handle and control our emotions. The philosopher Martha Nussbaum[7] noted, concerning our human emotions, that they can represent for us 'geological upheavals of thought'. They can indeed upon occasion be all powerful and dominating – but without them, however, we would be impoverished social beings. The father is rightfully angry and actually states that it is his First Nation status that enables him more fully to empathise with other marginalised people. Parents of chronically ill children he maintains are marginalised people. The cultivation of healthy emotions contributes therefore to our being fully human and fully aware of the world around us and the needs of other people. We need our emotions to drive and fuel our psychological well-being. Moreover, emotions themselves as reflected in our psychological make-up need to be periodically subjected to our discerning thought processes – otherwise we could become overly controlled and dominated by our emotions. The father comments about the need for balance in our perspectives, which he states comes easier to him because of his cultural heritage.

The father who is evidently attached to his daughter tells us that he perceives all people as having intrinsic value – because they are all members of the human family and the various differences among peoples are but reflections of the rich tapestry of our shared humanity and these individual differences are to be treasured. This ideological perspective on the human race he attributes as much to his own familial and cultural values as a First Nation Canadian, as to his Christian faith. Most healthcare workers would also say that they too strive not to discriminate between races, cultures, peoples of differing faiths or those manifesting various disabilities and medical conditions and so on; but in reality upon occasion they do so. For most professionals and officials working with children, especially children with disabilities and complex medical conditions, seeing a child and regarding that child as an integrated whole – representing in their fragile and sometimes fractured (wounded) personhood a unique but also *blessed* combination of a particular mind, body and spirit – is almost impossible. There is the real danger that because these children are on the margins of professional preoccupation they may also suffer from a lack of professional know-how and expertise – or as Christina M Bruhn[8] noted in her fascinating paper on the marginalisation of children with disabilities by professionals, a child's '. . . disability may impede optimal development, not only as a result of physical, emotional, or cognitive characteristics but also as a result of the social repercussions of having those characteristics' (p. 174). This is something that the father feels profoundly and for him the emotion is akin to the feeling of rejection and marginalisation experienced because of his First Nation status. Bruhn[8] continues to observe that the consequences of professional inappropriate response to these children can have serious repercussions for the children and their families. She observes that while most child welfare and medical workers have the best interest of children at heart, many professionals may never have received adequate training in identifying and responding to these particular children with these particular disabilities – something which the father also notes concerning workers in his daughter's school.

Healthcare professionals are often educated to work effectively and efficiently in one specific area of the human experience. This specific approach to medical work is probably the norm for most healthcare workers – but this fragmentation of the professional's perspective itself creates as many human problems as it helps in resolving. It is little wonder then that there are logistical problems with integrating aspects of care such that the care can be experienced by patients and their families as *holistic care*. To the frustration of many parents, as the father recounts to us, even legislative structures can hinder the promotion of an individual's well-being; not through inherent state malevolence but due to the inbuilt inflexibilities of social and legal systems; ironically, inflexibilities often brought about in the first place to avoid just such allegations of discrimination, favouritism, fragmentation and injustice!

The father is commenting here on essentially two main philosophical issues, the issue of justice as recognised by generations of political and moral philosophers and one often addressed by a reference to human rights. The second issue is that of the lack of inter-connectedness and interpersonal integration of all that makes us human and unique, that is, a lack of a respect for the idea of holism. This notion of holism, is a philosophical theory addressed by many contemporary philosophers, and is one which the father sees as crucial to the welfare of his daughter and one which if practiced would make all the difference to the quality of her life. It is also a value which as a First Nation Canadian he considers central to his identity.

There is a clash here of values and moral principles; between the father's moral expectations and needs and the healthcare workers' and schools' guiding principles. The philosopher John Rawls[9] in his brilliant mind experiment, demonstrated a particular need for and approach to social justice, which all families of children with life-limiting conditions and whose children are marginalised by society, can recognise and identify with. Sarah's father goes further, however, for he not only wants social justice for his daughter but also he wants us to primarily see her (and indeed *know her*) as a fun-loving little girl, not only to recognise her and refer to her as a young patient with an unusual syndrome in need of medical attention, adequate schooling and a realistic mobility allowance. He wants professionals to start practicing holistic care and while he himself is beginning to learn how to fight for compassionate justice, he is beginning to speak the language of moral engagement.

But what would Sarah have to say about all this? Does the father's story give us any insights into her mind? Has Sarah anything meaningful to say to us directly? As Gareth Matthews[1] the children's philosopher noted, any '. . . theory that rules out, on purely theoretical grounds, even the possibility that we adults may occasionally have something to learn, morally, from a child is, for that reason, defective; it is also morally offensive' (p. 67). So if we believe that we can learn something from Sarah herself – what might it be?

As with many children with complex medical, nursing and social needs, in order to hear what they have to say we may have to be extremely attentive to their articulations. The careful listening to these children may involve in addition to listening skills much observation on our part – as the children most probably will be articulating and commenting on their life using more than just one of their senses. Often deprived of the full use of speech they will make up for this loss with an even greater reliance on their remaining senses of hearing and touch, or they will develop even better and finer-tuned social and interactive skills, and various other talents like having an exceptional ability for music or painting, through which they will express themselves and so on. The father comments that '. . . Sarah builds bridges and exemplifies acceptance. The aforementioned qualities draw care and support to her and join those around her closer together and closer, ultimately, to Sarah.' Obviously Sarah is quite capable of manipulating the world around her to benefit her needs – a very useful interactive skill; and she is also apparently quite capable of communicating as so many other children, through painting and singing. The UNCRC[4] notes that a child's right to be heard (Article 12 and 13) is one of the more fundamental rights accorded to children and together with the right to the best and most appropriate healthcare (Articles 23 and 24) – Sarah should be assured the best integrated care available to promote her social and mental development.

In conclusion, while reading the father's tale, many ethical and philosophical ideas and concerns come to mind. Taking as our initial premise that the tale itself was a powerful moral tool for explaining Sarah's plight and then analysing several of the points raised within the tale – for their ethical significance – some moral aspects of Sarah's life have been illuminated. At Sarah's birth, her father stood on the path outside the hospital and philosophised – wondering what would become of him, his daughter, and their life together as a family? He considered what may lie ahead for him and his daughter on the shared path of their life. He did not know at that time what lay ahead; just as the poet Robert Frost[5] did not know what lay ahead of him as he looked down the two paths that he encountered in the woods. For the poet both paths looked equally enticing and not much seemed to differentiate them. He said that both paths

> . . . That morning equally lay
> In leaves no step had trodden black.
> Oh, I kept the first for another day!
> Yet knowing how way leads on to way,
> I doubted if I should ever come back.

We cannot go back on our life's paths and traverse down another – but we can share our life's paths' journeys with others – and that can make all the difference.

N.I.C.E. analysis

Needs

My parental role of advocate motivates me to identify and act to reduce complacency-induced injustices. I do not speak of behalf of those who can't but on behalf of a common pursuit of the fullness of humanity. What we *need* is to enliven a dialogue that considers that diversity is a positive human attribute that must be valued and extended to the realm of ability.

Interests

Our collective *interests* are to ensure that we never create a disposable sector of society for fear that we may one day be caught up in an indiscriminate definition of disposability. As a community member, I apply my energies to ensure that I celebrate the brilliance of humanity in a physical body that is sometimes less than whole.

Concerns

My *concern* is that the dialogue regarding paediatric palliative care is being left to chance through the perception that the best supports for children living with life-limiting conditions are a crutch, prescription or surgery. Support commensurate with need might better be sustained support that recognises the value of small flames as vital light. I am concerned that a voice of advocacy, in some jurisdictions, is failing to emerge because we don't know what to advocate for.

Expectations

My *expectations* are that those that experience the limitations of policy and perspective on children living with life-limiting conditions merge with those that champion diversity and democracy to use the vehicle created by the paediatric palliative care dialogue to advance the cause. The misconception that illness-oriented care is more suited to our children than wellness-oriented care presents barriers that need to be challenged.

From the above analysis please reflect on:

● The challenge that I promote is an incremental broadening of worldview paired with a measure of intensity in advocacy. The advantage of patience is sustainability while the disadvantage is complacency. The advantage of advocacy is profile while the disadvantage is alienation. I also employ the age-old vehicle for perpetuating what we value through stories. I'm convinced that there are many catalysts for change.

Action plan: next steps

To the policy-makers, the challenge is to create a less complicated and more dignified space for our children. For our neighbours and friends, the story needs to portray that Sarah's worth is no less than that of their own children. People are always ready for a hopeful story. Translating that into good public policy is the challenge.

REFERENCES

1 Matthews GB. *The Philosophy of Childhood.* Cambridge, MA: Harvard University Press; 1994.
2 de Wit HF. *Contemplative Psychology.* Pittsburgh, PA: Duquesne University Press.
3 Plato (1991 [Waterfield R, translator]). *The Republic.* Oxford: Oxford University Press.
4 www.unicef.org/crc/
5 Frost R. *The Poetry of Robert Frost.* New York: Henry Holt & Co; 1975.
6 Greenhalgh T. *What Seems to be the Trouble? Stories in illness and healthcare.* Oxford: Radcliffe Publishing; 2006.
7 Nussbaum M. *Upheavals of Thought: the intelligence of emotions.* Cambridge: Cambridge University Press; 2001.
8 Bruhn CM. Children with disabilities: abuse, neglect and the child welfare system. In: Mullings J, *et al. The Victimization of Children: emerging issues.* Binghampton, NY: The Haworth Maltreatment and Trauma Press; 2003. pp. 173–203.
9 Rawls J. *The Theory of Justice.* Cambridge, MA: Harvard University Press; 1972.

11

Hearing the voices of parents and carers

Bea Brunton

By 1985 I had achieved my dream and thought life was perfect as I was a stay-at-home mum raising two beautiful children, a boy and a girl. I loved every moment I spent with them and we were always so busy finding fun ways in which to learn. Ours was the house that everyone wanted to visit because we were always making, baking and creating! I never thought that 14 years later I would be writing about my son's life and death.[1]

To cut a long story short, my son, Simon, was diagnosed as severely deaf when he was 3 years old and diagnosed with a degenerative eye disease when he was 7 years old. This meant that we had a lot of dealings with doctors, consultants, hospitals and support services throughout his young life. This involvement greatly increased when, at 13 years old, he was diagnosed with a malignant brain tumour. The next two years were a huge learning curve for us as parents. The worst part was accepting that we were not 'in control' anymore. We had to hand the responsibility for our child's well-being over to a succession of other people and had to learn to care for him all over again.

BARRIERS

The first major barrier to getting any sort of care or support for Simon was that no one would believe us, his parents, when we tried to tell them there was something wrong. From the time we suspected that there might be something wrong with Simon's hearing to the time we found out that there was definitely something wrong we had numerous visits to our GP and health visitor, which spanned a period of 18 months. It was only when we got angry with the GP and insisted that he referred us to an ENT consultant did anything start to happen. This is a story I have heard from countless parents during the years since. We are accused of being over anxious parents. Even if that proves to be the case surely there is scope to investigate such concerns if they are causing the families concern, professionals shouldn't be so flippant in their dismissal of our worries. It was the same years later when we had to keep visiting our GP because of the severe headaches that Simon was getting. Thankfully some work has been done to identify a set of symptoms that should be flagged up for referral if a child presents with them. I believe this has resulted in a speedier diagnosis for some.

INFORMATION AND SERVICES

Parents often don't know where to go for help when seeking support and therefore I feel that information should be available from different sources. This seems to be a major focus for the *Better Care: Better Lives* strategy[2] and I am sure having more information will empower families. I do think the need for a navigator/mentor/key worker is vital as families often haven't the time, inclination or skills to find out what support is available to them, although I do think this is improving with the advent of the Internet, as long as families are accessing reputable online resources. In my work as the coordinator of PASIC (Parent's Association for Seriously Ill Children)[3] a charity that supports families of children diagnosed with cancer, I get opportunities to go along to workshops and conferences whose themes revolve around the different aspects of care for children, young people and their families. I'm not at all sure how I came to be at the *Better Care: Better Lives* strategy launch, but when I read the document of that name I felt that it was long overdue and would be a great step forward if only it could be delivered successfully.

PALLIATIVE CARE

People often don't know what palliative care is and even when I tried to find out there were many different explanations. The most common interpretation I have heard amongst those people that I have come into contact with is that it means care for someone who is dying. Perhaps this is because oncology families can quite suddenly need special care due to their child's illness reaching a more life-threatening stage or in the case of brain tumour sufferers their illness and subsequent treatment has left them with a devastating legacy. Their child wasn't born needing palliative care; this is something that has been thrust upon them, which may be the reason why many oncology families interpret palliative care as care for the dying. I must admit that was my impression at first. I have changed that view over time as I have learned that it is providing care to someone who is living with a condition which may impact on their lives and be life-limiting and life-threatening. Even then I think there may be some confusion as to the interpretation of life-limiting. Does this mean that it will affect only the length of life or that it will affect the quality of life as well? It is one thing to have such plans written on paper, but quite another to translate them into real-life terms for the families that need them.

As a parent reading the *Better Care: Better Lives* strategy[2] I felt that it was a wish list for parents of special children. These were such fundamental common sense ideas and I wondered why on earth they hadn't been recognised and acted upon before. As one parent commented at the launch, he could have written the document 20 years ago. Through talking to families on a cancer journey I have come to realise that there are huge inequalities in the provision of care for children, young people and their families. Where it works well, everything possible seems to be in place and where it doesn't work it fails the children, young people and their families abysmally. Whether it works or not largely depends on who is involved in setting up the care. This can be said of health, social or educational care.

Simon had been statemented for special educational needs throughout his life, but setting the needs out in a document and receiving them were two entirely different things. We still had to battle with the authorities to ensure that everything that should happen did happen. There were times that I felt that I just couldn't fight the system any more and felt very frustrated, but then I would pull myself together and think that if I didn't fight for Simon's rights then no one would. I pray that things have changed over the years, but through my work I still meet many parents who have to battle for services that should be more forthcoming. A particular problem seems to be working across disciplines and areas, especially if your child is treated in a specialist centre miles away from home. Getting healthcare services to communicate with social care services is sometimes a huge problem, especially if a family has to deal with different local authorities. So many times it seems that no one wants to take the responsibility of paying for a service, they would rather pass the buck and this can mean that the families are waiting for support far longer than they should be.

The professionals providing care should realise that they cannot put people into boxes, each person is an individual, each family unique and, as such, has very different needs. There might be lots of common ground, but the people who are assessing the care that is needed by an individual should listen to how they live their lives and work with them to find out what would make a difference in their lives. Often the smallest things can make the biggest difference. Some parents are opposed to having someone come in to their home and carry out personal care for their child, but they would welcome an offer for someone to carry out some basic tasks such as shopping, cooking or house work. Professionals should not assume that they know what is best for people. Only by living that life, either as the child, young person or the carers, can you possibly know what it is really like to endure the difficulties and challenges on a daily basis. Every member of the family is affected and needs appropriate support. Too often the care that is provided to families depends upon the person that is 'fighting their corner' and this can lead to huge inequalities of service. Hopefully the proposed guidelines will mean that teams of professionals will be working together to provide the best care possible for the individual.

I know that if I had to care for a child with care needs now, I would be able to find a lot more information and support than was available to us as a family when Simon needed care and support. The Internet can be a major source of signposting and also now people understand that they have a right to receive care and it is not just for the privileged few who can afford it. There have been huge improvements in the care and support available since our experience in the late nineties and I believe this is set to improve and that with willingness on behalf of the state and the agencies charged with providing care the lives of families caring for children will be greatly improved.

No parent wants to think about their child dying; of course we do in our darkest moments, but then we have to concentrate on what is and not what may be. I believe that it is vital to cultivate special moments for families whose children may be life-limited or life-threatened; it will ultimately be these things that families remember after their child has died. Care should concentrate on providing the best quality of life possible until such times as death cannot be discounted and end-of-life care initiated.

I wonder if anyone has ever dared ask families of children who died at home whether they wished that they hadn't chosen that option? I think for many the perception of the act of dying is very different to the actual experience of having to watch someone die, especially if it is not in a peaceful way. Speaking from my experience of dealing with oncology families I do think that more should be done to encourage the use of respite facilities, i.e. children's hospices so that families already have experience of these services should the need arise later for end-of-life care. Although I do know from our experience that there can be a very mixed reception to the topic of children's hospices amongst parents as they can be suspicious as to why the topic has been introduced especially when their child's care seems to be going well. When our Macmillan nurse suggested that we make use of Rainbows Children's Hospice,[4] I felt that they were trying to help us through a difficult time until Simon was well again, but my husband was very suspicious and thought that the suggestion had only been made to prepare us for the end. On reflection either of those things could have been true.

I believe that putting life into the *Better Care: Better Lives* strategy is going to rely on those involved being determined to see it work and willing to take on board that in the case of caring for children it is the parents of those special children that are the experts. The professionals need to be willing to listen to the parents and learn from them and they need to refrain from thinking that they know what is best for a child and its family.

Care pathways should not be 'set in stone', there should be some allowance for flexibility within those pathways as needs can change and professionals should be allowed to act upon those changes for the benefit of the families and not have to go 'back to the drawing board' and have to agree a new care plan before anything can be done to help the family.

NEED FOR SUPPORT WITH CHOICES AND DECISION MAKING

I believe the section 'My Life Would Be Easier If . . .'[2] (p. 9) is a real eye-opener and highlights the need to engage with children, young people and their families about what is important to them. During the launch one parent told the audience that his daughter had waited so long for a wheelchair that she had grown out of it before it was ever received. Gasps of astonishment and incredulity were heard and people were astounded that something like this could happen. I believe it happens more than we know. Sometimes the things that would make life a lot easier are so simple that they get overlooked. This is where the role of 'navigator' would be invaluable. A person who gets to know the family, but also knows what services, equipment, etc. are available, because the families often do not know what is available to them and they only find out by talking to other families and finding out what they have been able to access.

I believe that children, young people and their families want to be able to live ordinary lives, they don't want to be different, they want to do what other families take for granted like family holidays and days out, but so often these turn in to events which need military-style organisation. Help and support should be given to families to make a difference in their lives where they feel they need it. Each families' support needs will be different.

Choices – from my experience it was not always a good thing to be given choices about aspects of Simon's treatment. In fact I have found that the more choices there are the more difficult it is to make a decision.

I cannot read 'The vision' (p. 11) without thinking about the costs of services and who is going to pay for it. Is there going to be a heavy burden on the voluntary sector organisations to foot the bill, as in the case of research into childhood cancer or indeed cancer in general?

'The vision' states that:

> there will be full integration of services with a seamless transition of care between primary, secondary and tertiary healthcare settings, and close partnership working between healthcare, education, social services and voluntary sector organisations.

Sounds wonderful, but the bottom line is that you are dealing with human beings. I've witnessed situations where the outcome has depended upon who has the biggest personality or wielded the most power, regardless of who has had the better point of view. Simon was at a school with a hearing impaired unit attached to it and was fully integrated with his peers before his diagnosis of a brain tumour. He returned to that school after his treatment and many changes were made to accommodate his special needs, including a wheelchair. We thought all was going well until one summer holiday we learned that Simon would not be returning to that school, but would be starting at a special school in the September. This news was devastating to Simon and to us all. We only found out by accident when I had cause to contact the educational psychologist, who thought we already knew.

I would imagine that things are very different for families whose children are born with special needs. The need for care grows and adapts with the child and the families are already 'in the system', the need for special care has always been there. Families in an oncology setting often have these things thrust upon them after living seemingly ordinary lives. This can be a difficult transition for them and a time when they need a lot of different support. I know that at different times in Simon's life we had to deal with devastating news: first, that he was deaf; second, that he had a degenerative eye disease; and third, that he had a malignant brain tumour. The day after the diagnosis of his eye condition someone said to me 'Simon is the same little boy today as he was before the diagnosis'. I needed that reminder, after all, the tunnel vision and night blindness hadn't just happened, they were things that were the norm for Simon. It was my perception that had changed – that was what I needed help to come to terms with.

Information and data is important. I have been involved in some work as part of the 'Aiming High for Disabled Children' initiative[5] and was absolutely astounded to discover that there was not a database of disabled children. How can services be planned if you don't know the numbers of people you are planning for?

SERVICE USER AND CARER'S INVOLVEMENT

I do believe that parents and young people should be involved at a strategic level to help shape services. But I also realise that not all parents or young people should be involved as there is a need to be able to remove some of the emotion from the situation to be able to talk about it in practical terms, which professionals will take on board and not see as just another 'bleeding heart' account of a personal situation.

In my work for PASIC[3] I have had the opportunity to be involved in many workshops, committees, etc. that have sought parental involvement. For years I felt that this was only done to 'tick the boxes'; the professionals organising such events were told that they had to have parental involvement, but actually did not want it. They did not make parents feel welcomed or valued, they would often make it impossible for parents to attend due to short notice, lack of child care facilities or some such other reason. I have witnessed a change in many arenas over the years and most professionals, but certainly not all, are willing to listen to parents and take on board what they are saying and use that knowledge to implement change.

I do think that professionals do assume too much sometimes. They assume that they shouldn't mention certain subjects because they are too emotive; is that because they genuinely do not wish to upset the parents or is it because they don't know how to deal with the potentially emotional situation so they steer clear of it? We may get upset, but do not deny us our tears, just give us a moment and we will carry on. We want to help you to make things better for others even if it is too late for ourselves.

I think this avoidance is a symptom of conditioning by society; if a situation has the possibility to be emotional or difficult then just avoid it. This is just a short-term view and I believe can lead to huge problems later. I feel it is better to face something head on and get to grips with it, rather than put it off and have to deal with it later. Admittedly some parents are going to have to have more support than others to do this, but that shouldn't be a reason to avoid a subject.

A prime example of this in my work comes at such times as there is a transition between curative and palliative care in a cancer setting, when survivorship is no longer an option. I have come across many parents who do not know that their child is dying. One may question whether this is due to the parents not having been told or not having accepted the news. Have the consultants concerned in a child or young persons' care had the skills to communicate such news to parents or have they just presumed that the parents naturally know when a child has reached a point where cure is no longer an option? I think this is the biggest difference in dealing with oncology families; they hold on to the hope for cure, whereas families who are dealing with conditions that their child has been born with have never had the hope of cure, just the duty to ensure that everything is done in the best interests of their child to give them the best quality of life available.

I believe one of the biggest barriers to providing good quality, person-centred care is going to be attitude. The attitudes of those people who have the power to provide the care are going to be so important. There has to be a real willingness for agencies to work together for the good of the child, young person and their family. To forget about egos and territorialism and make the process of receiving palliative care as simple as it can be for families – they have enough challenges in life already without fighting for what should be their child's right to care. Give help when it is needed as quickly as possible, don't wait for a crisis to arise.

Commissioners and service providers need to champion the cause of palliative care and ensure that it is accessible to all who need it as swiftly as possible.

CONCLUSION

Services need to be designed around the needs of children, young people and their families and only by involving them in planning services will this happen.

Listen to the wishes of children, young people and parents and be willing, where possible, to consider making them a reality.

N.I.C.E. analysis

Please reflect on the issues raised in this chapter in relation to your own practice.

Needs

- To be believed and not just treated as over-anxious parents when we suspect that there is something wrong with our child.
- To be identified as a family with our own unique needs.
- To be given information at the time of diagnosis not just sent home to wait for further action to be planned.
- To be given the name of a contact person who can answer further questions.
- To be given sources of support and information available from other organisations.
- To be given ways in which to communicate that do not involve having to face up to someone.

Interests

- To help find ways of identifying strategies that can be used to ensure that children are diagnosed more rapidly.
- To use the experiences of families to educate those who plan and provide services.
- To establish better working relationships between children, young people, parents and professionals.
- Networking and finding further information and support that will benefit the families.
- To help ensure better communications in all areas.

Concerns

- That children are still suffering lengthy delays and misdiagnosis, i.e. migraine.
- That important treatment is delayed because of misdiagnosis.
- That once a care plan is produced it should be reviewed regularly to ensure that it is working as it should.
- Reviewing a care plan should not involve lengthy delays; if improvements are identified they should be initiated as soon as possible.
- That support services suffer a breakdown due to staff changes and shortages.

Expectations

- Education for the public as to what palliative care is.
- Banish the myth that palliative care is just for end of life.
- Assist families to live 'ordinary' lives; they don't want to be different.
- Work towards a standard of treatment that is available to all families regardless of geographical location.
- Ensure greater cooperation across disciplines, between hospitals and across county borders.

From the above analysis please reflect on:

- How you can be the person that is fighting for the best interests of the family and not just the person who is having what can be provided for the family dictated by the system.
- How you can best determine the needs of each individual in the family including siblings.
- The best ways to ensure that user/carer involvement is assured along each step of the planning pathway.
- How giving families multiple choices may, in fact, lead them to not being able to decide the best course of action.
- How communication can be improved between all the parties concerned in planning a care pathway.

Action plan: next steps

- Ensure that a family can have a voice when it comes to planning care pathways by exploring different ways of them being able to communicate their needs to those concerned. Some people might struggle face to face, but have no problem putting their needs into an email.
- Ensure that what is planned is delivered. Too often what is written is not what is delivered in real terms.

REFERENCES

1 www.btinternet.com/~b.brunton/index.html
2 GB Department of Health: www.positivelearning.co.uk/downloads/Better_Care.pdf
3 PASIC (Parent's Association for Seriously Ill Children) www.pasic.org.uk/
4 www.rainbows.co.uk/
5 Aiming High for Disabled Children www.everychildmatters.gov.uk/socialcare/ahdc/

12

Hearing the voices of siblings

Sally Blower

The hospice provides support for siblings of life-limited children and young people, both on a one-to-one and a group basis. Siblings of life-limited children may follow their brother or sister along a very long journey, which can often last years. This will involve countless hospital visits and periods of acute illness only for their brother or sister to improve again and be able to return home, but then again becoming very poorly. Apart from the rollercoaster of emotions that come with serious illness siblings have to often live on a day-to-day level of living with disability and the challenges this brings to the whole family.

Working with siblings there seems to be some common themes that keep coming up time and time again. 'Most young siblings experience lack of parental attention, isolation, ignorance about disability, difficulty coping with their experiences, and the financial impact of disability on the family. Many studies on siblings of children with a chronic illness indicate that siblings are at risk of negative psychological effects.'[1] The work in the hospice that we do with siblings certainly shows that this is in fact the case for many families to some extent or another.

Families are sometimes restricted to activities which they can access due to wheel-chairs, medical equipment and hoists, making day trips and holidays impossible for some people. The worry of being near to hospital should something go wrong also dictates where to go. For siblings this means that they are often not spending quality time together and doing activities that other families take for granted.

Even everyday activities can be difficult and their relationship with their brothers and sisters is perhaps not the type of relationship that their peers may have with theirs. This can make siblings feel different; at school they may be the only person in their class that has a brother or sister with a life-limiting condition. Sometimes this can lead to bullying from others; it can be a very isolating experience.

A big thing for lots of siblings is the fact that parents and other adults in their lives often have to devote lots of time to caring for their brother or sister. Siblings miss out on having parents' attention and can feel that all that matters is their brother or sister. Siblings will often understand why this has to be, but this doesn't stop them feeling a little resentful. Grace has explained some of her feelings in the writing below:

Being a sibling of my big brother Gregory has its good things and bad things, it can be very hard and can quite affect me, and for instance my life style is very different than any other people, such as friends. I have been bullied because of my brother's disability but I guess that shows who your true friends actually are. My two best friends are so good with Greg they come round my house and say hello Greg make him laugh have a play with him, make him smile it really makes me smile that I have them and that they actually understand what it's like, we are really close. Me and Gregory have a really close relationship as our family is a close family I always know how to make him smile when I hug him he will never let me go because he knows it's me. As you might know our family is a very musical family and I am also committed to singing and I sing to Gregory and it perks him up so much it's almost a miracle. My parents have to spend a lot of time with Gregory since he needs that special help, but I sometimes feel a little pushed aside but I understand that Gregory needs all the help and care he can get so I understand why that is. Being a sibling of Greg has made me grow up more, get more mature than others like my friends cause they don't have to think for themselves as they can just rely on their parents. So can I of course, but I try not to put so much pressure on them since they have so much to do since I have 2 other brothers as well as Gregory. The worst part of being Greg's sister is when he gets rushed into hospital it's most horrible feeling ever. All these thoughts go through my head like is he going to die? When will he get better? Will he ever get better? I get very emotional but try to be strong for the rest of my family. When things like this do happen my friends are always there telling me think positive just making you feel happier at that time. But when he gets better it's a relief. When he is in hospital and I'm really worried about Greg it sometimes affects my school work because my mind is just thinking about whether he will get better or not as he has a limited life. But we try to make the most of every moment with have with him. I am so glad I am Gregory's sister, I couldn't ask for a better brother. And it's great to go to sibling trips and meet people who know exactly what you're going through it kind of helps to have someone to talk to that will truly understand.

Written by Grace, aged 13

Grace conveys brilliantly some of what life is like to be a sibling and also shows that whilst it has its downsides we mustn't forget the positives that can come from having to deal with the challenges that are forced upon them. Siblings often find that they have to grow up quickly, but the bond that they may share with their sibling can make them have a greater understanding of disability and people's differences, giving them a better outlook on life.

The big message that comes across from many siblings is the love that they share and the wish to protect their sibling and care for them. Siblings can become carers sometimes through necessity, but often through wanting to help and be more involved. The picture by Katie shows perhaps how some siblings feel. She has painted her brother in the middle of herself and her younger sister (*see* Figure 12.1). Although Katie is younger than her brother she has placed a protective hand on his head.

The complexity of the relationships that the siblings have is perhaps unique. In other families the older children would sometimes feel protective of younger siblings

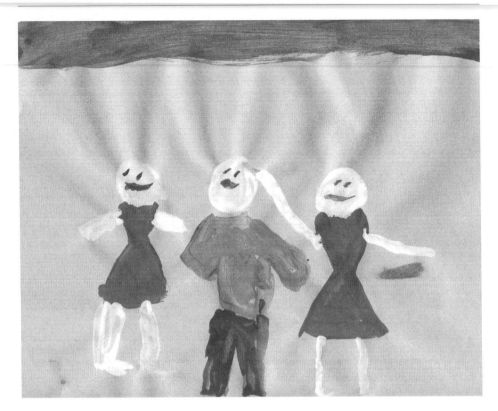

FIGURE 12.1 By Katie, age 7

whereas in families where there is a life-limited child the pecking order can be changed where the child may be younger, but expected to take on responsibilities that older children would normally do.

Not all siblings will feel the same and it will depend very much on their own individual situation. Factors such as their age, gender and cultural upbringing will make a difference as to what their thoughts and feelings are. Alex has painted a picture of himself and his mum on a recent sibling day (*see* Figure 12.2), which was held at the hospice. When a member of staff asked him to tell them about it Alex said that there wasn't room to put his sister. It may well have been the case, as he is only five, that his spatial awareness skills meant he had painted the pictures bigger than he thought. However, it may again illustrate the point that Alex has thoughts of just wanting to be with his mum. His sister requires lots of care and mum has to devote lots of time to providing this, as do lots of parents.

In the lives of life-limited children and young people there are also lots of professionals that are there to help with their care and they may receive respite, etc. Alex described his sister as lucky as she gets to do all the special things, such as coming to the hospice and getting presents, etc. Alex will have little input from these people and sees his sister getting what he thinks is special treatment. This can be difficult for siblings and in some cases can have effects on self-esteem.

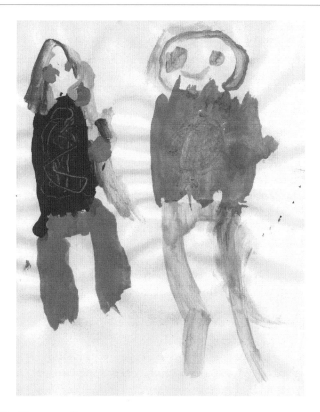

FIGURE 12.2 By Alex, age 5

At the hospice we provide groups for siblings to attend to gain support from peers and staff. The main emphasis of the sessions are for the siblings to have fun, but at the same time to be able to explore some of the issues that they may come across which can include self-esteem building. Therapeutic activities are offered and we try to answer questions that the siblings may ask about their brother's or sister's condition as often a lack of knowledge can be a cause of anxiety. Later on in the chapter, Will (a sibling) describes how not knowing what's going on in his sister's life means that he worries more. We hope by sharing things together and answering questions we can help to alleviate some worries.

The siblings are divided pre-bereavement groups into groups depending on their age. This means we are able to provide age-appropriate activities for the siblings for their developmental level. The groups are structured with Piaget's stages of development are in mind. He saw these transitions as taking place at about 18 months, seven years and 11 or 12 years. This has been taken to mean that before these ages children are not capable (no matter how bright) of understanding things in certain ways.[2] For this reason we have found separating the groups into the ages of 5–7, 8–10 and 11+ beneficial, allowing us to explain things to the siblings at a level they will understand.

Bereaved siblings of all ages attend the same group, however, again, siblings may be split into age groups once at the hospice to be able to deliver age-appropriate activities.

Bereaved siblings need to be able to express their feelings and have their voices heard. 'The psychological empowerment that arises when we validate and acknowledge the experiences of children draws on Bandura's concept of self-efficacy.'[3] 'A common finding in bereavement studies is that many parents and other adults are unaware of children's thoughts and feelings or the questions that children are left with.'[3]

The younger siblings will have craft activities and games in their groups; whereas for the older sibling groups we try to offer more project-based activities, such as producing a video or piece of music about their siblings and their feelings. Each group has four days offered to them per year. We also hold a weekend away and day trips to theme parks etc. We do this to enable the siblings to enjoy days out without the constraints of having their brother or sister around who as we have said may not be able to go on such trips. We also hope that these fun days will help to consolidate friendships that have been made. Siblings can get much support from their peers knowing that they are not alone.

Whilst there is a school of thought that siblings have very different needs before and after bereavement, we do mix bereaved siblings and non-bereaved siblings for trips out and weekends away. We feel that this enables those who are yet to be bereaved the opportunity to make friends or just be around those who have lost a brother or sister. We hope that this gives them the confidence to see that people can cope and move forward with their lives. Some bereaved siblings also seem to like the fact that they can help those who are worried, share their experiences of what has happened and what has helped them. We find that many siblings do keep in touch after the events and look forward to seeing each other next time, which is often a time of great excitement.

In sibling's lives, we as adults have the ability to learn by listening to sibling's stories and experiences, how we can help them. Will has written about how he would very much like to be included in decisions that are made about his sister Ellie. On talking with him he feels very strongly that most decisions made about Ellie's care and future have an impact on his life in some way and that he would like to know about them.

Me and My Sister

My sister is called Ellie and she is 14. Ellie has a condition were she has little control over her movements so she has to be in wheelchair all the time. Ellie can't talk very much but she understands everything you say. The way she communicates is a clever computer called a Dynavox which is a touch screen with a speaker attached. It acts like a keyboard and when Ellie has spelt out what she wants to say she will hit an area at the top and it will say the phrase out loud.

Many times I will get quite upset and angry at the way people treat Ellie and the way they talk to her. They think she is young because she can't walk and talk like us, but she still deserves as much respect as you or me. Ellie has a photographic memory and had an IQ test done. Even with 2 years of school lost due to operations she was age appropriate in all areas as well as above in some mathematical areas.

Ellie has been in hospital countless times for various reasons. Usually when Ellie is in hospital I will either stay at home with my dad or mum as they take it in turns to be with Ellie, or go over to my friend's house for the day or even over night. When this happens nothing feels quite right because I've got no one to tell how I feel. As well as missing Ellie I also miss my mum and dad because they're away too. I worry because I never know what's going to happen to her.

I would have loved to have a sister who can play sport and help me but we can't always have what we want. Unfortunately there is no cure for Ellie but I don't see there has to be one. I know I can't have an input in all the big decisions that happen but I would at least like to be asked about my opinion even if my wishes can't all be fulfilled.

By Will, aged 11

Will also expressed how he feels that people don't often think to tell him about what's going on and often what he is imagining is worse. Once someone has explained, he often feels better. Will acknowledged that it may seem unfair that he knows everything about Ellie, but expressed that as it affects all his family if it was the other way round he would be happy for Ellie to know about him too.

Will feels that if he is more involved he may be able to help Ellie too. As she has problems communicating he suggested that on occasions he might be able to help Ellie express her wishes too, but can't do this if he doesn't know what to ask her.

Together we talked about the future and how Will may see their relationship changing. He is extremely close to Ellie at the moment, but said that he feels as he gets older that may change. However, he feels he will always be there to look out for Ellie and be interested in what's going on. He still wants to be involved. Will feels that if he is not around to see Ellie as much he will worry more as he won't be able to see if she is happy, but by remaining involved he feels he can help himself to worry less and ensure Ellie is happy. When asked what he wished for the future Will said in his dreams it would be a 'normal life'; he said that he knows he can't have this so the next best thing is to be involved.

Hopefully the written pieces and pictures from the siblings have shown what life is like for them living with a brother or sister with a life-limiting or life-threatening illness. The hospice tries to support the siblings, but can't take away what is happening and make it 'better'. Hopefully by having the opportunity to explore and share their feelings it will mean that siblings can still actively take part in their own lives and achieve their full potential. Strohm (2002) observes that there is less risk of longer-term emotional problems if the ill child's sibling is surrounded by loving support, is allowed to be involved in the care of the ill child and is allowed to express his or her range of emotions.[4]

N.I.C.E. analysis

Please reflect on the issues raised in this chapter in relation to your own practice.

Needs

- Designated time for siblings to gain support.
- Raising awareness of siblings issues and needs through training.
- Involving siblings in decision making where appropriate.
- Sharing information with siblings honestly, regarding end of life issues if possible.
- Ensuring professionals include siblings in significant care decisions.
- To support parents to identify issues and problems and seek support.

Interests

- Training staff to raise awareness of siblings' needs.
- Ensuring siblings are not forgotten within the healthcare setting and the hospice.
- Communication with parents to help them identify what challenges siblings are facing.
- To provide group and peer support for siblings to share experiences.

Concerns

- Lack of resources and support for siblings.
- The challenge for professionals to have time and skills to involve siblings at some level in their deliverance of healthcare.
- Limited research and resources on sibling issues.
- Needs/confidentiality of the ill child versus that of sibling when including them in discussions.

Expectations

- Improved communication between professionals, parents and siblings.
- Increased awareness from all agencies regarding needs of siblings.
- Siblings feeling better supported and more able to express concerns and worries.

Action plan: next steps

- To encourage all agencies to involve siblings in healthcare discussions where appropriate.
- To continue to deliver group and 1:1 support for siblings at the hospice.

REFERENCES

1 www.sibs.org.uk/uploads/files/Sibs%20-%20Developing%20services%20for%20siblings%20 of%20disabled%20children.pdf
2 www.learningandteaching.info/learning/piaget.htm
3 Wright JB, Aldridge J, Gillance H, *et al.* Hospice-based groups for bereaved siblings. *Eur J Palliat Care.* 1996; **3**: 10–15.
4 Strohm K. *Siblings: coming unstuck and putting back the pieces.* London: David Fulton; 2002.

13

Transitions within the family

Jacqueline Newton

June 1993: we had our first child, a healthy baby boy just as we had hoped for. Life was perfect.

When Billy was 12–15 months old, we noticed a change; he lost the few words he had, seemed less interested in the world around him and would become fixated with certain toys and with his own hands, twisting and turning them. He slept all night and then would enjoy two naps a day. He was content and seemed happy. We were a little unsure of what he was doing, but he was our first child and I guess ignorance was bliss until Christmas Eve 1994 when the health visitor came to our house to do the 18-month assessment and told me right there and then that she suspected Billy had autism. Our whole world felt like it had fallen apart. I remember spending Christmas Day looking at his every move and, as he ran around flapping his little hands, thinking perhaps she was right. What a miserable time that was. Did we not have a healthy child any more? What would this mean for Billy and for us? One thing that would never change: he was Billy and we loved him. The three of us were the same three people but everything was suddenly very different. The experience was best described by Emily Perl Kingsley in her narrative 'Welcome to Holland'[1] when she compares it to planning a trip to Italy and you get diverted to Holland, a place you were never planning to visit.

Getting a diagnosis took a long time as Billy was so young; nowadays autism is diagnosed much earlier. He was almost three when we got a formal diagnosis by a community paediatrician, and I was six weeks pregnant with our second child. Our excitement over this expected new baby was also filled with worry as we had genetic counselling, but there were no answers, no special tests – just wait and see, and hope this time would be different, for all our sakes. It was a complicated pregnancy but Ellen arrived in December 1996, a wonderful Christmas gift.

Billy was now in a full-time special needs nursery, very nice but no real progress. He appeared to find the world around him such a confusing and frustrating place, but remained a sweet and loving little boy. We were determined to 'rescue' Billy and so began our journey. We read about 'Tomatis therapy', a programme of auditory stimulation over 30 two-hour sessions (the other end of the country though). Expensive, enjoyable, but it was not a cure for Billy. Then 'secretin therapy' at a clinic in London – not a cure either. We felt so helpless, but not resigned to just sit back and accept our destiny. At local support groups, the parents and carers were great but their children still had autism at 20. Our lives seemed to be mapped out.

In September 1997, we watched an episode of QED titled 'I want my little boy back'. Just a regular night in front of the TV became a life-changing experience. It was about the 'Son-Rise Programme' in Massachusetts, US. It was a very different way of teaching children with autism, more about reaching than teaching as we become the students of his world, going with him instead of against, hoping that he will become more and more motivated to explore and develop. All this takes place in a purpose-built playroom (our garage) with a team of volunteers led by parents, to work one on one with the child several hours a day. A loving and accepting attitude is the fundamental principle of Son-Rise, acceptance of ourselves as well as Billy's challenges. It was suggested that happiness is a choice; we can either give in to how difficult life is or turn it around in a practical way. After months of hospital visits all focusing on Billy's difficulties, at times it was hard to touch base with Billy for who he really was: our wonderful, cheeky son. The positive effect it had on the family on QED was what really touched us, and within days we were doing this really crazy thing and booking the trip. We were scared, excited, but just so relieved to be trying to do something to help him enter our world. The fundraising began – parachute jumps, marathons, endless raffles – but with family and friends we made it. Billy had his 5th birthday at the Options Institute, Massachusetts in June 1998 for a week-long therapy, us too. Ellen stayed home with family at only 18 months and it was a reminder of how we all took a back seat to Billy's needs; she was second child, not second best . . .

We returned home inspired and enthusiastic to work with our son. Our garage had been converted into the playroom, we had a team of volunteers and Jack had taken voluntary redundancy to lead the programme. We reversed our roles and I went back to nursing full time. Being a shift worker made it easier to fit work around our new lifestyle.

Then the seizures began. We were devastated, in total shock. By the time autism was diagnosed, we had worked it out anyway, but not this. How much more cruel could life get for our little man? There were practical issues as well as emotional ones. Billy was no longer able to go to the top of slides or/climbing frames, we couldn't leave him for a second in the bath or anywhere, we started taking the buggy with us everywhere 'just in case' and were too scared to take him swimming. It took us at least 12 months to get used to having that extra concern with us 24/7; we probably never really got used to epilepsy as it was ever-changing. You could no longer plan your life. Waiting times seemed endless when your child was suffering before your eyes. There were numerous medications and many, many hospital admissions. We had gotten used to the learning difficulties, but now we had a sick child. Just as Billy would respond to a drug, his seizures would take another form and we would have to start over. The drugs made him tired, the seizures made him tired. He would fall frequently and had bruises and bumps all over. All we could do in the moment of a seizure was hold his hand, talk to him and cry our silent tears.

Still we persevered in the playroom on the good days and at least we could work our programme around Billy; we had weekends and evenings unlike regular school. Good days were good, we greeted the autism gladly – to have him running around screeching, flapping and full of beans. We longed for the support of our Son-Rise mentors though, maintained in UK via telephone conference calls and sending videotapes of our playroom sessions to US. This wasn't a widely accepted mainstream way of doing things here, and was not without criticism from professionals, who told us 'not to aim too high', 'autism isn't curable'.

We decided to relocate to the US to be closer to our mentor, as his services weren't available in the UK. I was lucky enough to get a nurse travel contract, which would enable us all to live, and for me to work, in Miami, Florida, for a 20-month period. In hindsight, I think we wanted to be free from it all, from the constraints of socialised medicine, from a segregated education system for those with learning disability. A bonus was to find out we could access one of the world's leading paediatric neurologists at Miami Children's Hospital. We felt we had to grab this opportunity. Like most families, you would take your child to Mars if you thought it would help. As we toasted the millennium with champagne and looking forward to America, we could not imagine the storm looming. Billy went into status epilepticus, one seizure after another and had his first admission to PICU (Paediatric Intensive Care Unit), closely followed by a second admission.

All plans were cancelled.

Then, spurred on by thoughts of our American Dream, we sought a second opinion. This took a lot of courage although I don't know why. Billy responded to a different approach with his medication and there was only one admission for tests. With a treatment plan in place we left for the US in July 2000.

The move was pretty major for us but Billy just took it in his stride, enjoying the sunshine and the outdoor lifestyle immediately. He was probably the least phased-out of us all! Miami was just the craziest, vibrant place. We loved it and it became home. Twenty months turned into two years and then three. Billy learnt to swim! There were tears of joy as he had actually mastered something, what a big achievement for him. It wasn't reading or writing but we were very proud. He thrived in the warm sunshine, learnt to ride a bike, rollerblade, climb. All very slowly but steadily he managed. He had always hated the cold weather, and would just refuse to get out of his buggy. Our Saturdays had been brunch in Asda café, now he was walking the zoo or the beach. We were lucky enough to access a week at Island Dolphin Care, Key Largo, for dolphin therapy, which was incredible. After the first six months in Florida, when it was clear how much he loved the warm all around him, we scaled down our playroom sessions and actually sent him to the local mainstream school, where he had one-to-one teacher assistance. His Cuban teacher said she would show him she loved him first and then would teach him; it worked for all of us. Watching this amazing lady totally embrace her students, accepting where they were at, was a lesson in life for us, but it was no easy pushover. Soon she was getting Billy toilet trained, and he was sitting in class and contributing in his own way. Billy and Ellen were attending the same school. At age four she was way ahead of her brother academically but they ate lunch together, walked to class and it all seemed so 'normal' for the first time. The latin culture embraced us and we became part of 'la familia'. We were able to take Billy to dinner at restaurants, even to Disney World. He would act up sometimes but nobody really cared. It was a great feeling.

The epilepsy stayed with us of course, and was never easy, although for the most part he was kept out of the hospital. There always had to be a back-up plan in case he had a bad day, so that Ellen's disruption was kept to a minimum, but she really didn't know any different anyway. She got used to going to an event with just one parent or not at all. She never complained. Siblings of children with special needs are themselves so special . . .

Another special sibling, Rose, was born in May 2003, our family was complete. Billy had surgery to have a vagal nerve stimulator implant[2] soon after, which gave us a year of reduced seizures. This was a very special time for us, filled with happiness and wonderful memories. We had total acceptance of where we were at in life and similar dreams for the future as anyone else.

Sadly, this was all taken away so suddenly on 14 December 2004. Billy died as a result of SUDEP (Sudden Unexpected Death in Epilepsy). He was 11½. No explanation, no reason why now, after all he'd been through. Blind grief tore through our bodies. Our souls were sucked out. You now know what a broken heart feels like . . . but too painful to even begin to describe. We were alive but felt dead inside. How we managed to stand or just breathe I can't remember; just that it was incredibly hard to do or even care if you did. I do remember saying to a friend 'I can't' to which she replied 'you have to', and we did; we had our two little girls.

So we did. We slowly, very slowly, faced each day. I don't know how, but I do know why. The girls had lost their brother, their parents were broken and lost, but they would not lose them too. Days turned into weeks, into months; I can't remember so much except *pain*. The loss of a child physically hurts to your very core, to a place you never felt before. You never knew that place or that pain existed. You wish you didn't know now. You go through the motions of living not knowing if that person is really you. The girls still smiled at me and called me 'Mummy', so it must be me. I am still here.

I quit nursing for months, Jack had to go back to work after two weeks, numb and still reeling. It was exhausting even getting out of bed in the morning, to face another day without him. We had lost Billy. The centre of our family life, our core, was gone. His needs had been our focus for so long that now I struggled to even make a sandwich or change a nappy. This was a different way of life – different parenting that we weren't used to – parents instead of parent/caregivers. We missed him so much; we missed the way of life we used to wish we never had. If love could have saved him, he would have lived forever.

Ellen had been the youngest child, then the middle, was she now the eldest? She yearned to be one of three again, but only if Billy was one of them. One night she dreamt of her big brother, he was happy and smiling and talking in a deep voice. She said she now knew what his voice sounded like . . . I had a similar dream on the same night. He was free – from the pain of seizures, from the restrictions of this life.

The love for your child does not diminish, it is a continuing bond, just as it is with your children living. No less, no more. His life and love lives on within us. It does not fade. We threw ourselves into raising money for epilepsy treatment and research in a legacy to Billy; his struggle could not be in vain. A memorial charity gala in May 2006 raised over $100 000. Whoever expects to be doing such things for a child that's supposed to be alive? We attended a group for bereaved parents, seeking solace in total strangers but in whom we understood each other. Randomly chosen parents just like us that never expected to be in that room. What an awful club to be joining, but in our depths of despair it helped that we weren't alone. We soon saw, as new folk joined, that Billy wasn't alone either . . .

As Rose got older she inherited the loss; she wished she was a baby again so her brother would be here . . . Photographs and home video gave her the memories she was missing. Her love for her brother is as deep as all of ours (*see* Figure 13.1).

We moved back to the UK in March 2008, different in so many ways apart from the obvious. Being back with family and friends we had barely seen in years meant re-grieving for Billy all over. All the 'firsts' to do all over again with them. We had reluctantly got used to life in Miami without Billy present, and now we had to do the same in the UK. It was harder than we had imagined. Painfully, I get two Mother's Days now, the UK one and then the US one in May, as Rose was a Mother's Day baby, so will always be remembered as such. Life goes on though, tough as it is, and you learn to walk alongside and live alongside your grief. I have a job to do raising two beautiful daughters, for which I am truly grateful. I do believe that one day Billy will be in my arms once more. Until then I hold him close within me.

My son.

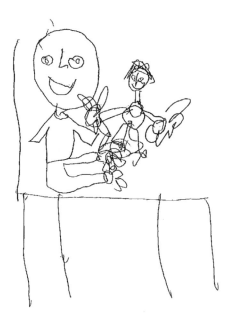

FIGURE 13.1 'I sat on Billy's lap when I was a baby before he died and went to heaven . . .' Rose, age 5

N.I.C.E. analysis

Please reflect on the issues raised in this chapter in relation to your own practice.

Needs

- Parents need choices and control over the situation.
- Parents need to feel their choices are accepted even if not supported by doctors.
- Think outside the box of conventional treatments.

Concerns

- It is difficult to go against advice.
- Fear of 'upsetting' professionals but it is 'my' child.
- Fear of seeking a second opinion.

From the above analysis please reflect on:

- The impact on the WHOLE family.
- Loss is experienced on many different levels.
- When your child with additional needs dies, you lose the only lifestyle you understand, as well as your child.

REFERENCES

1 www.our-kids.org/Archives/Holland.html
2 www.epilepsy.org.uk/info/vagal.html

SECTION 3

Minimising crisis points in paediatric palliative care

Susan Fowler-Kerry

With advances in medical science, technology and pharmacology we have created the opportunity for numbers of children with complex health needs to have significant increases in their life expectancy. These changes have contributed significantly to the long-term survival of a new cohort of children with life-limiting and life-threatening conditions who in a previous year would have died much earlier. What should be a good news story, however, has caused and will continue to cause serious strain on a healthcare system that has not planned nor kept stride with its own advancement. The result is the phenomena called 'transition care'. This section of the book provides a glimpse into the transition dilemma.

Governments must understand that an investment in children and their families represents a significant investment in the future productive capacity of society.[1] Children with palliative care needs should become our moral touchstone, and like all others must not be denied a fair chance at a standard of living that includes good education, protected environments, economic opportunity and healthcare that includes paediatric palliative care services.

As we attempt to move decision making in healthcare onto a firmer, more quantitative base, it is equally important to pay scrupulous attention to sources and truth. So perhaps the most important research question should be 'how do you know that?' Contained within each author's account is their answer to that very question, 'how do you know that?'

REFERENCE

1 Coffey C, McCain M. *Commission on Early Learning and Child Care for the City of Toronto: final report*. 2002. Available at: www.torontochildren.com (accessed 17 February 2010).

14

Pathways in palliative care

Rita Pfund

INTRODUCTION

A major framework to aid the development in palliative care of children and young people in the UK has been a series of pathways introduced by the Association for Children's Palliative Care (ACT) in 2004, 2007 and 2008.[1,2,3] A further pathway for neonates has also just been published by ACT (2009),[4] and is being adapted to local use through both Children's Palliative Care and Neonatal Regional Networks in the UK.[5] These pathways have been embraced in the UK strategy 'Better Care: Better Lives' (2008).[6]

In this section of the book we will look at the ACT Care Pathway[1,2,4] in greater detail. Ferguson (Chapter 15) will give a more theoretical overview of the background of working with pathways in the organisation of care, and also consider similar systematic frameworks available outside the UK. Wolff and Browne (Chapter 16) will give a very practical account how working with the ACT Care Pathway, adapted to local requirements[7] can make a real difference to the care families receive and the care teams are able to provide.

WORKING WITH THE ACT CARE PATHWAYS:[1,2] THE ACT CARE PATHWAY

The ACT Care Pathways provide the structure that enables healthcare professionals to meaningfully organise care for life-threatened and life-limited children and young people and their families. Some of the salient points are summarised below, but readers are strongly recommended to access the complete text.

Ladyman in Elston[1] explains that the ACT Care Pathways represents a pathway for engaging with the needs of the child and their family, which can be used to ensure that all the pieces of the jigsaw are in place, so that the family has access to the appropriate support at the appropriate time.

This document was written to complement the children's National Service Framework in the UK (NSF),[8] specifically guidance presented in the NSF Standard 8 on Disabled Children and Young People, and those with complex health needs.[8]

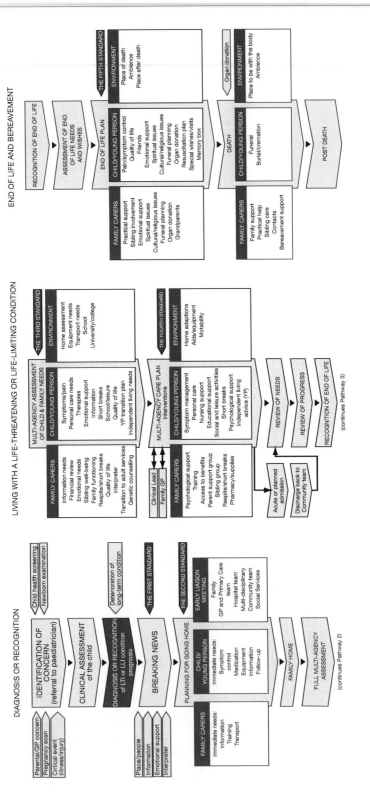

FIGURE 14.1 ACT Care Pathways

The ACT Care Pathway[1] has three stages (*see* Figure 14.1):

1   Pathway 1: diagnosis or recognition
2   Pathway 2: living with a life-threatening illness (LTI) or a life-limiting illness (LLI)
3   Pathway 3: end of life.

Five sentinel standards

Each stage begins with a key event of vital significance for the family.

The template sets out five sentinel standards along the pathway that should be developed as a minimum for all families, with the aim of achieving equity for all families wherever they live. The stages identify the weakest points for many families in their pattern of care. Elston[1] identifies them as the points at which there are frequently difficulties with communication and integrated working by professionals, and they are therefore key actions that should be given the highest priority. They include the following:

1   the prognosis – breaking bad news
2   transfer and liaison between hospital and community services
3   multidisciplinary assessment of needs
4   child and family care plan
5   end-of-life plan.

The template is intended to be a generic one for developing individual care packages, with the primary intention of providing the means for essential components that could underpin more detailed local pathways. Elston[1] emphasises that those at local level will need to develop their own pathway and delivery plans to take account of existing local services, available resources and geographical area.

Using the pathways to their full potential might include mapping where on the pathways individuals find themselves at any one time. Browne[9] states that this can be enlightening, as it is possible that the child, either parent or the professionals involved might not share the same perspective on this. This is illustrated by Friedrichsdorf *et al.* (Chapter 20) and Rooney (Chapter 3) on reflection on their case studies, but also by Brunton (Chapter 11):

> A prime example of this in my work comes at such times as there is a transition between curative and palliative care in a cancer setting, when survivorship is no longer an option. I have come across many parents who do not know that their child is dying.

TRANSITION PATHWAY

Chambers[10] explains that this pathway aims to facilitate the development of care pathways for young people with all types of LLI–LTI in all settings. It promotes equity of care.

Like the original pathway[1] it has three stages (*see* Figure 14.2):

➤   recognising the need to move on
➤   moving on
➤   end of life.

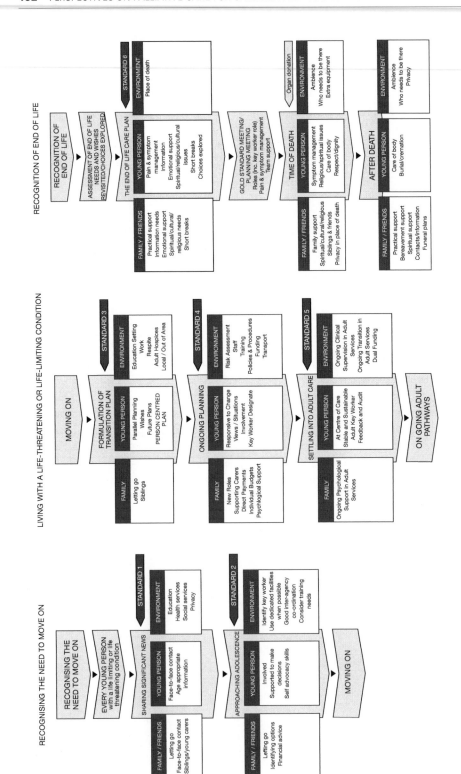

FIGURE 14.2 Transition Pathway

Six sentinel standards

1   sharing significant news
2   approaching adolescence
3   proactive planning
4   multi-agency care plan
5   multi-agency support
6   end-of-life care.

ACT[2] set out the principles for the development of Integrated Care Pathways (p. 9).

➤ They must be developed and 'owned' locally by a multidisciplinary team.
➤ They can cross organisational and inter-agency boundaries.
➤ They include a plan of anticipated care for an identified group.
➤ They make the patient the focus and allow for variation when appropriate.
➤ They incorporate evidence of research-based standards or guidelines.
➤ They include systems for rigorous record keeping.
➤ They include measurements of outcomes and promote continuous quality
   improvement.

A Pathway Assessment Tool[11] allows for audit of the process of care, and as evidence of good practice is being reviewed with parents as demonstrated by Gill (Chapter 9).

INTEGRATED CARE PATHWAYS[12]

In a wider context, integrated care pathways (ICPs) according to the Department for Education and Skills and the Department of Health 'are a tool and a concept that embed guidelines, protocols and locally agreed, evidence-based, patient-centred best practice into everyday use for the individual patient'.[11]

   An ICP aims to have the right people doing:

➤ the right things
➤ in the right order
➤ at the right time
➤ in the right place
➤ with the right outcome

all with attention to the patient experience.

CURRENT AWARENESS OF PATHWAYS

To stimulate a dialogue and to establish the current awareness of the pathways for this book we asked all our contributors about their understanding of pathways and how they work with pathways. The responses we received were revealing.

   Some parents were aware of the availability of pathways in the care of their children. One parent commented that:

> Care pathways should not be 'set in stone', there should be some allowance for
> flexibility within those pathways as needs can change and professionals should be

allowed to act upon those changes for the benefit of the families and not have to go 'back to the drawing board' and have to agree a new care plan before anything can be done to help the family.

This does not instil confidence that they are seen as a tool or help, rather they might be viewed as a hindrance.

A different parent interpreted the pathway in relation to the life path of his child: what do we see if we see a child with complex health needs?

The image of the child and family on this path, central to the entire field of palliative care for children and young people, has prompted us to examine the philosophical backbone of our interpretation of our role in relation to the children and young people we care for (*see* Chapter 10). This served as a stark reminder that it is the child and the family that has to be central to any policy, service or educational provision.

The story told by Brunton (*see* Chapter 11) of someone's daughter who had waited so long for a wheelchair that she had grown out of it before it was ever received is testament to how badly systems such as pathways are needed. This is not just to ensure that service provision stays on track, but also to remind professionals at the most fundamental level to award families the respect and dignity to have the tools to care for their children. It is also an audit tool at the commissioning level to serve as evidence that these tools are needed.

As we see in Chapter 16, where the pathway is followed through, it can work. However, the practical difficulties families encounter, highlight that we have not yet reached a state where this is possible across the board.

Brunton (*see* Chapter 11) tells us:

> Getting health care services to communicate with social care services is sometimes a huge problem, especially if a family has to deal with different local authorities. So many times it seems that no one wants to take the responsibility of paying for a service, they would rather pass the buck and this can mean that the families are waiting for support far longer than they should be.

Pathways provide explicit standards[12] which help to reduce unnecessary variations in patient care and outcomes. This is particularly important in a field that currently reports great variations of service provision. This is a phenomena explained by Rooney (*see* Chapter 3) in a UK context and also experienced globally.

Where pathways have been implemented successfully, as described by Wolff and Browne (*see* Chapter 16), they ensure coherent implementation of end-of-life plans. This might necessitate intricately involved arrangements that make it possible for individual children to be taken home or to their children's hospice in case of sudden collapse.

Revisiting the philosophy of ICPs Middleton *et al.*[13] define them as a multidisciplinary outline of anticipated care for patients with a similar diagnosis or set of symptoms. Whilst this is somewhat at odds with the spectrum of children and young people encountered in the field, the next items in the definition are more helpful.

➤ The ICP document specifies the interventions required for the patient to progress along the pathway.

➤ It places them against a timeframe measured in terms of hours, days, weeks or milestones.

➤ They are 'patient-focused' as they view the delivery of care in terms of the 'patient's journey'.

➤ They seek to improve both the coordination and the consistency of appropriate care – that is, what is suitable for each individual patient and in relation to the clinical evidence base and/or consensus of best practice.

➤ The ICP can act as the single record of care, which each member of the multidisciplinary team requires to record their input on the document.

As readers embark on this next section of the book, 'Minimising crisis points', and perhaps linger over the details provided in an 'end-of-life plan', and the 'wishes and choices' section within this (Chapter 16), we would like to remind you of a comment by Brunton (Chapter 11):

> . . . People who are assessing the care that is needed by an individual should listen to how they live their lives and work with them to find out what would make a differ-ence in their lives. Often the smallest things can make the biggest difference.

N.I.C.E. analysis

Please reflect on the issues raised in this chapter in relation to your own practice.

Needs

● To engage with pathways as integral elements of the palliative care strategy.

● To recognise the potential with which pathways can enhance the care of children, young people and their families.

● To customise and interpret pathways to local use.

Concerns

● Reluctance to engage with pathways.

● There are many different 'protocols' in place between paediatric and adult services.

Interests

● To share current experience with pathway across networks.

● To learn from each other's good practice.

● To avoid reinventing the wheel by sharing good practice, but retain the ability to customise pathways to local requirements.

Expectations

● Pathways serve as tools for service commissioning, and through this as tools to ensure families receive the best possible care wherever they live.

● Pathways serve as a tool for quality assurance and audit.

● The implementation of pathways will significantly improve care of children, young people and their families.

From the above analysis please reflect on:

● What progress is made in your area of care in relation to the implementation of pathways?
● What are the barriers to the implementation of the pathways and how are they being addressed?
● What are the views of children, young people and their families in relation to following a care pathway?

REFERENCES

1 Elston S. *Integrated Multi-agency Care Pathways for Children with Life-threatening and Life-limiting Conditions.* Bristol: ACT; 2004.
2 Association for Children's Palliative Care. *The Transition Care Pathway.* Bristol: ACT; 2007. Available at: www.act.org.uk/ (accessed 17 February 2010).
3 Association for Children's Palliative Care and Children's Hospices UK (2008) *A Practical Guide to Commissioning Children's Palliative Care Education and Training: planning and developing an effective and responsive workforce.* Draft consultation document. Bristol: Association for Children's Palliative Care; 2008.
4 Association for Children's Palliative Care. A neonatal pathway for babies with palliative care needs. Bristol: ACT. Available at: www.act.org.uk/ (accessed 1 March 2010).
5 East Midlands Children's Palliative Care Network. Neo-Natal Palliative Care Workshop. Leicester; 22 January 2010.
6 UK Department of Health *Better Care: Better Lives.* 2008. Available at: www.dh.gov.uk/en/Publicationsandstatistics/Publications/PublicationsPolicyAndGuidance/DH_083106 (accessed 1 March 2010).
7 Wolff T. *Nottingham Integrated Care Pathway for Children with Life-limiting and Life-threatening Conditions.* Nottingham: Nottingham University Hospitals; 2006.
8 NSF: all the documents for the National Service Framework for children can be accessed via the Department of Health website. Available at: www.dh.gov.uk/PolicyAndGuidance/HealthAndSocialCareTopics/ChildrenServices/ChildrenServicesInformation/ChildrenServicesInformationArticle/fs/en?CONTENT_ID=4089111&chk=U8Ecln (accessed 17 February 2010).
9 Pfund R. *Palliative Care Nursing of Children and Young People.* Oxford: Radcliffe Publishing; 2007.
10 Chambers L. ACT transition care pathway. Conference presentation. Cardiff, 18 April 2007. ACT UK Conference: Transition: Onwards and upwards?
11 www.act.org.uk/page.asp?section=114&search=Pathway+assessment+tool
12 UK Department for Education and Skills and the Department of Health. *Evidence to Inform the National Service Framework for Children, Young People and Maternity Services.* London: Department for Education and Skills and the Department of Health; 2005. p. 217.
13 Middleton S, Barnett J, Reeves D. What is an integrated pathway? *Evid Base Med.* Available at: www.medicine.ox.ac.uk/bandolier/painres/download/whatis/What_is_an_ICP.pdf (accessed 20 February 2010).

15

Use of clinical practice guidelines and critical pathways

Linda Ferguson

Janine Smyth, a new nursing graduate with six months of practice experience as a Registered Nurse on a large surgical unit, has recently moved to a small rural facility. She is a baccalaureate graduate with a strong emphasis on evidence-based practice and is challenged by the lack of educational resources available to her. In this new facility, she works with a nursing assistant and a care aide to provide care for 15 patients with a variety of nursing and medical needs. The nursing director of the facility is available to her on an on-call basis by telephone. She has come to rely on the Internet resources available to her via the nursing unit computer.

During a recent evening shift, she was notified that a 6-year-old child from the community was being admitted to the facility for palliative care. The physician told her that this child had been diagnosed with osteosarcoma, was palliative and was being admitted for assessment and treatment of uncontrolled pain. Her mother and grandmother, her primary caregivers, would be accompanying the child. Janine had no experience with children requiring palliative care, and limited experience with palliative care of adults. Janine immediately used the computer to seek clinical practice guidelines for the care of children in palliative care and the treatment of pain. She admitted the child, provided care guided by the clinical practice guidelines and engaged the mother and grandmother in the care of the child. Nonetheless she was not satisfied with the quality of care she was able to provide and consulted a more experienced colleague the next day.

EVIDENCE-BASED PRACTICE

An evidence-based approach to the care of patients is widely accepted as a practice norm. Evidence-based practice (EBP) was initially founded on the premise of the 'conscious, explicit, and judicious use of the current best evidence in making decisions about the care of individual patients,'[1] an exclusive focus on research evidence that has since been negated. EBP is achieved through the use of the best available evidence to support specific practices, applied with the judgement of the practitioner and consideration of patient preferences and values,[1-3] and available healthcare resources.[3] EBP is a widely accepted approach, and has many benefits for patient outcomes: yet there are a number of challenges associated with such a practice.

The nature of the evidence available to support practice is the first consideration, particularly in nursing. The hierarchy of evidence, reflecting the strength of that evidence, from the strongest to the weakest, privileges scientific evidence from tightly controlled clinical trials. Although we have some evidence at the strongest level, particularly in terms of drug trials, there is a limited amount of what is categorised as the gold standard in terms of palliative care, especially with children. Qualitative data concerning patient approaches and strategies for care have often been under-valued. In addition, individual practitioners often experience time constraints in finding and analysing high quality evidence. DiCenso *et al.*[3] identified a hierarchy of *preprocessed evidence* that provides strong bases for practice, including as the strongest form of evidence, *systems of evidence* such as practice guidelines, clinical pathway, and evidence-based textbooks. Synopses of systematic reviews, and single systematic reviews are also considered good sources of evidence for practice. This system of evidence, clinical practice guidelines, was the type that Janine accessed to prepare her for care of her newly admitted patient and family.

CLINICAL PRACTICE GUIDELINES

DiCenso *et al.*[3] defined clinical practice guidelines (CPGs) as 'systematically developed statements or recommendations to assist practitioner and patient decisions about appropriate healthcare for specific clinical circumstances. They [guidelines] present indications for proper management of specific clinical problems'. Clinical practice guidelines may be one of the most effective means of addressing variations in clinical practice and the difficulties of interpreting large volumes of scientific studies about particular care issues. CPGs are tools that can bridge the gap between published peer-reviewed scientific evidence and clinical decision making.[4] A Cochrane review demonstrated that the use of clinical practice guidelines did improve patient outcomes,[5] as did a systematic review of interventions to support research utilisation in practice.[6]

The development of clinical practice guidelines is dependent on the use of strong research evidence to support particular practices. Reviewers select original literature about research projects, or if possible, systematic reviews on the specified topic. Evidence-based recommendations are developed through committee consensus and consideration of clinical moderating factors, and then submitted for independent review. Following modifications as necessary, CPG recommendations are implemented and tested in specific clinical settings, finalised and ultimately implemented in a specific setting, jurisdiction or country. A review period is planned for the updating of the guidelines, based on more recent evidence. CPGs are often limited to specific geographical areas, to allow for differences in culture, baseline risks, preferences of certain individuals and local availability of interventions.[7]

CPGs are generally made available to the general healthcare professionals through repositories such as the 'National Guideline Clearinghouse' (www.guidelines.gov), sponsored by a US government department known as the Agency for Healthcare

Research and Quality. Another source of Best Practice or Clinical Practice Guidelines is the Registered Nurses Association of Ontario (www.rnao.org), a Canadian professional nursing association. The Association for Children's Palliative Care (ACT) provides documents in support of the care of children in palliative care (www.act.org.uk). The National Institute for Clinical Excellence (NICE) (www.nice.org.uk) in England also maintains a publicly available collection of guidelines, as does the New Zealand Guidelines Group (NZGG) (www.nzgg.org.nz). The Cochrane Library of the Cochrane Collaboration also makes systematic reviews available free of charge, often through health region computer systems or library systems (www.thecochranelibrary.org), or PubMed Clinical Queries (www.pubmed.gov). In addition, various professional associations or societies such as the American Academy of Pediatrics (www.aap.org) and the Association of Women's Health, Obstetric and Neonatal Nurses (AWHONN) (www.awhonn.org) also make clinical practice or best practice guidelines available to members and non-members.

The advantage of *preappraised* or *preprocessed* information such as is provided on all of these websites is that it has been peer-reviewed, evaluated, consolidated with other relevant evidence, synthesised and formulated into practice ready directives or technical reports that can be applied to individual patient situations.[8] Various consensus statements are also developed, using best available evidence and the opinions of experts, with feedback from interested parties. One such consensus statement was produced by the National Institute for Health State of the Science Conference on Improving End-of-Life Care.[9]

Specific CPGs may be particularly useful to those practitioners working with children and families in palliative care. CPGs for care of patients in palliative care[10] are available at the Institute for Clinical Systems Improvement or the National Guideline Clearinghouse (www.guidelines.gov). Palliative Care for Children Guidelines are available at the American Academy of Pediatrics website (www.aap.org). Guidelines for the assessment and management of pain and the management of cancer pain in adults and children are available through the RNAO (www.rnao.org). The Cochrane Library (www.thecochranelibrary.com) has several systematic reviews related to palliative care, including drugs for treatment of fatigue,[11] haloperidol for treatment of nausea and vomiting,[12] constipation in palliative care children[13] and medically assisted nutrition.[14]

In addition, a number of clinical practice guidelines related to paediatric palliative patients are also published in various journals: assessment and management of fatigue,[15] neurological symptoms,[16] pain management,[17] community-based care,[18] psychosocial and spiritual needs,[19] depression and anxiety,[20] gastrointestinal issues,[21] compassion fatigue in paediatric palliative care providers,[22] withdrawal of mechanical ventilation[23] and family support.[24] Guidelines for communicating with children and families are available from the American Academy of Pediatrics.[25]

Implementation of clinical practice guidelines requires more than the commitment of individual practitioners such as Janine in the above example. Implementing guidelines on an agency or jurisdiction basis requires forethought and planning.[26] The appropriate guideline must be selected for the setting, recognising the cultural, geographical, and population-specific practices that need to be acknowledged, and at times, modifications are necessary.

Stakeholders in the process, including practitioners, patients, families, administrators and in some cases, self-help or special interest groups, must be involved in the adaptation of guidelines, the plans for implementation, and the identification of outcomes and evaluation. The needs of all stakeholders must be addressed in the planning process, along with consideration of resources needed to implement the guidelines successfully. RNAO[26] identifies the process of assessing environmental readiness, the likelihood that the implementation at that time will be received and implemented as planned. With all these factors in mind, an implementation plan for a unit or agency must be devised, along with the plans for evaluation of the effectiveness of that implementation. This planning process can be lengthy and time consuming but may be the best alternative for effective implementation of evidence-based guidelines for practice.

CRITICAL PATHWAYS

Critical pathways, also called critical paths, clinical pathways and care paths are defined as 'management plans that display goals of patients and provide the sequence and time of actions necessary to achieve these goals'.[27] The intent of these pathways is to reduce variation in care, manage resource utilisation, and improve patient outcomes, thereby improving the quality of healthcare. Critical pathways are developed out of clinical practice guidelines and the evidence on which they are based, and can be viewed as a quality management tool. Well-developed clinical practice guidelines are a necessary condition to precede the development of critical pathways, a condition that may be lacking in many areas of practice.

In paediatric palliative care, the Association for Children's Palliative Care (ACT) has produced a critical pathway for the provision of care in palliative care settings.[28] This document identifies aspects of care to be highlighted at particular points in the child's illness, and identifies goals or outcomes of care. An assessment tool accompanies the critical pathway to determine how effectively goals have been attained.[29] The critical pathway is intended as a guide to action but also functions as a standard of practice against which practitioners can measure the care a patient has received. Areas for needed improvement become readily apparent.[3,8]

Use of clinical judgement in application

Janine was able to access and quickly read the American Academy of Pediatrics[30] statement on palliative care for children prior to admitting the child and her family to the nursing unit. She tried to incorporate the principles of care as she had read them but was dissatisfied with the outcome. She also felt the family, although very distressed and concerned for the child, was somewhat dissatisfied with care as well. She resolved to discuss the care of this child and her family with more experienced colleagues.

Although the CPGs provide general direction, application of the guidelines requires critical analysis and clinical judgement on the part of care providers.[31] As Janine discovered, CPGs provide an evidence-based approach to care, which may or may not be acceptable to the patient. In order to determine the appropriateness of the evidence to the patient's situation, the practitioner must understand the patient's circumstances and illness trajectory to determine the appropriateness of the evidence in the specific situation.[31] As Benner and Leonard[31] stated, 'expert clinical decision making is a much more nuanced and multidimensional process than the straightforward application of evidence' (p. 164) and reflects the difficulty of applying population-related research to individuals. To add complexity to the situation, every patient is different, with a different set of circumstances, medical history, personal relationships, hopes, dreams and aspirations, and thus, different patterns of responses. That the patient is a child increases the complexity and adds the patient's family as an integral part of the child's world. In addition, how the guidelines are applied, reflecting the practitioner's skill and experience, also influence patient response.

Clinical judgement is multi-faceted and develops through experience.[32] Clinical judgement includes practice or procedural knowledge, formal or declarative knowledge, holistic practice, saliency, skilled know-how, moral commitment to the well-being of the patient and knowledge of the patient.[32-35] As Carper[36] indicated, nurses have scientific knowledge, along with personal knowledge, aesthetic knowledge, and moral knowledge, all of which combine to constitute professional knowledge. Clinical judgement includes reasoning across time about the patient due to knowledge of the person, the condition, and of changes in the person or condition.[31] This professional skill develops through experience,[33,35] and reflection on patient outcomes and professional interventions that may not have achieved the desired outcomes. This reflection can be enhanced through interaction with and discussion with other more experienced and expert clinicians.[32,37]

Clinical judgement is the attribute of an expert practitioner that allows the practitioner to make reasoned decisions about the application of CPGs and critical pathways in ways that benefit the patient. In addition, in order to deviate rationally from CPGs and critical pathways, one must have the confidence in practice that comes through experience and the procedural and declarative knowledge one gains through experience.

CONCLUSION

In the scenario at the start of this chapter, a relatively inexperienced nurse applied clinical practice guidelines to the care of her clients. Her application of these guidelines likely reflected a direct application, a characteristic of one who does not yet possess the depth of practice knowledge or the experience with the specific patient or other patients like this child to adapt the guidelines in a more expert practitioner manner. Her recognition of the limited effectiveness of the guidelines in this situation would likely add to her practice knowledge for future patients. Additionally, as she gains more knowledge of the specific child and her family, her application of these guidelines would likely be more efficacious and beneficial to the patient. Nonetheless, this inexperienced nurse's use of the guidelines was admirable in the face of an unknown patient care situation, and reflects a commitment to EBP through the use of the CPGs.

N.I.C.E. analysis

Please reflect on the issues raised in this chapter in relation to your own practice.

Needs

- Developing skills in information access and processing.
- Supporting families in seeking the quality of care to meet the needs of their children.
- Developing competence in nursing informatics and computer use, to access online information.
- Well designed research in the area of paediatric palliative care, to thoroughly identify care concerns, needs and effective care strategies.
- Involvement of families in the decision making in the care of their children.
- Ensuring the development and availability of clinical practice guidelines and best practices.

Interests

- Ensuring that safe evidence-based care is available to children and their families.
- Encouraging experienced healthcare professionals to share their practice or experiential knowledge with newer practitioners.
- Create effective teams of professional healthcare providers, families and children as appropriate.
- Ensuring that values and beliefs of children and their families are incorporated into plans of care.
- Healthcare providers have the motivation and time to access clinical practice guidelines.
- The experiential knowledge of experienced healthcare providers is incorporated into care.

Concerns

- Availability of well-researched evidence to support practice.
- Difficulties in researching some of the aspects of care that contribute to the quality of care and satisfaction of children and their families.
- Evidence for practice may take precedence over children and their family's preferences.
- Difficulty in accessing good evidence and best practices.
- Outdated research evidence may be accessed.
- Practitioner's skill in assessing the credibility of the evidence.

Expectations

- All caregivers are committed to the well-being of children and families in palliative care.
- Caregivers seek best practices and best available evidence to support their practice decisions.
- Families, and where feasible, children are involved in determining appropriate courses of action.
- The values and beliefs of children and their families are foremost in the provision of culturally sensitive and appropriate care.
- Modifications in routines are necessary to meet children and family needs.

Action plan: next steps

- To ensure that best available evidence and best practices in palliative care are available publicly to caregivers, professionals and families.
- To ensure that children's palliative care teams share professional knowledge among team members and families.
- To support professionals in their determination to apply best evidence for practice with due consideration of family and children's needs and preferences.
- To support safe but holistic care for children and their families in paediatric palliative care.
- To support research endeavours that continue to develop the evidence to support caring effective and safe practice in paediatric palliative care.

REFERENCES

1 Sackett DL, Straus SE, Richardson WS, *et al. Evidence-based Medicine: how to practice and teach EBM.* London: Churchill Livingstone; 2000.

2 Muir Gray JA. *Evidence-based Healthcare.* New York: Churchill-Livingstone; 1997.

3 DiCenso A, Guyett G, Ciliska D. *Evidence-based Nursing: a guide to clinical practice.* Mosby: Elsevier; 2005.

4 Slutsky J. Using evidence-based practice guidelines: tools for improving practice. In: Melnyk BM, Fineout-Overholt E, editors. *Evidence-based Practice in Nursing and Healthcare.* Philadelphia, PA: Lippincott Williams and Wilkins; 2005.

5 Thomas LH, Cullum NA, McColl E, *et al.* Guidelines in professions allied to medicine. *Cochrane Database Syst Rev.* 1999; **1**(1): CD000349. 1: CD000349. (Reprinted 2009, Issue 1).

6 Grimshaw JM, Shirran L, Thomas R, *et al.* Changing provider behaviour: an overview of systematic reviews of interventions. *Medical Care.* 2001; **39**(8 Suppl. 2): PPII-2-II-45.

7 DiCenso A, Ciliska D, Dobbins M, *et al.* Moving from evidence to action: using clinical practice guidelines. In: DiCenso A, Guyett G, Ciliska D, editors. *Evidence-based Nursing: a guide to clinical practice.* Mosby: Elsevier; 2005.

8 Melnyk BM, Fineout-Overholt E. *Evidence-based Practice in Nursing and Healthcare.* Philadelphia, PA: Lippincott, Williams and Wilkins; 2005.

9 Improving End-of-Life Care. *NIH Consensus and State-of-the-Science Statements.* 2004; Dec 6–8: **21**(3):1–28.

10 Institute for Clinical Systems Improvement (ECSI). *Palliative Care (Clinical Practice Guidelines).* 2008. Available at: www.guidelines.gov (accessed 17 February 2010).

11 Radbruch L, Elsner F, Krumm N, *et al.* Drugs for the treatment of fatigue in palliative care (protocol). *Cochrane Database Syst Rev.* 2007; **4**: CD006788.

12 Perkins P, Dorman S. Haloperidol for treatment of nausea and vomiting in palliative care patients (protocol). *Cochrane Database Syst Rev.* 2006; **4**: CD006271.

13 Friedrichsdorf S, Wheeler DM, Collins JJ. Prevention and treatment for constipation in chronically ill children or children undergoing palliative care (protocol). *Cochrane Database Syst Rev.* 2005; **3**: CD005453.

14 Good P, Cavenagh J, Mather M, Ravenscroft P. Medically assisted nutrition for palliative care in adult patients (review). *Cochrane Database Syst Rev.* 2008; **4**: CD006274.

15 Ullrich CK, Mayer OH. Assessment and management of fatigue and dyspnea in pediatric palliative care. *Pediatr Clin N Am.* 2007; **54**: 735–56.

16 Wusthoff CJ, Shellhaas RA, Licht DJ. Management of common neurologic symptom in pediatric palliative care: seizures, agitation, and spasticity. *Pediatr Clin N Am.* 2007; **54**: 709–33.

17 Friedrichsdorf SJ, Kang TI. The management of pain in children with life-limiting illnesses. *Pediatr Clin N Am.* 2007; **54**: 645–72.

18 Carroll JM, Torkildson C, Winsness JS. Issues related to providing quality pediatric palliative care in the community. *Pediatr Clin N Am.* 2007; **54**: 813–27.

19 McSherry M, Kehoe K, Carroll JM, *et al.* Psychosocial and spiritual needs of children living with a life-limiting illness. *Pediatr Clin N Am.* 2007; **54**: 609–29.

20 Kersun LS, Shemesh E. Depression and anxiety in children at end of life. *Pediatr Clin N Am.* 2007; **54**: 691–708.

21 Santucci G, Mack JW. Common gastrointestinal symptoms in pediatric palliative care: nausea, vomiting, constipation, anorexia, cachexia. *Pediatr Clin N Am.* 2007; **54**: 673–89.

22 Rourke MT. Compassion fatigue in pediatric palliative care providers. *Pediatr Clin N Am.* 2007; **54**: 631–44.

23 Munson D. Withdrawal of mechanical ventilation in pediatric and neonatal intensive care units. *Pediatr Clin N Am.* 2007; **54**: 773–85.

24 Davidson JE, Powers K, Hedayat KM, *et al.* Clinical practice guidelines for support of the family in the patient-centred intensive care unit: American College of Critical Care Medicine Task Force 2004–2005. *Criti Care Med.* 2007; **35**(2): 605–22.

25 Levetown M, Committee on Bioethics of the American Academy of Pediatrics. Communicating with children and families: from everyday interactions to skill in conveying distressing information. *Pediatrics.* 2008; **121**: 1441–60. Available at: www.aap.org (accessed 17 February 2010).

26 Registered Nurses Association of Ontario (RNAO). Toolkit for implementation of guidelines. 2002. Available at: http://ltctoolkit.rnao.ca/ (accessed 17 February 2010).

27 Every NR, Hochman J, Becker R, *et al.* Committee on Acute Cardiac Care, Council of Clinical Cardiology, American Heart Association. Critical pathways: a review. *Circulation: Journal of the American Heart Association.* 2000; **101**: 461–5.

28 Association for Children's Palliative Care (ACT). *Act Integrated Palliative Care Pathways for Children and Young People with Life-threatening or Life-limiting Conditions and their Families.* Available at: www.act.org.uk (accessed 17 February 2010).

29 Ibid.

30 American Academy of Pediatrics. *Palliative Care for Children.* American Academy of Pediatrics; 2000. Available at: www.aap.org (accessed 17 February 2010).

31 Benner P, Leonard VW. Patient concerns, choices, and clinical judgment in evidence-based practice. In: Melnyk BM, Fineout-Overholt E, editors. *Evidence-based Practice in Nursing and Healthcare.* Philadelphia, PA: Lippincott, Williams and Wilkins; 2005.

32 Benner P, Tanner CA, Chesla CA. *Expertise in Nursing Practice: caring, clinical judgment, and ethics.* New York: Springer; 1996.

33 Higgs J, Bithell C. Professional expertise. In: Higgs J, Titchen A, editors. *Practice Knowledge and Expertise in the Health Professions.* Oxford: Butterworth Heinemann; 2001.

34 McCormack B, Titchen A. Patient-centred practice: an emerging focus for nursing expertise. In: Higgs J, Titchen A, editors. *Practice Knowledge and Expertise in the Health Professions.* Oxford: Butterworth Heinemann; 2001.

35 Higgs J, Titchen A. Framing professional practice: knowing and doing in context. In: Higgs

J, Titchen A, editors. *Professional Practice in Health, Education and the Creative Arts*. Oxford: Blackwell Science; 2001.

36 Carper BA. Fundamental patterns of knowing in nursing. *Adv Nurs Sci*. 1978; **1**(1): 13–23.

37 Boshuizen HPA, Schmidt HG. The development of clinical reasoning. In: Higgs J, Jones M, editors. *Clinical Reasoning in the Health Professions*. 2nd ed. Oxford: Butterworth Heinemann; 2000.

16

Minimising crisis points in paediatric palliative care: the ACT care pathways in action

Toni Wolff and Jackie Brown

INTRODUCTION

From the time of diagnosis of a life-limiting or life-threatening condition, through the variable length of time living with the condition until the death and bereavement, there will be many potential crises for the child and family.

Often the diagnosis is made in hospital, and without a robust discharge planning process including good communication with community professionals and prompt provision of equipment, drugs, oxygen, etc. a crisis is likely to occur as soon as the child gets home.

During the variable length of time the child is living with a life-limiting condition, which will be many years in some cases, there needs to be an appropriate and coordinated team of professionals around the child and family. Crisis prevention relies on a comprehensive and ongoing multi-agency assessment of all the current and anticipated needs of the child and family. From the assessment comes the multi-agency care plan, which is reviewed regularly, according to the rapidity of change of the child's condition and family circumstances.

This care planning process needs be coordinated by a lead professional and supported by a key worker, who may be one-and-the-same person.

The family must be fully involved in the care planning process and invited to all review meetings. Ideally the multi-agency care plan is family held, going with the child wherever he or she goes, i.e. school, short break unit, hospital or home.

Once the child comes to the end stages of a life-limiting condition the changing medical condition triggers the need for the care plan to include the personal resuscitation plan and the wishes and choices of the family regarding the death, according to their cultural, religious needs and preferences.

'End-of-life' or 'advanced care' planning requires a team approach with the care team working in partnership with the child and the family to ensure good care.

There are no clear rules apart from working together in the best interests of the child. Judgements on benefits of interventions versus burden to the child are subjective and rarely evidence-based. Professionals will have their own beliefs and opinions and it is therefore essential that they work as part of a team and in partnership with families to try to ensure that any influence they bring is as objective as possible.

Finally, despite the best laid plans and intentions, there will always be unforeseen emergencies. Whether or not these develop into a crisis depends on the resilience of the family and the capacity of the support team to respond swiftly and flexibly.

The following case scenarios will be used to illustrate good practice as recommended by the Association for Children's Palliative Care – Integrated Care Pathway,[1] and to consider issues with reference to the UK Department of Health strategy to improve children's palliative care, *Better Care: Better Lives*.[2]

NIDA'S STORY

Nida was born in hospital prematurely, at 35 weeks gestation. There had been no concerns during the pregnancy until her mother went into premature labour. However, when she was born Nida was very floppy and made little effort to breathe. She was intubated in the labour suite, transferred straight to the neonatal unit, and put on a ventilator.

On the neonatal unit Nida was found to have a rare metabolic disorder. She remained very floppy and did not suck, so she was tube fed.

She was weaned off the ventilator with difficulty but continued to require oxygen at 0.2 L/min to prevent respiratory distress.

Nida's mother and father were first cousins of Pakistani origin and Muslim faith. They had previously had a little boy who died at three months of age in Pakistan.

Mother spoke English well, but father's English was poor.

The medical team on the neonatal unit told the parents that Nida had a life-limiting metabolic condition and it was likely that she would die in the first months of life just as her sibling had done. Both parents were present and mother acted as interpreter for father. Nida's parents accepted what they had been told and her mother said she wanted to take Nida home for Ramadan which started in two days' time.

The neonatal team arranged for home oxygen and contacted the community nursing team.

Nida was home for three days and then had increased breathing difficulties because of a respiratory tract infection. Her mother called a 999 ambulance and Nida was taken to the paediatric emergency department.

Her neonatal notes were not available and the discharge summary had not been typed. She was admitted to the paediatric ward and intravenous antibiotics were commenced.

Mother wanted Nida to stay in hospital because she herself was exhausted because of the two-hourly tube feeds round the clock and frequent suction of respiratory secretions that Nida had been requiring.

Over the next few days Nida's respiratory symptoms worsened. She had extensive infection in both lungs. The consultant paediatrician spoke to her mother, who was living on the ward with her, and they agreed to give Nida a small dose of morphine as she was experiencing such respiratory distress. Nida died peacefully that night in her mother's arms.

Nida's father was angry. He said the morphine had killed Nida and he wanted to know why she had not been ventilated. She was ventilated at birth and he believed she should have had every possible medical intervention to try to keep her alive.

The parents subsequently separated.

USING THE ACT CARE PATHWAY[1] TO CARE FOR NIDA (ACT PATHWAY 1) (*SEE* FIGURE 14.1)
First standard
Breaking the news

> Every family should receive the disclosure of their child's prognosis in a face to face discussion in privacy and should be treated with respect, honesty and sensitivity.
> Information should be provided both for the child and the family in language that they can understand.[1]

The initial disclosure of a life-limiting condition often affects the way communication between the family and professionals continues. Disclosure must be honest, timely and sympathetic.

Each parent's support needs have to be considered individually and they often respond to the news differently. It should not be assumed that they will be able to support each other at such a difficult time.

Unless both parents speak English well an interpreter is needed. Because of the high emotional impact it is not advisable to rely on a family member, particularly not one of the parents to interpret for the other.

Parents should also be given information in writing as soon as possible (translated if necessary) with a contact phone number for further information and support if needed.

Issues
Training for doctors to give bad news is part of the core competencies of their training; however a doctor needs more than just knowledge of how to do it.

The doctor must have a high level of social communication skills and empathy, which enable him or her to give bad news at the appropriate pace and with the appropriate detail for people with different levels of understanding and emotional distress. These skills are very difficult for some individuals to acquire and this needs to be considered when junior doctors are being advised on their career path.

The national advanced communication skills training programme is available to senior practitioners through the regional cancer networks in the UK.[3]

The 'Right from the Start' template to support good practice in breaking news to parents is available on www.scope.org.uk/early years/rfts.php and further support with local audit, training and development of policies is also available from Scope.[4]

Even when skills and policies are in place, it is still very hard to provide a consistently high level of practice when breaking the news that a child has a life-limiting condition. The diagnosis is often made while the child is in a busy ward or neonatal unit where the senior paediatrician is also looking after all the acutely ill children and new emergencies. Yet he or she needs to arrange to meet with both parents and a support worker, sometimes plus an interpreter, in a place of calm and privacy for one or more hours without interruptions. There is likely to be the need for several meetings with the same senior clinician to discuss the child's medical needs and best care plan. Many hospital paediatric and neonatal departments have adopted a 'hot week' system that does allow the same paediatrician to dedicate themselves to the inpatient needs for up to seven days at a time.

There may be a problem with availability of interpreters particularly at short notice and for uncommon languages. An interpreter ideally needs at least 48 hours' notice and an idea of what will be said as they may need to prepare themselves.

The availability of written materials translated into other languages is very limited. However, it is often possible to get a particular piece of information, such as a written leaflet, translated or spoken on to a recording for people who do not read.

The Contact a Family directory[5] is a very useful source of contact details for specific support organisations and brief written information on disabilities and rare disorders of childhood (www.cafamily.org.uk).

Second standard
Planning for home

> Every child diagnosed in the hospital setting should have an agreed transfer plan involving hospital, community services and the family, and should be provided with the resources they require before leaving hospital.
>
> ACT 2004[1]

The transfer or discharge plan requires a comprehensive assessment of the needs of the child and family.

The hospital team will have a detailed understanding of the child's medical needs and likely future problems. This information needs to be clearly shared with parents, carers and the receiving community team, ideally in a face to face meeting and then with written care plans.

The equipment and facilities needed to care for the child at home must be considered in the light of what is available and practically do-able by the family. This is likely to require a home assessment visit by an appropriately trained professional. A community children's nurse will be able to assess the facilities for nursing procedures and a paediatric occupational therapist will consider equipment and housing issues.

A safe and comfortable way of transporting the child home is often forgotten until the last moment.

Issues

All of this planning and training of carers takes time. Yet delay must be avoided. Everyone wants the child home as soon as possible, not only to give the child and family the best quality of life, but also to avoid inappropriate use of an acute hospital bed. However, if support is not in place there is a strong risk of the child bouncing straight back into hospital again in a crisis.

More than one parent/carer needs to be trained and assessed as competent in all the child's care needs before discharge. This can be provided by nurses on the ward. However, a senior and experienced clinician should consider the child's whole care programme in the light of the family circumstances. Hourly suction of respiratory secretions and two-hourly nasogastric tube feeds may be doable in hospital supported by a team of nurses on shifts, but is not sustainable by two parents, particularly if either needs to go to work.

The hospital team has to lead on discharge planning but often there is no specific person in the hospital team with the skills, experience, authority or time in their job plan to do it. The child's named ward nurse or even the hospital consultant will have had limited experience of discharge planning for a child with a life-limiting condition particularly if there are complex health needs. This person needs to be able to coordinate the assessments, reports, and care plans working in partnership with and advocating for the family. They need knowledge of the wide network of community professionals and how to contact people quickly. They also need clerical support to invite professionals to the discharge planning meetings, produce minutes and care plans and distribute them.

Getting all the appropriate professionals around the table at the same time is very difficult particularly at short notice. Generally the only way to get senior paediatricians from hospital and community to a meeting table together quickly is for them to agree to a meeting time between themselves by telephone.

In summary, all paediatric inpatient units need a specifically identified professional whose job it is to coordinate the discharge planning of all the children with complex needs and/or life-limiting conditions from that unit.

ALTERNATIVE SCENARIO FOR NIDA

The children's community nursing team had an Asian link worker/family support worker. She was contacted as soon as the neonatal team realised that Nida was likely to have long-term disability or a life-limiting condition. She spoke several Asian languages. She met both of Nida's parents and accompanied them when the disclosure of Nida's metabolic condition was made. She acted as interpreter and also provided emotional support. She subsequently took on the key worker role and arranged the discharge planning meeting. She continued proactive contact, visiting the home within 48 hours of hospital discharge.

At the discharge planning meeting Nida's mother said she wanted to take her home for Ramadan in two days' time. However, it was clear that Nida needed two-hourly tube feeds throughout the day and night, as well as frequent suction of her mouth and throat, plus continuous oxygen. Her problems were likely to worsen over time.

Her father had not learned to feed her and there was no extended family support. Clearly the parents were not going to cope for long without a short break or continuing care service.

The community nursing team ordered the oxygen concentrator, oxygen saturation monitor and suction machine for home. All were available promptly. Because she had a life-limiting condition Nida was able to be 'fast tracked' through the assessment process to access a continuing care service which offered care in the home.

The neonatal consultant liaised with the community paediatrician to ensure Nida's medical care was continuous. They met together with the parents and the Asian link nurse acting as interpreter as well as advocate to agree the emergency care plan and personal resuscitation plan. Potential emergencies, particularly the likelihood of respiratory infections, were discussed, plus the choices of interventions and who would be available to support the family depending on whether they wanted to stay home or come into hospital. The parents' different beliefs and wishes for Nida were explored with support from their local Muslim imam. The lead paediatrician was identified as the community paediatrician who took the responsibility of the medical care plan from the point of discharge.

Nida went home with a comprehensive written care plan including emergency/personal resuscitation plan. There was a parent-held copy and copies were faxed to all professionals who would potentially be involved in supporting her including the general practitioner, the 'out of hours' medical service and the paramedic ambulance service. A copy was also kept in the local paediatric emergency department.

Because all equipment, information, support and care plans were in place promptly Nida was able to go home and stay home even as she deteriorated.

JAMES' STORY

James presented with a wobbly gait and frequent seizures when he was three years old. A diagnosis of Batten's disease was made by the paediatric neurologist and the anticonvulsant medication that he was given helped control the seizures.

He is now four years old. He has been managing in mainstream nursery with the support of the physiotherapist and is about to start mainstream school. However, he is losing his speech and has choked a few times while eating. Education staff in nursery have spoken to the staff in the proposed primary school and they say they can't take James because of the risks of choking and seizures and he will have to go to a special school where there will be nursing support on site.

James' school placement will be delayed by the special educational needs assessment (SEN) process and paperwork which will take at least six months.

James' mother is exhausted. James is having seizures in the night and he needs constant supervision. She is a single mother and she has three other children. A social worker has been trying to visit but contact has not been successful.

CARING FOR JAMES WITH ACT PATHWAY 2[1] (*SEE* FIGURE 14.2)
Third Standard

> Every family should receive a comprehensive multi agency assessment of their needs as soon as possible after diagnosis or recognition, and should have their needs reviewed at appropriate intervals.[1]

Fourth Standard

> Every child and family should have a multi agency care plan agreed with them for the delivery of coordinated care and support to meet their individual needs. A key worker to assist with this should be identified and agreed with the family.[1]

Feedback from parents with disabled children and children with additional health needs has long highlighted the issue of numerous appointments with many different professionals who don't share information and the need for coordinated multi-agency assessment and support in partnership with parents.

The Vision in *Better Care: Better Lives*[2] includes 'an early, inclusive, joint (health and social care) assessment of need' and 'care that is planned and delivered in full consultation and partnership between the child and family, and service providers.'

The ACT Care Pathway[1] and *Better Care: Better Lives*[2] both suggest a key worker/ lead professional will be responsible for ensuring joined up and coordinated service provision for children with life-limiting and life-threatening conditions.

The National Service Framework for Children (Standard 8) requires English local authorities and NHS trusts to ensure that families caring for a disabled child with high levels of need have a key worker/care manager to oversee and manage the delivery of services from all agencies involved in the care and support of the child and family and to ensure that the family has access to appropriate services.[6]

Issues

But what is a key worker/lead professional and how do you get one? And how can they ensure a holistic multi-agency approach in partnership with parents?

Multi-agency assessment

Most life-limiting conditions of children will be identified by a health team often in a hospital setting. The prompt and holistic assessment of health and social care needs of the child and family requires there to be an immediately available multi-agency team, who know and trust each other's opinions, meet together regularly to discuss shared cases and use the same paperwork.

In many parts of the country children's social workers have been moved out of their previous hospital bases. The social care element in specialist teams for various life-limiting conditions of children is often provided by a charity-funded family support worker. The funding for these posts is not secure and is inequitable.

When there is no family support worker in the team, one of the health professionals will need to start a CAF (see below)[7] to gather the information required to enable a referral to a specialist social care team. The paperwork for this feels like cumbersome bureaucracy to specialist health professionals who will not have had the training or the additional time to complete such an exercise when it seems perfectly obvious that the child will need a full core assessment from social services.

The Common Assessment Framework (CAF)[7] is an assessment tool which professionals working in children's services should be using to identify and record the additional needs of a child and family in a systematic way. The idea is that this will help to ensure that all the needs of the family including siblings will be considered and that the same information in a common language will provide the information required to support appropriate referral to all the support agencies that the family needs.

It will usually be a professional in universal children's services such as a health visitor or teacher who will begin a CAF[7] with the family's permission once they perceive the child and family are going to need multi-agency support.

In the case of a child with a life-limiting condition that already has a key worker it will be the key worker who starts the CAF to gather the information required for a referral to specialist teams in other agencies, particularly social services.

The Children Act 2004 (Section 10)[8] gives local authorities a duty to improve the well-being of all children in their area, particularly considering the five *Every Child Matters*[9] outcomes. The associated guidance says that all local authorities should implement the CAF to support coordinated working by 2008 and most local authorities have invested in CAF trainers and implementation programmes.

Multi-agency support

For a disabled child with a life-limiting condition in England, the Early Support programme is the UK government recommended system to provide family-centred, coordinated support.

The Early Support materials are free to any family with a disabled child in England. They give information on both general disability and specific conditions and include the family file which helps families share information about their child, lists the professionals involved and helps develop and hold the multi-agency care plan.

The programme requires a 'team around the child' approach with families having a chosen lead professional and/or key worker, and the system also supports key worker training.

The Early Support definition of key worker is taken from Care Coordination Network UK (CCNUK) key worker standards 2004.[10]

The role of the key worker is defined as:
1 providing information
2 identifying and assessing the needs of all the family members
3 providing emotional and practical support
4 assisting families in their dealing with agencies and acting as an advocate if required.

However, CCNUK[10] takes the position that all disabled children with complex health needs will need a key worker service which will also include the role and function of the lead professional.

The lead professional role is defined as:

1 act as a single point of contact
2 coordinate the delivery of actions agreed by the practitioners involved
3 reduce overlap and inconsistency in services.

www.everychildmatters.gov.uk[9] also stipulates that:

> Lead professionals need the knowledge, competence and confidence to:
> a Develop a successful relationship with the child and family and communicate without jargon.
> b Organise meetings and discussions with different practitioners.
> c Use the common assessment framework and develop support plans based on outcomes.
> d Coordinate the delivery of effective early intervention work and ongoing support.
> e Work in partnership with other practitioners to deliver the support plan.

The key worker mentioned in the ACT Care Pathway[1] and Better Care: Better Lives[2] does indeed seem to encompass this fuller key working role; being responsible for ensuring joined-up and coordinated service provision whilst also providing proactive practical and emotional support.

Key workers can be designated or non-designated

A designated key worker is employed and paid specifically to carry out the key working role for a number of families. A non-designated key worker is one of the professionals already working in the team around the child who agrees to undertake the key working role in addition to the professional role in which they are already employed. Whilst there are a few designated key worker services in the UK, currently it is usually the case that a family with a child with a life-limiting condition will have a non-designated key worker, if they have a key worker at all.

Not surprisingly, professionals have been reluctant to agree to take on the key working role without additional resources and training. Therapists in particular often see this as a nursing role, and indeed it is often the child's community nurse who will act as key worker. However, many children with life-limiting conditions have no community nurse involved in their care until the very end stages of the condition.

It is also not always appropriate for one person to take on all the coordination responsibilities. It may in fact be more appropriate for one member of the team around the child to visit proactively to provide practical and emotional support, i.e. the 'key worker' role whilst another professional ideally who has clerical support and sufficient authority calls the multi-agency meetings (in liaison with the key worker and family) and monitors the multi-agency action plan, i.e. the lead professional role.[11]

Implementation of early support

The Early Support programme[12] was launched in 2004 for children with disabling conditions aged 0–5 years, but its implementation across England has been patchy and slow. The provision of regional Early Support coordinators and further promotion of the process with recommendation of its use for disabled children and young people up to 19 years of age under Aiming High for Disabled Children 2008,[13] has given a boost to wider implementation. However, it is still far from being universally used in England, even with preschool children.

The statutory requirements for 'special educational needs' reviews and 'Looked after child' (LAC) reviews continue to lead to a school-aged child with a life-limiting condition having lots of reviews by separate agencies with separate agendas, time scales and paperwork.

In summary, the CAF, the Early Support programme, lead professional (and key worker systems) are all promoted as solutions to the problem of providing coordinated multi-agency working, but the implementation of each is patchy across the UK. Even when a local area is implementing all of them, there is often confusion about how they work together.

ALTERNATIVE SCENARIO FOR JAMES

As soon as it was clear that James had ongoing disability, even before his specific diagnosis was made, his health visitor recognised the need for multi-agency working to support this family. With his mother's permission she began an assessment of need using the CAF tool. She took on the role of lead professional to call regular multi-agency planning meetings and introduced the Early Support programme providing James' mother with the family file and information pack.

At the first multi-agency coordination meeting it was clear that James and his family were going to need emotional and practical support as well as coordination of services. James' mother chose the community children's nurse to be the ongoing key worker. She had been there when the neurologist told her the diagnosis and was visiting the home regularly to give information and emotional support regarding Batten's disease and the seizures.

As soon as the feeding problems began the key worker liaised with the paediatric neurologist and arranged a referral to the speech and language therapist. She brought forward the date of the next multi-agency planning meeting in nursery. Those professionals already involved attended as well as the mother. The social worker was invited with the mother's permission. The information already available on the CAF and in the Early Support family file informed the subsequent core assessment and provision of a short break service. The speech therapist's assessment showed that James had a safe swallow as long as fluids were thickened. The meeting resulted in a written multi-agency care plan, including emergency care plans regarding seizures and feeding.

School staff had training from the children's community nurse regarding James' seizures. The clear description of James' needs and detailed care plan supported the application for funding for additional teaching assistant support in mainstream school through the local education department special educational needs budget. James moved up into mainstream school successfully.

James' changing needs would continue to be monitored and planned for by regular multi-agency planning meetings every six months or every school term depending on the rapidity of his decline.

MARY'S STORY

Mary was a five-year-old girl with very severe neurodisability following birth asphyxia. She had severe spastic quadriplegia, epilepsy and cortical visual impairment. She had an unsafe swallow and was totally gastrostomy fed. She recognised familiar voices and smiled, but she had little head control.

In the first two years of life Mary was frequently admitted to hospital with seizures and chest infections and was ventilated on the paediatric intensive care unit on two occasions. Then for two years she had been relatively well with fewer seizures and fewer chest infections.

She had devoted care from her parents who gave her chest physiotherapy and suction of her mouth and throat several times per day. They had been reluctant to let anyone else care for Mary, but she had recently started to attend special school and she was also starting to have a home-based short-break service.

However, for the past nine months she had been having increasingly frequent and prolonged chest infections and had been admitted to hospital for two or three week periods every six to eight weeks. Her cough was weak, and one of her lungs was not clearing in between infections. She had been prescribed home oxygen and prophylactic antibiotics.

During one of her most recent admissions Mary's clinical condition during her chest infection led to the medical team on call liaising with the paediatric intensive care unit team, but she was not ventilated. 'Intensive care should be avoided' was written in the notes.

Mary's parents knew that these were life-threatening chest infections, and that Mary's quality of life was now much poorer. She was spending more and more time in hospital and they knew she suffered when doctors struggled to resite the intravenous infusion into her veins, but they wanted her to be given every chance to pull through each episode.

They saw different doctors in the emergency department and on the ward each time she was admitted to hospital and each time they discussed the best plan of care for that particular episode, but they did not want to discuss the possibility of limiting the intervention in any way. She had been seen in the paediatric respiratory clinic but her regular outpatient follow-up was with a community paediatrician who had known her since she was a baby.

Mary was admitted to hospital with a chest infection. Initially she seemed to be responding to the intravenous antibiotics, but then one evening, without warning, she had a sudden cardio/respiratory arrest. As she saw the heart rate drop on the monitor the nurse called the emergency medical team and cardiopulmonary resuscitation was started. She responded initially and was being taken round to the paediatric intensive care unit, but arrested again on the way and this time resuscitation was unsuccessful. Both parents were resident in the hospital and present throughout these events. They were, of course, very shocked and distressed.

Mary was taken into a cubicle on the paediatric intensive care unit (PICU). The nurse from the children's ward was still with her and was also very distressed as she had known Mary for many years. Because she was so upset, it was the PICU staff that helped the parents wash and dress Mary. Mary was then taken down to the mortuary and the parents collected their belongings from the ward. They were shocked and angry and barely spoke to the nurses on the ward who were also upset.

Mary's parents didn't want to return to the hospital the next day so the community nurse collected the death certificate and took it out to them. They visited Mary's body on several occasions before the funeral but did not come back up to the ward. They refused all offers of contact from nursing staff, bereavement team and paediatrician. They subsequently sent a formal complaint that Mary had not been given appropriate care in her last illness. They particularly felt that she should have had intravenous antibiotics sooner, and been transferred to the intensive care unit for ventilatory support.

The nurse who had been with Mary when she arrested was off sick with stress for six weeks.

CARING FOR MARY USING THE ACT CARE PATHWAY 3[1]
(*SEE* FIGURE 14.3)
Standard 5

> Every child and family should be helped to decide on an end of life plan and should be provided with care and support to achieve this as closely as possible.[1]

Recognising the end of life

Mary had severe neurodisability and was having life-threatening episodes which could not be successfully prevented or cured by medical interventions (ACT group 4).[14]

It was recognised by her medical team and her parents that Mary was likely to die, but to her parents the thought of losing her was too awful to contemplate.

Discussion

The need for an emergency medical care plan including the personal resuscitation plan can be a way to start the process of end-of-life planning.

1 Shortly after an acute life-threatening event, families are eager to talk about what happened with their medical team and make a clear plan of what to do if it happens again.

2 A change in condition, particularly a deterioration, can trigger a discussion of where things are going and what is likely to happen next, including the possibility of sudden life-threatening events.

3 The current care plan needs to be reviewed and the new care plan can incorporate the emergency care plan, and the personal resuscitation plan.

4 The death of another child with a similar condition may prompt a family to consider their wishes and choices for the death of their own child.

5 Transitions to new places of care such as nursery, school, short break unit or when the child or young person may be left in the care of a non-family member at home, raises the need for an agreed, written and universally appropriate emergency care plan including personal resuscitation plan.

In each of the above situations the care team can approach the family to suggest making a plan jointly so that everyone knows what to do in a potential emergency, so that the most appropriate care is given to their child.

The process of drawing up the plan

The process of drawing up the plan can be lengthy or short depending on whether both parents and the lead paediatrician are of the same opinion about the most appropriate care.

The discussions need to take place in privacy and where the parents feel comfortable, confident and unhurried.

The first meeting may lead to a complete plan that all are satisfied, describes fully the best care for the child or may lead to a draft for further consideration and discussion.

Staff at school or short break unit will need to be consulted about the practicalities of delivering the most appropriate care when the child is away from home.

The availability of out of hours support needs to be considered.

Who should be present?

Ideally both parents would be present to discuss the plan, but this is not always practically possible and one of the parents may take a draft plan away to discuss with the other. It will often be appropriate to incorporate the views and preferences of an older child, but initially parents will find it difficult to talk in front of the child and are likely to want to introduce the topic themselves after their discussions about the likely future scenarios and the options available to them as a family.

The doctor brings medical knowledge and experience of other similar cases, and/ or knowledge of the current medical literature. Knowledge of that particular child's medical problems and previous medical history is essential, and therefore it is most appropriate for the child's lead paediatrician to provide the medical input. Ideally he or she has known the child and family for some time and therefore from the family perspective, he or she can have a clearly valid and trusted opinion on what medical care is appropriate and in the child's best interests. The doctor will have his or her own cultural and religious beliefs and must consider how much these are influencing their judgment. It is important that the doctor works in a team, sharing their views with colleagues.

The parents bring knowledge of their child and their perception of the child's quality of life plus awareness of their particular practical circumstances, cultural needs, aspirations, wishes and choices.

Usually it is helpful for one other person who knows the child and family well to also be present. This will often be the community children's nurse, special school nurse or family support worker. Ideally they will have a detailed knowledge and understanding of the family circumstances and culture and be able to provide long-term emotional and practical support. This person may be needed to act as advocate for the parents. They may be able to contribute to the discussion regarding potential support available outside hospital and outside usual working hours.

The discussion

The doctor will be coming to the discussion with a view on what he or she believes is the most appropriate medical care for the child, however it is vital that he or she is highly sensitive to and genuinely values the parents' perceptions of their child's needs and quality of life and their expectations.

The first thing the doctor needs to do is to find out where the parents are in their own minds; what is their understanding of the situation and plans for the future?

You have to start on the same page!

Then the doctor needs to share with the parents the current medical situation and their predictions of what the future medical problems will be, particularly regarding potential life-threatening events and the pros and cons of different possible interventions.

It is essential that the paediatrician is honest about their level of expertise and ready to seek more expert opinions from others when necessary, for example a respiratory paediatrician, or paediatric intensive care specialist.

Families may fear that their child will be denied interventions because of their disability and that the medical professionals may be protecting resources for other children who they may value more highly.

It is the doctor's role in this situation to help make the best plan of care for their patient, this child or young person; he or she is not protecting resources, but considering always the best interests of the child before them. On the other hand a doctor cannot guarantee that a ventilator will always be available and appropriate. It is best to say invasive ventilation 'would not be appropriate' or 'may be appropriate'.

The medical care plan cannot be considered in isolation. The child and family's wishes regarding place of death will be highly relevant. The services available to support the family outside hospital have to be discussed in detail and honestly. The family's views regarding post mortem examination, organ donation, care of the body after death and funeral plans need to be considered (*see* 'The Wishes and Choices checklist' on p. 221 and Figure 16.2).

Talking to young person themselves

The views and wishes of the young person themselves must be included if they can be ascertained. As already mentioned, the parents are likely to have views on the best way to approach the child and may want to lead the discussion themselves with or without the medical team. It may be helpful to agree the phrases to be used with the child/ young person with the parents in advance such as:

➤ When you're ill next time what do you want to happen?
➤ Do you want to come in to hospital or stay home?
➤ Who do you want to look after you?

Documenting discussions – family-held care plans

As already mentioned, elements of the 'end-of-life plan' are often documented in different places, e.g. the medical case notes, DNAR [Do not resuscitate] forms, community nurse records.

Ideally the whole picture can be incorporated into a single family-held plan which will be followed wherever the child is, whether at home, hospital, short break unit or school.

In England, young children with severe disability should have the Early Support materials blue family file.[12] This blue family file should always be with the child and should already contain the list of professionals involved, medication and equipment, therapy programmes and intervention targets. Thus the ideal place for the emergency care plan/personal resuscitation plan for a disabled child is at the front of this family file. It should go with the child into school and short break service, and in an emergency, into hospital.

The family may also be willing for a copy of the 'wishes and choices' to be in the file or they may prefer to keep it more privately until needed.

The value of a template

The documentation needs to be easily found and clearly recognisable to all carers and professionals who might be involved in that child's care in a gradual or sudden deterioration.

Examples of templates used in Nottingham are shown at the end of this chapter.

The personal resuscitation plan

At the beginning of the personal resuscitation plan (*see* Figure 16.1), there needs to be an introductory statement to put the plan in context such as the child's diagnosis and that they are in the late stages of a life-limiting condition.

The particular signs that indicate that the child or young person is deteriorating need to be described in detail. This is often very specific to the individual child and is often best recorded in the parents' own words.

The required interventions need to be very clearly and unambiguously stated so that medical and non-medical people know exactly what to do. Ideally these will be selected from a prewritten list of set phrases which are clear but in a language that conveys respect and is acceptable to families. This also avoids interventions being recommended which are not always practically achievable, such as 'bag and mask until parents arrive'.

Any system for documentation of 'end-of-life plans' needs to incorporate a system for the plans to change over time as the child's condition changes and the choices of the family change. It is therefore vital that the plans are not photocopied and that the distribution list for the plan is an integral part of the plan itself.

The Wishes and Choices checklist

For many families, although their head acknowledges that one day their child is going to die, their heart does not always allow them to explore this in depth – it is often their way of coping and we do not have the right to take 'hope' away, although we should never give false hope. However, it is important that families are aware that throughout the end stages of their child's illness, or earlier if they wish, the opportunity will be offered to discuss and document any of their wishes, choices, fears or worries and that when and if they feel it would be helpful, it can be arranged at any time. Documenting these thoughts and wishes ensures that everyone knows what has already been discussed with the family, making sure they will not be asked by 20 different people the same difficult questions, over and over again at each contact.

The Wishes and Choices checklist is a tool to support and document very difficult discussions. The professional, often the key worker, approaching these issues must be known and trusted by the family. Some parents will only want to discuss one or two aspects or choices, whilst another family will want to have everything planned in great detail early on in their child's illness. The professional must be highly sensitive to the family's feelings and be able to stop and re-visit the issues as often as is necessary.

The tool documents what each family member understands about the child's illness, including the child themselves and any siblings. It can be used alongside other resources and workbooks such as 'Beyond the Rainbow', which helps children share their thoughts and feelings about the illness they or their sibling have.

This will help professionals avoid making the wrong assumptions or disclosing something unintentionally, but it can also help pick up and give the opportunity to put right any misunderstandings or misconceptions. It can be updated as the child's condition and understanding changes. It documents what has already been put in place, such as a personal resuscitation plan and ambulance notification, etc. It considers the emotional support needs of the family documenting who is already involved but also suggesting other local resources.

Practical support issues are also considered such as financial, transport, housing and who is taking the lead in helping the family with these issues, which might get in the way of the family enjoying the precious time they have together. The document then goes on to look at the choices the family have around the child's death. These will need revisiting as the family's wishes and ability to discuss these choices change, possibly as their child's condition deteriorates. Many families do not want to consider their child's death – sometimes in the belief that if it is spoken out loud it will make it happen. Families should never be forced to look at these issues and need to be reassured that their feelings are entirely natural, but for some families considering these choices earlier and making everyone aware of them, allows them to be put to one side so that they can enjoy the time they have together.

It is also important to acknowledge that although something has been written down it is not 'set in stone'; the documentation is only there as a means to communicate the family's thoughts at the time. Events around the child's death may cause these thoughts to change.

The child's own wishes should be taken into account and included whenever possible and at no time should the family be offered something that is not practicable.

The document can be very empowering for families, knowing it is there 'just in case' and also helps to look at building memories and keepsakes whilst the child is still alive. The whole family may want to do their hand and footprints together, choosing their own colours, etc., making a mess together. Families can record their memories and create a life book. How much nicer to share their memories with the child who is dying rather than afterwards, and it allows the child's own memories to be included.

The form also looks at issues such as organ and tissue donation and post mortems. These are very difficult areas to discuss whilst the child is still alive, but often allow a limited time scale for decision making if they are not considered until after death. It encourages the family to be proactive. So often they are not asked about these things, with the intention of protecting the family from painful thoughts; however if we do not ask we have effectively made the decision for them, disempowering them. It is far better for them to say 'no thank you' than to hear them say later 'if only I had been asked'.

It is important to clarify with the donor coordinator beforehand whether any tissues could be used after death, including donation for research purposes, as again this ensures families are not offered something that is not actually possible. The practicalities also need to be considered, such as transport to the hospital for donation if the child dies at home.

Practicalities, such as where the family wish to be, and who they wish to be there can also be considered and prepared for, wherever possible.

The wishes and choices should also take into account the family's cultural and religious needs. It is always important not to make any presumptions but to ask. However it is often something that worries staff and may sometimes be difficult to arrange if left until the last minute, particularly if the family wish to take their child's body out of the country immediately after death.

Many parents will have never planned a funeral before, let alone that of their child, and they will find it particularly difficult to do at a point of intense grief. This may lead to regrets about the service or events later. It may be helpful for families to have some idea about the options available to them beforehand and a young person may in fact wish to plan their own funeral.

There are many options such as:
➤ which funeral director
➤ the place of rest before the funeral
➤ embalming
➤ burial or cremation
➤ burial site
➤ if cremated what to do with the ashes afterwards
➤ where and who to hold the service
➤ what type of service, coffin, and vehicle?
➤ what time of day?
➤ music
➤ flowers, announcements, donations
➤ clothes for the child and friends and family
➤ themes.

It is hoped the Wishes and Choices checklist is very much an empowering tool for the family. As previously stated, it is not intended to be paperwork that staff and family are forced to complete, but is part of the child's care plan and is seen as something that is helpful to complete, but can then be put to one side, allowing the family to carry on and enjoy their time with their child as much as possible, knowing their wishes and choices have been documented and that the professionals are clear on what the family wish to happen, if and when the time comes.

Status of the plan

In the system described above, the central element of the 'end-of-life plan' is the family held 'personal resuscitation plan', which is a medical care plan and has the legal status of such. The consultant paediatrician must sign it and confirm that it has been agreed with the family. It is usual and often empowering for the parents to sign it to confirm their agreement. But occasionally parents cannot bring themselves to sign. They may feel that by signing they will somehow hasten the child's death. In this case it is good practice for another member of the team to confirm the family's agreement and sign the plan. The family can change their minds at any time and therefore there is no fixed renewal date. The plan does not time expire.

In an emergency situation the on call medical team need to give the child the most appropriate medical care. However, they may never have met the child before and previous medical records may not be available quickly. It is extremely helpful when the child and family bring a personal resuscitation plan with them, giving the background information and the best management in the opinion of the child's lead consultant paediatrician and the family. The doctor in the emergency department still has to make a judgement and act in the best interests of the child. Occasionally the particular circumstances may not have been considered or the family may have changed their minds, but even then the plan gives useful information on what has been discussed with the family already.

End-of-life plans and child death review process[15]

Since April 2008 all child deaths in the UK have to be reviewed by a local child death overview panel. It is expected that this will give local and eventually national information on why children die and will lead to ways to prevent children's deaths. As part of this process there are local rapid response teams, including police and social workers who need to gather information quickly when a child dies unexpectedly.

An unexpected death is defined as 'the death of a child that was not anticipated as a significant possibility 24 hours before the death, or where there was a similarly unexpected collapse leading to or precipitating the events that led to the death.[16,17]

There is a risk that the death of a child with a life-limiting or a life-threatening condition will be inappropriately investigated. Local safeguarding boards have put systems in place to alert the rapid response team when a child dies. Ambulance staff may be under instruction to take the body of any child found dead at home to the hospital emergency department for post mortem examination and the place of death may be made a crime scene. A personal resuscitation plan in the home provides written confirmation that the child is at risk of a life-threatening event, plus contact details to allow rapid liaison with the child's palliative care team. This should help avoid inappropriate activation of the rapid response team.

Feedback from families about end-of-life planning

Families report that it is emotionally difficult to talk about the death of their child but they find making a personal resuscitation plan empowering. They want to discuss the options with someone they know and trust. They say it is helpful to have clearly in writing what everyone needs to do.

Issues with reference to Better Care: Better Lives[2]

Although we now have templates and systems for making end-of-life plans with children and families, the choices available are limited by resources particularly the lack of children's community nursing services capable of providing emergency and end-of-life care outside hospital, 24 hours a day.

Because of the small numbers and unpredictability of the work load it is hard for small nursing teams to justify having a senior nurse on call 24 hours per day, seven days per week. However, without a pre-arranged on-call rota the nursing service cannot respond when a child suddenly deteriorates and needs a home nursing service.

In some regions, community nursing teams combine out of hours to provide on-call cover to a larger population. The down side of this is that it makes it less likely that a child and family will have support from a nurse they know and trust. Some teams have combined the children's community nursing service and the home-based short break service to provide a larger, skill-mixed caring team to call upon in an emergency. Disabled children with life-limiting conditions are often receiving a service from both teams.

Additional government health funding for children's palliative care and short-break services was not ring fenced and many primary care trusts in the UK have not chosen to develop these services.

The proposed ACT mapping initiative[18] and minimum data set will eventually lead to standardised data collection across the UK, which may then stimulate further service development.

Meanwhile regional children's palliative care networks[19] are bringing teams together, and linking with regional cancer and neonatal networks, leading to sharing of good practice, and the development of care pathways and increased training opportunities.

ALTERNATIVE SCENARIO FOR MARY

Mary's parents were reluctant to agree in advance to any limitation of intervention and could not contemplate her death.

They did, however, see the need for an emergency care plan so that each time Mary was brought to the emergency department medical staff would have information on what was the best care for her. Also, staff at school and at the short-break service wanted a medical care plan including an emergency care plan to follow when the parents were not there.

Mary's community paediatrician discussed her case with the respiratory paediatrician in the hospital and then met with both her parents at home to draw up a personal resuscitation plan (PRP). Mary's parents described the first signs that would indicate that her chest was deteriorating. The plan included when to call an ambulance and listed the interventions that worked well for Mary, including warm humidified oxygen and chest physio as well as intravenous antibiotics. The paediatrician put on the plan that ventilation would not be appropriate. The paediatrician also spoke about the possibility of a sudden deterioration and what level of attempted resuscitation would be appropriate. This was of course very upsetting for Mary's parents to talk about, but they agreed that suction to clear the airway and a trial of bag and mask or 'mouth to mouth' respiratory support would be appropriate, but that it would not be appropriate to try to resuscitate Mary from a cardiac arrest.

The consultant signed the plan. Mary's parents accepted that it was a useful plan but didn't want to sign it. The parents kept a copy with Mary at all times and copies were distributed to school nurse, home-based short breaks team, paediatric emergency department and hospital case notes. Mary continued to have chest infections and was admitted on several more occasions. Each time, the parents brought the PRP with them and showed it to the admitting medical team even though they hadn't signed it.

During one of these admissions another child with severe disability died on the ward. Mary's family knew this child and his family and were very upset. Mary's named nurse on the children's ward sat with them. They started to discuss what might happen if Mary died. Mary's mother said she wanted to have Mary at home when she died, but she couldn't contemplate not bringing her in for hospital treatment just in case it saved her life. The nurse was able to explore various options with them and documented this with their agreement (Wishes and Choices, *see* Figure 16.2). The parents said they felt better having talked it through 'just in case' but asked that it was not talked about again.

A few months later Mary was in hospital with a chest infection. She seemed to be responding to the intravenous antibiotics but then without warning, one evening, she had a sudden cardio/respiratory arrest. The parents were present and the nurse seeing the heart trace drop on the monitor encouraged Mum to hold Mary while she gave five inflation breaths with bag and mask.

Mary died in her mother's arms.

Mary was moved into a cubicle. The nurse helped her parents to wash and dress her in her favourite pink pyjamas. Her brother and grandparents came in and they spent time chatting and listening to her favourite music. When they were ready, the family accompanied Mary to the chapel of rest. They collected their belongings and were told that the child bereavement team would contact them in the morning, but to telephone the ward in the meantime if they needed to.

The child bereavement team met with the ward nurses in the morning and talked through the events and also discussed the 'Wishes and Choices' checklist. Although all the nurses were sad, they felt Mary's death had been calm and dignified.

The child bereavement team telephoned the parents and arranged to meet them on the ward later that day, to collect the death certificate, register the death and to see Mary in the chapel of rest. Meanwhile the necessary paperwork was completed, including the cremation form, and the child death review team was notified. Later that day Mary was collected by the funeral director and was taken home. She stayed in her bedroom until her funeral. Her family were visited and supported by the community nurses who had known Mary.

The parents attended a follow-up medical appointment with the paediatrician a few weeks later. Although devastated by the loss of their child, both parents were satisfied that the medical care had been appropriate and were glad to have been with Mary on a familiar children's ward with nurses who they knew well when she died.

LAST COMMENTS

The ACT Integrated Care Pathway gives those working to support children with life-limiting and life-threatening conditions clear standards with which to audit and improve their services. The strategy document Better Care: Better Lives[2] provides a framework for the further development of comprehensive services for this client group. Inspired by these documents, providers and commissioners are coming together in regional children's palliative care networks throughout the UK to map the needs and to collaborate to improve services for children with life-limiting and life-threatening conditions and their families.

PLEASE KEEP VISIBLE AT THE FRONT OF MEDICAL RECORDS AT ALL TIMES
DO NOT PHOTOCOPY

Children's Centre
xxxxxxxxxxxxxxxxxxxx
xxxxxxxxxxxxxxxxx
xxxxxxxxxxxxxxxx
xxxxxxx

Consultant: Dr White, Consultant Paediatrician
☎ xxxx xxxxxxxx
Email: xxxxxxx@xxxxxxxx

PHOTO

Personal Resuscitation Plan for Child / Young Person
Created 23.04.09 Amended _______

1.

Name: Mary Smith
Hosp no: K12345678
DOB: 12.09.2003
Address: 65 Redbrook Grove
Nottingham

2. Background

Mary has very severe neurodisability following problems at birth. She has cerebral palsy, epilepsy and all nutrition is by gastrostomy.

She suffers from frequent chest infections which are life threatening.

Mary has a suction machine and also continuous oxygen at home.

3. Resuscitation Plan

3.1. In the event of a **sudden collapse** with respiratory and or cardiac arrest:

Mary may have sudden breathing difficulty due to problems clearing her respiratory secretions.

1. Comfort & support child and family
2. Suction upper airway
3. Oxygen for comfort face mask/nasal cannulae
4. Airway management including oral/nasopharyngeal airway if it helps
5. Mouth to mouth / bag & mask ventilation ~~whilst heart beat present~~ trial of five inflation breaths
6. Endotracheal tube & ventilate would <u>not</u> be appropriate
7. ~~External cardiac compressions/defibrillation/adrenaline~~
8. ~~Advanced life support including inotropic drugs and *iv* access~~

Personal Resuscitation Plan for date – Page 1 of 6

Dr Wolff – Version 3 (Jan 2009)

FIGURE 16.1 Care plan for Mary

Name: Mary Smith
Hosp no: K12345678
DOB: 12.09.2003
Address: 65 Redbrook Grove
Nottingham

3.2.   This child is at risk of generalised tonic clonic seizures:

Rescue anticonvulsant regime is:

Buccal Midazolam (Epistatus) 5mg (0.5ml) for generalised tonic clonic seizures lasting longer than 5 minutes.

3.3 Transfer to

Transfer to the paediatric emergency department. Mary is well known to Dr White at Queen's Medical Centre.

Paediatric intensive care unit would not be appropriate.

Ambulance staff can call ahead to alert receiving staff that child has a specific resuscitation plan.

3.4 Who to call
if at home:

999 ambulance and show this plan, also call community nurse on 07968342581.

If at school or short break unit:

999 ambulance   and parents on 07898554721

If in hospital:

Emergency medical team   and parents on 07898554721

3.5 Ambulance directive   yes

FIGURE 16.1 Care plan for Mary (continued)

> Name: Mary Smith
> Hosp no: K12345678
> DOB: 12.09.2003
> Address: 65 Redbrook Grove
> Nottingham

4.   Emergency Care Plan

4.1   In the event of a gradual life threatening deterioration:

> Mary has frequent chest infections. She will have a cough and fever. Her secretions become green and she breathes faster and harder.
>
> She will need admission to hospital for intravenous antibiotics and chest physiotherapy.

1. Comfort & support child and family

2. Suction upper airway

3. Increase her oxygen for comfort via face mask/nasal cannulae

4. Airway management including oral/nasopharyngeal airway if it helps

5. Mary is already taking antibiotics -- Azithromycin three times per week

6. She will need *iv* fluids

7. She will need *iv* antibiotics

8. Endotracheal intubation & ventilation ~~would~~/would not be appropriate

9. Other symptom relief:

> Mary will benefit from humidified oxygen and chest physio.

4.2   Transfer to

> Paediatric Emergency Department

Ambulance staff can call ahead to alert receiving staff that child has a specific resuscitation plan.

PLEASE KEEP VISIBLE AT THE FRONT OF MEDICAL RECORDS AT ALL TIMES
DO NOT PHOTOCOPY

Name: Mary Smith
Hosp no: K12345678
DOB: 12.09.2003
Address: 65 Redbrook Grove
Nottingham

5.   Plan for review

The patient or parent / guardian can change their mind about any of these options at any time

6.   The plan has been revised   **date**   day month year

7.   The plan has been discussed with

Child or young person

Mother   √

Father   √

Guardian

Other people

FIGURE 16.1 Care plan for Mary (continued)

**PLEASE KEEP VISIBLE AT THE FRONT OF MEDICAL RECORDS AT ALL TIMES
DO NOT PHOTOCOPY**

> Name: Mary Smith
> Hosp no: K12345678
> DOB: 12.09.03
> Address: 65 Redbrook Grove
> Nottingham

8.   Consultant's agreement

I support this Personal Resuscitation Plan

Name & signature   _(signature)_   date | 25 | 4 | 09 |

9.   Child or young person's agreement

I have discussed and support this Personal Resuscitation Plan

Name & signature   date | | | |

10.   Parent or Guardian's agreement

I / We have discussed and support this Personal Resuscitation Plan

Name & signature   _(signature)_   date | 25 | 4 | 09 |

11.   Team's agreement

I / We have discussed this PRP with the child or young person / parent or guardian

Name & signature   date | | | |

PLEASE KEEP VISIBLE AT THE FRONT OF MEDICAL RECORDS AT ALL TIMES
DO NOT PHOTOCOPY

Name: Mary Smith
Hosp no: K12345678
DOB: 12.09.03
Address: 65 Redbrook Grove
Nottingham

12. Copies of this PRP are held by

Parents / guardian	☒ at home address and at	As above
With patient at all times	☒ contact details	C/o Parents as above.
School	☒ contact details	C/o School Nurse Hillcrest Primary School
Respite care	☒ contact details	C/o Named Nurse The Cottage Short Break Unit
Hospital	☒ contact details	C/o Dr White's Secretary Queen's Medical Centre
GP	☒ contact details	
Community Nurses	☒ contact details	
Local Notes (CDC or community)	☒ contact details	CDC and Community records, C/o School Nurse
Dr Wolff – Audit File C/o CDC (with parents consent)	☒ contact details	

Personal Resuscitation Plan for   date – Page 6 of 6
© *Copyright Nottingham University Hospitals NHS Trust & University of Nottingham*
Dr Wolff – Version 3 (Jan 2009)

FIGURE 16.1 Care plan for Mary (continued)

Nottingham University Hospitals **NHS**

NHS Trust

Wishes And Choices

Child Profile   ** All patient and family information on this form is fictional**

Name of Child: *Mary Smith*   ~~Male~~/Female

Preferred Name: *Mary*   Date Of Birth: *12.09.2003*

Hospital Number:

Address: xxxxxx   Ethnicity: *White British*

Spoken Language: *English*

Religion: *C of E*

Religious Observances: -

Family Profile

Mother's Name: *Gloria Smith*   Father's name: *John Smith*

Spoken Language: *English*   Spoken Language: *English*

Is interpreter required: ~~Yes~~/No   Is interpreter required: ~~Yes~~/No

Are Parents: Married / ~~Partners / Single / Divorced / Separated~~   Any contact: Yes/No

(If not together: Ensure both addresses for contacting parents are recorded)

Mother's Address / Telephone number: Father's Address / Telephone number

As above   *As above*

Child lives with: *Both parents*

Person with legal responsibility for the child: *Parents*

Names and ages of siblings: *Jake Smith age 11   20/2/98*

Significant others e.g. Grandparents, Foster carers:

Name of Family key worker: *Yvonne Smalley*

Name of Child's Consultant: *Dr White*

©Copyright Nottingham University Hospitals NHS Trust and University of Nottingham
Jackie Browne – Gillian Bishop – Sally Robbins (January 09)

FIGURE 16.2 Wishes and choices

Nottingham University Hospitals **NHS**

NHS Trust

Significant People/Organisations Involved

Name	Base	Contact Number

FIGURE 16.2 Wishes and choices (continued)

Nottingham University Hospitals
NHS Trust

Is an Emergency Care Plan/Personal Resuscitation Plan in place?   **Yes/No**

If yes where are copies held:
Parents and with Mary at all times
School, respite care, hospital, GP, community nurses, local notes and
community paed.

Brief details of plan:
If Mary were to collapse suddenly she would receive:
Comfort and support, suction and oxygen, airway management and 5 bag and mask
breaths.
ETT and ventilation, advanced life support and external cardiac massage would not
be appropriate.
If 999 called she would come to ED, but admission to PICU would not be appropriate.
If gradual deterioration as above and also IV fluids, IV antibiotics, humidified
oxygen and chest physio.

Is the plan registered with EMAS?   **Yes/No**

Has 'out of hours' Emergency GP/ NHS Direct Special Note been completed?   **Yes/No**

Practical Support Needs/Issues

For example does the family have any: housing, financial, employment, respite care, educational, play, complementary therapy or transport needs/issues etc?
Family are happy with the amount of respite they receive from children's
centre.
Mary attends school when well enough and family are very happy with the
support there.
House is adapted to meet Mary's needs.

Keepsakes and memory activities

Have the family been offered the opportunity to obtain keepsakes whilst the child is well?
Lock of hair: ☐ *obtained for all family members*
Footprints: ☐
Handprints: ☐ *handprints of Mary and Jake taken together*
The family may like keepsakes of <u>all</u> family members to be taken in various ways.

The family may also consider compiling life/memory books/diaries whilst the child is still able to contribute themselves
Thinking about this.

Nottingham University Hospitals **NHS**
NHS Trust

Family's Level of Understanding and Emotional Support Needs:

Please give consideration to the family's emotional needs and how they are coping with the situation they find themselves in. It may be helpful to consider what support systems are in place and their individual and joint coping strategies. Are other support agencies involved? What information/resources are available?

What is the child's understanding of their condition?
Mary is unable to talk or communicate, although she recognises familiar voices and smiles
*Parents do not want death to be discussed in Mary's presence.

Support/information?

What do the parents understand about their child's condition?
Parents are aware that Mary has a life-limiting condition and that this could mean a slow deterioration or a sudden collapse. This has been discussed with them and they have completed a PRP.
They do not wish to discuss this again unless they raise the subject or Mary's condition deteriorates and necessitates further discussion.

Support/information?
Choices' booklet given – will look at it when they are ready.
Have visited hospice – aware of services, but do not wish to use at the moment – feel it is too far away.
Aware of child bereavement team and will meet if and when necessary .
Happy to talk to community nurse.

What do the sibling's understand about the situation?
Jake is aware that Mary is poorly and may die.
School is aware of the situation.

Support/information?
Supportive teacher and school nurse available for Jake to talk to.
Attends sibling group.
Has completed workbooks with butterfly worker.

Agencies that may be able to help include:
Hospice: xxxxxxxxx☐ *family aware not using at the moment.*
Child Bereavement Team : xxxxxxxx☐ *family are aware but do not want to meet yet.*
Butterfly Project : xxxxxxxxx☐ *Using for sibling support.*
Specialist Social Worker
Specialist Nurse
Hospital/Community Psychology Teams
GP/School/ Counselling services☐ *School nurse.*
Support Organisation for child's specific condition
There are many useful leaflets and workbooks available to help families.

FIGURE 16.2 Wishes and choices (continued)

Nottingham University Hospitals

NHS Trust

Specific wishes and choices around the time of death

It is important to take the child's wishes into account where possible.
Circumstances and events around the child's condition and death may cause these wishes and choices to change, so these should be revisited as often as necessary, according to child and family's needs.

Where would the family prefer their child's death to take place, if choice is a possibility at the time?
(At home, in hospital, hospice other)
Would like to be at home – but scared as they feel they want everything done –
so feel hospital would be best.
Feel hospice is too far.

Who would the family like to be with them at the time of death?
(Immediate family, extended family, community nurse, specialist nurse, support worker, GP, religious/cultural representative etc)
Nurses know to them.
Contact community nurse and community paed asap
Possibly chaplain if in hospital

If at home, who will certify death?
Community paed.

What do they wish to happen immediately after the child dies?
(Keep the child at home, collection by funeral director, hospice, embalmed and returned home, cultural or religious observances etc)
Not sure at the moment – would depend on situation.

How soon would family like equipment/drugs to be collected from the home?
Would like to be asked at the time.

Do the family know which Funeral Director they would use?   Yes/~~No~~
If yes name of Funeral Director and contact number:
Grants telephone –
Used them when maternal grandma died.

Do the family wish to contact the Funeral Director before the child's death to discuss any questions?
Not at the moment.

Do the family know if they would have a burial or cremation?
Cremation.
Funeral information sheet given: Family will look when ready.   Yes/~~No~~

Would the family like any help with planning the funeral before or after death?
~~Yes: Before~~
Yes: After
~~No~~

Nottingham University Hospitals

NHS Trust

Tissue Donation

Following a death some families may wish to consider donating organs or tissue for the purposes of transplantation or research. If this is requested by the family then the key worker should contact the On-call Donor co-ordinator (via QMC Switchboard). They will then give the family all the advice and information to help them reach an informed decision.

Corneas can be obtained up to 24 hours after death

Heart valves can be obtained up to 48 hours after death.

Unless the child is attached to a ventilator on PICU, it would not be possible to donate any organs for transplantation, although donation for research purposes may be possible.

Because of the short time frame whenever possible it is helpful to have explored this choice beforehand.

Discussed: Yes/ No

If yes, do the family have any thoughts:

Do not feel this is appropriate for them as a family. Appreciate offer.

Post Mortem Examinations

Some families may express an interest in having a post mortem after the death of their child. This may help answer questions and may help with the planning of any future pregnancies etc. In this situation please contact the pathology team at QMC tel.

Discussed: Yes/No

If yes, do the family have any thoughts:

Do not want a post mortem – feel Mary has been through enough already and they know all about her condition.

Copies of this document are held by:

Family   ☑

Key worker   ☑

Hospital Case Notes   ☑

Dr White   ☑

(For audit purposes if family give permission)

Signed: **Date:**

Print name and designation:

If you would like any assistance in completing this form then please do not hesitate to contact the Child Bereavement Team at QMC Tel: xxxxxxx

FIGURE 16.2 Wishes and choices (continued)

Nottingham University Hospitals
NHS Trust

Special wishes and memories can be recorded here along with any other additional information:

N.I.C.E. analysis

Please reflect on the issues raised in this chapter in relation to your own practice.

Needs

- A child needs the best possible care plan at the end of life.
- Parents, and sometimes the dying child/young person himself, need to know what is going to happen and make plans.
- Knowledge is empowering.
- Families want to understand their choices and have as much control as possible.
- Families want to discuss the options in advance with someone they know and trust.
- Nurses attending a dying child feel more confident when there is a clear care plan endorsed by the consultant paediatrician and parents.

Misconceptions

- *'Families don't want to discuss their child's death'*
  - ▶ Nobody wants to talk about their child dying, but families are often ahead of the doctor in having thought about what will happen and starting to make plans.
  - ▶ Families find making the plans difficult, but are often relieved to have done it and to feel that they and everyone else will know what to do.
- *'You can't have these discussions with parents of some faiths and cultures'*
  - ▶ All families may not want to talk about an 'end-of-life plan' but all will value a family-held emergency care plan, detailing symptoms and signs of deterioration, what to do and who to call. They will want to be sure that all potentially helpful interventions are promptly given.

Concerns

- Starting the discussions at the right time.
- Professionals tend to shy away from these discussions, feeling they will be too painful for children and families.
- Some paediatricians prefer to keep focused on interventions and believe the child or family will raise the issue when they are ready to talk about it.
- It may be difficult to recognise when a child is entering the end stage of life. Children in ACT groups 3 and 4 in particular may be close to death and then pull through many times over many years.
- Lack of user-friendly tools to help the discussions and document decisions.

Expectations

- It is expected that personal resuscitation plans will replace 'Do Not Attempt Resuscitation' orders for disabled children.
- It is expected that the plans provide mutual support for doctors once some families have them, allowing all members of the team to follow them, working in partnership and sharing uncertainty.
- It is expected that the template will provide a tool that helps doctors to initiate and document discussions.
- That there is parallel planning for life and death.
- 'Role out' so all stakeholders are clear about personal resuscitation plans.

Concerns (continued)

- Most UK health organisations use 'Do Not Attempt Resuscitation' orders to document end-of-life decisions. These forms are not appropriate. Children, families and professionals need positive care plans about what to do, not 'do nothing' orders.
- However, care plans written in the medical case notes may stipulate things that are not practically possible in all situations, and are not always readily available in an emergency.

Barriers to implementation

- How do we make sure that the personal resuscitation plan is always available?
- Once plans have been made and agreed by the medical team and family how can we ensure that they are always available and followed, no matter where the child is?
- Can everyone follow them?
- Clarification of the legal status of the plan.
- What happens if people change their minds?

Action plan: next steps

- We have used the templates and care pathways above to support 'end-of-life care planning' for disabled children with life-limiting and life-threatening conditions. Feedback from families and nurses has been very positive.
- The templates help professionals, paediatricians, nurses and family support workers to open the discussions and document decisions. The documentation is then family-held and has the status of a medical care plan.
- All of the local disability paediatricians and paediatric neurologists have used the system, and the use of personal resuscitation plans is being rolled out across the region via the Regional Paediatric Palliative Care Network.
- The next steps will be formal evaluation of the system.

REFERENCES

1 Elston S. *Integrated Multi-agency Care Pathways for Children with Life-threatening and Life-limiting Conditions.* Bristol: ACT; 2004.

2 UK Department of Health (2008) *Better Care: Better Lives*. Available at: www.dh.gov.uk/en/Publicationsandstatistics/Publications/PublicationsPolicyAndGuidance/DH_083106 (accessed 17 February 2010).

3 www.cancerimprovement.nhs.uk

4 Right from the Start Template. Available at: www.scope.org.uk/early years/rfts.php (accessed 17 February 2010).

5 Contact a Family Directory. Available at: www.cafamily.org.uk (accessed 17 February 2010).

6 NSF: all the documents for the UK National Service Framework for children can be accessed via the Department of Health website: Available at: www.dh.gov.uk/en/Healthcare/Children/DH_4089111 (accessed 17 February 2010).

7 CAF practioners' guide: guidance on carrying out common assessments. Available at: www.ecm.gov.uk/caf (accessed 17 February 2010).

8 www.opsi.gov.uk/acts/acts2004/ukpga_20040031_en_1

9 www.everychildmatters.gov.uk/

10 Care Coordination Network UK. *New standards for Key Working 2004*. Available at: www.ccnuk.org.uk (accessed 17 February 2010).

11 *The Lead Professional: Practitioners' Guide Every Child Matters: Change for Children Programme* Available at: www.dcsf.gov.uk/everychildmatters/about/ (accessed 17 February 2010).

12 Early Support Programme. www.earlysupport.org.uk

13 www.everychildmatters.gov.uk/socialcare/ahdc/

14 www.icpcn.org.uk/page.asp?section=0001000100080004&itemTitle=What+is+Children%92s+Palliative+Care%3F

15 www.everychildmatters.gov.uk/socialcare/safeguarding/childdeathreview/

16 Fleming PJ, Blair PS, Bacon C, *et al. Sudden Unexpected Death in Infancy. The CESDI SUDI Studies 1993–1996*. London: The Stationery Office; 2000.

17 www.londonscb.gov.uk/files/resources/cdop/rcpch_guidance_on_child_death_review_process.pdf

18 www.act.org.uk

19 www.act.org.uk

SECTION 4

Supporting transitions

Susan Fowler-Kerry

Section 4 of this text provides glimpses into the transition dilemmas that occur within the hospital setting. The act of transferring or moving a patient from one clinical setting in the hospital to another is an everyday, normal occurrence for hospital staff. This mundane act may not be perceived as so by parents of a child with a life-limiting or life-threatening diagnosis especially when the transition is largely due to the physiological decline of the child. How families cope with any type of changes varies greatly among people, and it is simply not possible to catalogue or predict all possible responses. However, through the narrative accounts within this text, parents paint many different pictures depicting a state of existential limbo, which results from a distortion in their role as parent and in their time world, where normal parenthood involves concentrating on and investing in the present as a way of preparing for the future. How then does a parent prepare or contemplate a future when their child is critically ill or dying and how can staff reduce the stress this causes?

There is no doubt that each and every family's lives have been forever transformed as a result of their child's diagnosis. So, how do we as healthcare professionals make changes within and among service delivery units so as not to further disrupt their lives? Healthcare sectors along with policy makers must understand that there should be no breaks in the continuity of care provided to these children and their families. As we attempt to move decision making in health onto a firmer substantiated base, it is equally important to pay scrupulous attention to the sources of truth, which includes both traditional quantitative and qualitative perspectives.

Transitions within acute care settings: the chaplain's perspective

Paul Weeding

This chapter seeks to recognise some of the difficulties that families may experience when they have a child with a life-limiting condition and who are in transition from one intensive care area to another within an acute hospital setting. These transitions can take place in a number of ways – from the home to acute hospital setting, within the acute setting from one intensive care to another or to the ward, from home to hospice and any combination in between. Many different staff will be offering support in one way or another, but this contribution is written from the perspective of those who seek to offer spiritual and pastoral care and who are in the main chaplains. Since the contributor is a chaplain working in an acute hospital setting, much of what is written reflects that context. In looking at the spiritual and pastoral care that is offered, consideration will be given to the way that fits in with the Nottingham Integrated Pathway for children.[1]

There are many ways in which chaplaincy can offer support to children and families, but perhaps those mentioned below are some of the key ones:

➤ religious rites and ceremonies
➤ communication
➤ relationships between staff and parents
➤ engendering a realistic sense of hope.

It is a natural instinct when faced with a child who is in a life-limiting situation for parents to want to do all that is within their power to help that child. For some that will mean turning to a higher power in the hope of help for a child both in this life, and also some assurance that if the child dies that life will continue beyond death. This desire for God's help, however God is understood, is independent of religious affiliation. Many parents who have the most nominal links with faith groups will nevertheless want some form of religious rite or ceremony.

In talking with several colleagues it is clear that much of the spiritual and pastoral care that is offered to families is similar across the different religions. Paradoxically, having a definite faith in God and religious beliefs does not necessarily make things easier (as some might believe). However, all religious rituals and services, if done in an appropriate way, will bring some comfort. Caution is always needed in advising which ritual or service may be appropriate within any particular religion, as culture always has a large part to play.

Different faiths' attitude to suffering does affect the way in which pastoral care is offered. For instance, generally Islam teaches that life is full of challenges and that suffering is seen as being both one of those challenges and the will of God. This is not seen as a negative thing or a punishment, but rather that any suffering we have in this life is counted as a bonus in the life to come. Many non-Muslim parents and families would find this concept very difficult to understand. However, for many Muslim families it helps them to make sense of what their child and they themselves are going through/ have been through. For them this is a spiritual way of offering support.

Later in this chapter I will discuss in a little more depth the question of hope, but chaplains always have uppermost in their minds, when preparing to offer a religious rite, not to give an unrealistic hope for the child's future prognosis. As a chaplain from the Christian faith I am always keen to stress to parents there is nothing magical about Christening/baptism. That said, results of research by Robinson *et al.*[2] have shown how much many families have appreciated religious rites even when the child has then subsequently died.

It is widely known that families form a bond with staff, even over quite a short period of time, and especially in acute areas, where staff to patient ratios can be one-to-one. The move to a different area can be fraught with difficulties, not least building a rapport with new staff. Chaplaincy involvement can be helpful in providing continuity between areas, so that the same chaplain who knows something of their history from one area can continue to support them in another. Inevitably issues can arise where families are unhappy with changes/differences. Sometimes it may just be simply a matter of letting off steam, or explaining some of the differences in care. But if this is not sufficient, then with parents' permission chaplains may bring to staff's attention their concerns. They may not want to mention it to staff for fear of upsetting them or affecting their child's care, so it can be helpful for a third party to intervene. Equally staff may be struggling to convey certain information or expectations to families, and chaplains again can be helpful as a trusted third party.

Perhaps a case example can illustrate this.

Baby Fizz was brought into hospital on the children's intensive care unit after a dramatic decline and major breathing difficulties. Much later it was discovered she had a rare genetic condition with a very poor prognosis, but at that stage there was no clear indication of diagnosis. Chaplaincy was introduced at an early stage and parents were very happy to have our support. After several weeks baby Fizz was moved onto one of the children's wards. For the parents this was a very difficult time as they had no diagnosis for what had so dramatically and adversely affected their child and had already spent a considerable time away from home, which was some distance away.

The transition from intensive care to the ward was stressful as it often is for many parents, with the challenge of getting used to much lower staffing levels. But for the parents of baby Fizz things were made that much more difficult because although she was out of immediate danger things were not simply gradually getting better. This added pressure inevitably meant that at times there were communication problems between staff and parents. Chaplaincy was able to help assure parents and to help overcome some of these problems. Over many weeks the parents struggled with not having a diagnosis for baby Fizz's condition. Eventually a diagnosis was given and the baby's condition stabilised sufficiently that they were able to go home, albeit on the basis that they did subsequently have to return again when the baby's condition worsened.

Here was an example of chaplaincy being involved with a family for a number of months and from an early stage. As the family moved from intensive care to children's ward, to home and then back again, chaplains were able to be there on the rollercoaster ride that is the experience of having a child in hospital long-term. At times when the parents felt like they were never going to get out of hospital with their child we were able to give a right sense of reassurance. We were some of the consistent staff faces who journeyed with the family up to and including baby Fizz's death and were able to offer support afterwards. As it stands, the pathway would not have brought us in until the last stages of the baby's life, when our effectiveness would have been seriously reduced.

At this stage it is worth recognising the stress involved with nursing children in intensive care areas. Staff may have a very short time to get to know patients and families before being involved in life or death situations. Very naturally the first port of call for staff will be their colleagues, who know their situation better than most. After this we recognise as chaplains that we can offer staff support, which is both confidential and one step aside from their immediate departments.

The area of hope is a major issue for parents and staff. No staff wish to remove hope from parents, but it needs to be hope based on a right understanding of the child's situation. This is a paradox and a mystery as so often we come across children whose families have been told with the best of medical information that they will only live a very short time and then lo and behold they pull through at least for that time (though many sadly die later). This hope can often be linked with trust.

Perhaps a case example can best illustrate this.

Baby Jason was born with a variety of complications and spent some time in different intensive areas of the hospital. There were a number of issues that arose with parents. An early procedure that did not go as well as planned caused his parents to lose some trust in medical staff. This was exacerbated in the parents' minds when told on more than one occasion (rightly so) that Jason would very likely die, only for him to recover. In addition, the parents viewed Jason's general state as far more positive than medical staff were trying to reflect back to them. This mismatch was causing a lot of stress.

A number of support staff were called in to offer help to the parents and improve communication. Chaplaincy had already been involved because of the parents' request for Jason to be christened, and worked alongside other staff to reassure the parents that all that could be done was being done. Here was an ongoing conflict. In an ideal world the end-of-life section of the pathway would allow an agreed plan by staff and parents as to how to care for baby with pain relief and minimum interventions. However, in baby Jason's case his staff were wanting to agree on a palliative care approach, but his parents were determined that maximum support be given whatever the long-term outcome and however poorly he became.

As Jason moved from one intensive care area to another one within the hospital, the mismatch between parents and staff of how best to care for Jason continued. Staff asked if we could help parents to see how much Jason was suffering and how poor his future would be. Coming back to this theme of hope, I tried to share with parents the Christian hope of life that continues beyond death. In other words, that there is more than simply this life on earth and that therefore, although incredibly painful, it is possible to begin to let go and not seek to offer maximum support at all times. Again referring to research done in the US by Robinson *et al.*[2] it has been recognised how important and beneficial a belief in a life after death has been to parents.

It is very difficult to say how much chaplaincy input made a difference alongside all the hard work of so many other staff. But I do believe that the time we spent with parents built up a level of trust, so that when things reached crisis point we were in a position to guide and help them. In terms of what I might have done differently, I can only reflect that giving a realistic sense of hope is walking a tricky and very sensitive path. If at times I drew back from confronting parents with some of the realities of their situation, it was because I realised how vulnerable they were.

Out of the total number of children with life-limiting/threatening conditions that we are in contact with, only a small percentage of these would actually be on the Nottingham Pathway. This is partly due to the acute hospital setting where children have very suddenly come into intensive care because of a dramatic/catastrophic event. Obviously in these situations the children will not be on the pathway, but may suddenly find themselves at the end-of-life stage. Also I am aware that it is still early days for the Nottingham Children's Pathway[1] and its use has been relatively small. As time goes on I am sure its take up and use will increase greatly. All this is by way of saying that at present it is difficult to assess the effectiveness of the Pathway in providing appropriate spiritual and pastoral care.

One of the key questions for the future as the ACT Care Pathway's[3] use begins to pick-up and increase, is at what stage/s is spiritual and pastoral care best provided? In both of the children's cases that have been previously mentioned, chaplains were able to have a positive impact because we had met family early on. This meant that when things became very difficult we already had a good relationship with them.

Having reflected on the chaplain's role in the pathway at Nottingham and looking at what is happening nationally, it does seem that often spiritual care is only incorporated at the end-of-life stage, when really it would be much more helpful to be brought in earlier if parents/families would value us. At this point I have to put my hands up and acknowledge that myself and another colleague were consulted about and contributed to the Nottingham Pathway. I think perhaps we should have been requesting that the offer of spiritual and pastoral care be made at an earlier stage and written in the pathway to that effect. Here I refer to Feudtner,[4] who undertook a national survey on the spiritual care needs of hospitalised children and their families. Of course this then begins the question of how staff introduce our service. Certainly staff are very geared up to offering chaplaincy support at the end of life, but maybe not so much at an earlier stage. This may at times be due to a confusion about our role, with staff perhaps thinking that we focus our time on the dying and those with a definite religious affiliation. Whilst this will be a part of spiritual and pastoral care, by far the greatest amount of chaplains' time is spent addressing the spiritual issues of the living, who have no particular religious affiliation.

To talk about spiritual care is to talk about what gives human beings their sense of worth, purpose and hope, without which all of us become less than we should be. This is so much more than simply religious affiliation and goes to the very heart of what it means to be human. At or around the time of breaking the news to families of a child's life-limiting condition, all of the above senses will have taken a big knock and it may be they would value someone to talk to in confidence. The take-up of our service is then very dependent on how it is introduced. If fellow staff are confident to advise families that this is a confidential and non-judgemental service that others have found helpful regardless of faith, then the response is more likely to be positive. This in turn is affected by how comfortable staff are with their own spirituality. Some research has been done revealing that the more comfortable staff are with their own belief system the more easily they will be able to identify spiritual issues in families and refer them onto chaplaincy. As staff change, there is the ongoing challenge to explain our role and not allow ourselves to be stereotyped in ways that will reduce the uptake of the service. I refer here to two pieces of research: one by Armbuster *et al.*[5] on paediatricians' beliefs about spirituality and religion in medicine; and the second by Grossoehme *et al.*,[6] who examined paediatrician characteristics associated with attention to spirituality and religion in clinical practice.

Talking to other chaplains working with children and families it is apparent that much of the way our service is introduced, and when, is dependent on staff's attitude to spiritual and pastoral care. In other words there are not many times when it is written into procedure to contact chaplaincy or to offer spiritual and pastoral care. This is unlike other disciplines that will routinely be called on at different stages in the care of a child, and whose work is written down within a care plan and monitored. Again this backs up the argument for the need for spiritual and pastoral care to be written in the pathway at all three major stages, so that chaplains are routinely consulted, even if it is to simply verify that our service is not required.

It may have been noticed by the reader that the majority, if not all, of the references in this chapter are to American journals and research work. Despite considerable effort and consultation with other chaplains, it seems there is very little written in the United Kingdom about how chaplaincy is able to work alongside other disciplines in providing spiritual and pastoral care to families with children who are receiving palliative care. Maybe this will change in the near future.

N.I.C.E. analysis

Please reflect on the issues raised in this chapter in relation to your own practice.

Needs

- To recognise the resource available to both families and healthcare professionals through the chaplaincy service.
- To integrate chaplaincy into the multidisciplinary care provision for children and young people with life-limiting illness.
- To engage the chaplaincy team at the beginning of Act Care Pathway 1.

Misconceptions

- Professionals supporting children, young people and their families might need to address their own perspective on spiritual matters to avoid letting their own perspective determine whether they should make a referral to chaplaincy services.

Concerns

- There is a very limited body of knowledge currently available in respect of spiritual support of children, young people and their families.
- There seems to be misconceptions amongst healthcare professionals about the role chaplaincy might play in the care of vulnerable families.

Expectations

- That the spiritual needs for children, young people and their families are met.
- To recognise how chaplaincy can support families and staff alike over and above religious affiliation.
- Improve the body of knowledge pertaining to spiritual support of children and young people and their families.

From the above analysis please reflect on:

- How is chaplaincy currently integrated in your area of work?
- Are there any barriers to the successful integration of spiritual support?
- Are there advantages/disadvantages in integrating chaplaincy as part of the multidisciplinary team?

Action plan: next steps

- To establish clear communication channels between children, young people and their families in relation to their spiritual needs.
- This might require a re-evaluation of attitudes and values held by individuals in respect of their own spiritual stance and how this might differ from that of the families we care for.

REFERENCES

1 Wolff T. *Nottingham Integrated Care Pathway for Children with Life-limiting and Life-threatening Conditions.* Nottingham: Nottingham University Hospitals; 2006.
2 Robinson MR, May M, Thiel M, *et al.* Matters of spirituality at the end of life in pediatric intensive care. *Pediatrics*, 2006; **118**: e 719–29.

3 Elston S. *Integrated Multi-agency Care Pathways for Children with Life-threatening and Life-limiting Conditions.* Bristol: ACT; 2004. Available at: www.act.org.uk/landing.asp?section=40&sectionTitle=Help+for+professionals (accessed February 2010).

4 Feudtner C, Haney J, Dimmers MA. Spiritual care needs of hospitalized children and their families: a national survey of pastoral care providers' perceptions. *Pediatrics.* 2003; **111**: e67–72.

5 Armbruster CA, Chibnall JT, Legett S. Pediatrician beliefs about spirituality and religion in medicine: associations with clinical practise. *Pediatrics.* 2003; **111**: e227–35.

6 Grossoehme DH, Ragsdale JR, McHenry CL, *et al.* Pediatrician characteristics associated with attention to spirituality and religion in clinical practise. *Pediatrics.* 2007; **119**: e117–23.

Transitions at the beginning of life: psychological support

Ian Woodroffe

This chapter examines the multiple loss world of the family who has a pre-term baby on a Neonatal Intensive Care Unit (NICU) or a Special Care Baby Unit (SCBU). The concept of the assumptive world is examined as is the idea of a family emotion/death culture. Multiple loss is explained and a brief conclusion to the section considers helpful strategies for family-centred care of parents with multiple loss and possible bereavement. The UK's strategy *Better Care: Better Lives*[1] presents a vision that there should be 'universal provision of emotional, psychological, spiritual and bereavement support for the family (including siblings) carers and wider community'.

This part of the chapter puts that vision in the context of the experience of parents following a pre-term birth.

INTRODUCTION

Most people live their lives as if nothing serious will go wrong. We know at a cognitive level that things do go wrong, but at an emotional level we go about our daily lives as if our world, and the world of those around us, is safe and secure. I would probably not get out of bed in the morning if I thought that a serious accident would happen that day and that I was likely to lose both my legs.

This assumption that the world is safe and secure is what in psychological terms is known as our 'assumptive world'.[2] If we apply the concept of the assumptive world to the reproductive part of life, most potential parents will assume that becoming pregnant should be without too much difficulty, maintaining a pregnancy is usual and that the safe delivery of a full-term baby will go according to plan. That may be said to be the assumptive world of the parent and family with regards to reproduction.

What is known is that when the assumptive world is tested or shattered then there is a psychological reaction to that shattering. The psychological reaction will differ according to the context of the shattering, and the emotional experience of the shattering of the assumptive world will be like the emotional experience of grief and loss. If the shattering of the assumptive world is very unexpected then it will take a long while before the world is trusted again and the experience of safety is experienced again. So for an example, if two people are in a long-term relationship and the relationship is unexpectedly ended by one party, it may take a long time before the 'injured party' trusts another individual enough to enter into a close relationship again.

If the assumptive world is shattered too violently it may be that the safe and secure assumptive world is never fully restored. There are very long-term consequences of being in a terrorist event such as the 'The Twin Towers' or the bombing of the London Underground. The consequences may produce post-traumatic stress disorder (PTSD) with the full diagnostic symptoms of DSM-IV.[3] Even if the symptoms of the shattering of the assumptive world do not lead to fully diagnosed PTSD then there will always be consequences to the shattering experience for the individual, which either will be contained or in some way expressed. The concept of post-traumatic stress symptoms is well researched.

What enables some people to 'internalise' and contain the experience and others react very differently is a complex issue as the multiple variables that govern the response are numerous.[4] One such variable may be the individual's family emotional culture; this can be illustrated by the consideration of the 'family death' culture.

THE FAMILY DEATH CULTURE

Very small children learn about loss and separation at a very young age often by observing the behaviour of the people around them. They may be aware of how loss and death are dealt with by the family long before they can talk about the experience for themselves.

Case one

Peter is a young boy aged five who is strongly attached to his goldfish. Each morning he feeds his goldfish and talks to it before going out of the house.

One morning he comes downstairs to feed the fish and finds that it is not swimming but floating upside down and Peter at once recognises that something is wrong. He experiences a sensation of sadness that begins to be expressed by some tears. Peter's parents immediately try to distract him away from the sadness. There is a promise that the goldfish will be flushed down the toilet and that a new fish will be purchased immediately to replace the fish that has died. Peter is told that 'big boys do not cry' and that he can have a treat in the form of food or some other distracting behaviour.

As a result of this experience it is possible to suggest some 'seeding' of responses in Peter. It is possible that Peter will have internalised the fact that it is not reasonable for males to cry when they are sad. It is possible that Peter has learnt that sad moments can be pushed aside by distractions or treats and that in order to move on the object that is lost is replaced as soon as possible.

The seeding influences of this culture are possibly that Peter learns to 'hold in' his emotions at sad times and he learns that one behaviour around sad moments is that of distraction. He may also learn that what is lost can apparently be replaced quickly and there is no need to worry about what has gone. Such influences may inform Peter's response to loss and grief when he is an adult.

Case two

Consider the scenario that Peter is growing up in a different environment. This environment deals with the situation in a different way.

Peter discovers that his goldfish is floating upside down when he comes to feed it in the morning. He asks his parents what is wrong with the goldfish and they tell him that it is dead. They explain that all living things die and that when they die people who were attached to them often feel sad. Peter receives a hug and is told that when people are sad they often cry and that is a natural response to the sad situation; in fact, he notices his dad is upset as well. It is explained to Peter that the goldfish will be buried at the bottom of the garden in a grave and that the grave will be marked with some flowers, or with a symbol. If the family has a religious belief the grave may be marked with a religious symbol.

The seeded influences of this culture are possibly that Peter understands that living things die, that there is an appropriate emotional reaction to the sad situation and that there are rituals for the saying of 'goodbye' and the disposal of the remains. As stated above, these influences may inform Peter's response to loss and grief when he is an adult.

If we consider Case One and Case Two, we could predict that the adult Peter may deal with the loss, grief and death situation differently depending on the family culture around loss and emotions.

Support workers in grief and loss often observe that families deal with loss and grief differently. One of the 'determinants' that influence this different response may be the family death culture.

You may like to consider whether what sort of culture around loss and death existed in your family as you grew up. Was the culture one in which emotions were freely expressed regardless of gender or was the culture one in which emotions were not expressed?

It would be reasonable to suggest that the influence of these factors will be very much at the centre of the adult reaction to the trauma situation in the NICU.

THE JOURNEY OF MOTHER, FATHER AND FAMILY

In the world of the NICU, the focus is, and quite correctly, on the baby that has been born and on the family response to the present moment of fragility. It is easy for the staff to miss the whole story of the complete pregnancy journey for it is probably deeply buried in the mother's notes somewhere but not easily accessible. The previous pregnancies will hopefully be recorded in the nursing care plan, but the details of the beginning of the journey are likely to be absent.

There may not be any recorded details of the struggle that existed to become pregnant in the beginning. There will almost certainly be no information about the emotional distress that may have been experienced by the couple with regard to infertility issues. There may be no reference to the sleepless nights that couples may have had following a scan that had 'a slight indication' that there were genetic abnormalities that would have to be checked later. There may be no reference to the struggle that some go through trying to decide to continue the pregnancy or terminate based on the information that has been imparted to the parents by the medical profession.

If any of these scenarios have been part of the pregnancy journey, then already long before the baby is born there have been complicated emotional responses of grief and loss that will have had consequences for the parents. The loss of the 'perfect dream' of having a family and believing that all will be exciting is obviously a huge loss.

If the pregnancy continues, the months will contain anxiety since the assumptive world of pregnancy and child bearing has been questioned by the life events. None of this information may be accessible to the staff on NICU. The fact that all this information may be vital in order to understand the parents is often overlooked.

With an understanding of the shattering of the assumptive world, the family culture around emotions and the possible pregnancy difficulties, it is time to consider the multiple loss context that parents find themselves in when they enter the world of neonatal intensive care. These losses will be on top of any losses that have been experienced during the pregnancy journey as explained above.

LOSSES BEFORE THE PARENTS EVEN STEP INTO THE NICU
The lost weeks of the pregnancy
A preterm baby may be admitted to the NICU from 23 weeks gestation in the UK. For the parents this will be a shock however well they have been prepared. They will be very aware of the fragility of the baby, not just by the physical appearance, which may be shocking for them to see, but also because of all the statements that will have been made by the medical staff. The parents may have received multiple messages about the percentages of babies that survive at that gestation and messages about the likelihood of disability, etc. The overall effect of that communication will have made the future of their baby very fragile.

For the mother there may be all kinds of thoughts about the loss of the 17 weeks of pregnancy. She will be aware that because of the early age the organs of her baby will not be fully developed and she may well reflect that if she had been able to 'hold onto' her baby for longer then the life expectancy might be improved. She may feel a real sense of guilt for not being able to 'hold on'. She may blame herself for the early birth and may microscopically examine her life up to the birth to try to find a reason for the early birth. Such feelings of guilt, blame and responsibility for the event are driven by her emotional state. Any amount of cognitive reasoning with the mother will not necessarily help. At one level she knows the reasonable, at the emotional level of her understanding she is trying to make sense of the situation that she finds herself in and cannot believe. The shock and the suddenness of the situation will give rise to emotional responses that are similar to a sudden loss or death situation. She may feel that it is all a nightmare that she cannot relate to and may have a sense of numbness.

Dreams of a perfect birth
The dreams of the perfect birth never considered that anything would go wrong and certainly did not contain the prospect of a birth just over halfway through the pregnancy. All that the parents had learnt from other parents and from any prenatal

education has been lost in the confusion, panic and terror of the preterm birth situation. All the preparation that may have been done in preparing the nursery, beginning to buy items for the baby now seems to have been premature and in some cases almost futile. The very fact of having been so prepared can for some parents make them feel that they 'tempted fate'.

The early photographs that are seen to be such a joyful communication for all the family are no longer shared in the same way. A tiny preterm baby wired up for observation and whose face may not be visible due to tubes and wires does not evoke the same photographic enthusiasm for the parents. For some it is even difficult to see any beauty in their baby.

Control over the birth process

Being in control is an important feature for most people's existence. When we are not in control there is often an anxiety. The intensity of the anxiety may depend on the situation and the individual concerned. Mothers who have spent time in their pregnancy at classes which, by various techniques, have taught them how to control the labour and the pain will certainly feel out of control if halfway through the pregnancy when suddenly told that they must have an emergency caesarean section. The cognitive part of the parents will know that the procedure may be important but the emotional consequences may be overwhelming. Such a way of going about things was not in the dream and certainly was not in the birth plan if one had been written. Mothers may feel strongly that all control has been taken away from them. The loss of control and the frustration can, for some, be increased if they are conscious during the procedure. If the baby is immediately taken away for resuscitation or taken to NICU then even having any control over the first few moments of the baby's life has also been taken away. There is an enforced abandonment of control. All parties are cognitively aware that this may be for 'the best' for the baby but the psychological consequences for mothers can be complex.

Bonding and attachment

The early moments following a birth can be very powerful and significant and there is recognition of the 'critical period' described by Herbert[5] where the infant moves up the mother's chest to find a place of security and safety. It is known that this primitive movement stimulates the lactation in the mother in order to provide nourishment for the offspring. The early moments of the first cuddle provide a strong emotional moment of reality, of the new life that has been created and often the joy is inexpressible save through the medium of tears from both parents.

A not unusual scenario in NICU is that Mum may have come in for an appointment and then been told that she is to stay in hospital. The result is that Mum may have a caesarean section within 24 hours and the baby is taken to NICU. It may be that Mum has been shown baby (although even that sometimes does not happen) but there will be no opportunity for a cuddle at birth. This is another dream moment lost for the mother. The important moment of post-birth bonding and attachment has been detrimentally effected. The effect is often so powerful that when the mother visits the Unit for the first time they may have great difficulty believing that this is their baby.

As a mother recently said, 'All the babies looked the same. I could have believed that any of the babies were mine.'

It is very unlikely that many mothers would have seen a pre-term baby so when a mother describes her baby as 'looking like a roast joint' it is clear to all that attachment and bonding has been affected. If, as can be the case, it is up to 4–12 hours before the mother even sees her baby, the loss of the early bonding is compounded.

The father may attempt to provide a progress report for the mother but even in that process he may have to weigh up and censor the amount he tells his partner. That very process may undermine his ability to bond as he has been catapulted into the protector/caring role of mother and baby. The practice of sending a photograph from NICU to the mother may be helpful to the mother but it has never been evaluated whether the images cause more fear in the mother rather than pleasure.

The lack of early pre-term bonding is a serious loss which not only affects the moments in the NICU but has the potential to affect the long-term relationship between mother and child.[6,13] The same of course can be said of fathers and the rest of the family unit. There is serious coordinated work to be done with the parents on bonding and attachment. The latter part of this section reflects on these issues.

Possible loss of breast feeding

As a result of the trauma and surgical procedure it may be that mother's milk production is affected. At the start of her child's life the reality may be that the baby cannot feed. The mother will certainly not be able to breast feed in the way she hoped for, if that had been her intention. The best the mother may be able to do is to find a corner somewhere (not so easily done in some places) and use a breast pump. The sense of failure may be compounded by only being able to produce a small amount of breast milk in the early stages.

Confidence as a mother

If, for the mother, the sum total of the pregnancy has been problems in the pregnancy, a surgical procedure and then an early pre-term baby in NICU, with all the compounding factors of that experience, there is a very strong possibility that her confidence as a mother has been undermined. This loss of confidence can seem to be at the very root of her femininity and her ability to play her part in the reproductive process and her role as a woman and a mother, which may have been a powerful longing for some time. At a deep level she may feel that she has let her partner down and somehow let society down. Her very sense of being a 'useful human being' could be questioned and that process has psychological consequences for her, some of which could lead to depressive tendencies.

THE BIRTH OF A STILLBORN BABY OR THE DEATH OF A TWIN

The birth of a stillborn baby ranks as one of the top stressors for parents. Often the procedures leading up to the stillbirth are traumatic before the event. Mothers may know that they are to deliver a stillborn baby. They know that they have to go through the same labour as any other mother yet there will be a dead child. Thankfully most maternity services are aware of the trauma that will be caused for the family and for the staff and have support services in place. Long-term bereavement counselling from suitably trained counsellors may be necessary. Again there needs to be a strategy and care pathway written – not to do so could constitute a lack of duty of care.

The death of a twin for parents when the surviving twin is on NICU is one of the most complex grief scenarios. How can you remain hopeful for the twin that is struggling in NICU and grieve for the twin that has died. Many parents find the handling of this difficult situation almost impossible. The research into the grief process will indicate that it is impossible for grief to be expressed at the same time as hope.

That means that when the parents are on the Unit they may not be able to think about the dead twin who may still be in the mortuary. Many parents recount how guilty they feel not thinking about one of their babies because they have to focus on the other. If they focus on the dead twin (and they may have to because of funerals, etc.) then they find it impossible to think of the live twin. Parents need to be assured that they will not be able to hold both the grief experience and the hoping in the palm of one hand. They may need to be assured that the grief for their dead baby may be processed at sometime in the future. If that is the case and that is the information that is given to parents, then again it is a duty of care issue for the Unit to provide long-term bereavement care for the parents. If that is not possible from the Unit resources (a bereavement counsellor, etc.) then a referral must be made to an outside bereavement service and the referral must be recorded in the medical notes. To discharge parents from a Unit without the necessary support offer in place would be an act of neglect carrying all the consequences of that neglectful action.

A MIRROR HELD TO THE ENTIRE TRAUMA

It is suggested that traumatic experiences lead to emotional responses and the emotional responses can give rise to certain behaviours. The question is, in the NICU situation can we have some understanding of the responses and therefore be prepared for, and have an understanding of, the behaviours that may be exhibited? In fact, can we write our strategies and our care pathways for truly family-centred care based upon the research of the loss world of the parents? Such a strategy would demonstrate understanding to the parents and may provide genuine therapeutic benefit.

In 2006 I systematically asked parents to describe their experience of being in NICU. I asked for one word from the mother and one from the father to describe their experience, their feelings and their behaviours. The words listed in Boxes 18.1–18.3 are words of the service users.[7] (Boxes 18.1–18.3 are reproduced by kind permission of the editor of the *Journal of Neonatal Nursing*.)

These are the words that parents have used to describe the experience of coming onto NICU:

Box 18.1

Unattached	Lonely	Scary
Unreal	Hell on earth	Nightmare
Devastating	Terrifying	Guilty

The feelings described by parents on a NICU:

Box 18.2

Frustration	Isolation	Fragility
Panic	Despair	Confusion
Disorientation	Exhaustion	Worry
Anger	Helplessness	Guilt
Resentment	Fear	Numbness
Excitement	Hope	Pride
Thankfulness		

Emotional states will affect the behaviours of the individual. As a result of the feelings that are expressed in Box 18.2 it can be predicted that certain behaviours will be exhibited within the NICU environment.

Behaviours that might be observed as a result of the emotions experienced:

Box 18.3

- Withdrawal
- Tearful
- Angry with staff partner (God, if faith system)
- Defensive
- Resigned numbness
- Needing knowledge
- Needing control
- Demanding
- Thankful
- In awe
- Supportive of other parents

If the staff in a NICU and SCBU were to be ever-mindful of the experiences and feelings of parents as described in Box 18.1 and Box 18.2 then serious communication breakdowns between staff and parents might be minimised.

In my work with parents it seems that it is often the insensitive remark by a doctor or a nurse that causes great distress and certainly demonstrates a lack of understanding of the inner traumatic world of the parent. Anybody who has ever been in a nightmare scenario and feels helpless and disorientated will know just how vulnerable parents can feel. With that understanding a behaviour of 'withdrawal' on behalf of the parents will be understood and not judged.

EVEN MORE MULTIPLE LOSS

The combined experience of some, or all, of the losses mentioned above will almost certainly contribute to a sense of trauma and multiple loss for the mother and father. As part of a risk assessment this trauma and multiple grief response could be anticipated. In some cases the trauma may be so severe that some months after the birth a diagnosis of PTSD is confirmed. In this case the mother will exhibit symptoms of restlessness, flashbacks, hypervigilance, extreme anxiety, etc. Sometimes PTSD may not be diagnosed, but post-traumatic stress syndrome is confirmed.[8,9] Such diagnosis will have a disabling consequence on the life of the mother leading to a non-functioning existence for her and those around her.

It is estimated that, in the UK alone, traumatic births may result in 10 000[10] women a year developing PTSD. Also, as many as 200 000 more women may feel traumatised by childbirth and develop some of the symptoms of PTSD according to the Birth Trauma Association.[10]

The multiple grief experienced by the preterm birth and having a baby on Neonatal Critical Care may mean that the parents, but particularly the mother, is unable to process any emotional experiences and may have a profound inability to absorb more information, particularly if it is of a distressing nature either for the present or for the future.[11,12]

The experience of multiple grief leaves individuals numb and in a similar emotional state as the recently bereaved – numb and unable to rationally comprehend what has gone on; many describe the state as one of detachment and 'as if in a dream/nightmare'. The sense of realty of the events is unable to be understood. This is likely to mean that it will be difficult to absorb and process any other information that is given particularly if it is perceived to be bad news.

There is a potential complexity to this multiple grief since the experience will not take place in isolation to the other life experiences of the parents. It is unusual in the NICU situation for the staff to know much about the previous loss history of the parents. The previous losses in the obstetric history may be known but it is unlikely for family losses to be known. Those losses may be deaths, relationship breakdown, redundancy and other life events that create a loss reaction.

It is understood in grief theory that the grief of the present moment reawakens the grief experience of the past. That means that emotions from past losses may become real in the present situation. Emotions from previous loss events will contribute to the experience and behaviour of the individual in the present.[13,14] For example if a parent has been subjected to the multiple grief situation of a preterm baby on NICU and had experienced the death of a significant parent recently then the feelings of the loss of that parent will be activated.

For the greater understanding of the psychological state of the parent it is strongly suggested that staff discover the previous losses and family support systems as this knowledge becomes essential to provide the necessary components of psychological family-centred care. One method for documenting this important information is the Family Tree.[15]

A Family Tree is the tool that is often used in palliative care but is not often used in the NICU and SCBU environments. The Tree is an ideal multidisciplinary tool that clearly demonstrates in pictorial form the past losses within the family and much more. If the Tree is placed in the front of the medical notes then it is available to speech and language therapists, dieticians, counsellors, etc. who will be able to use the information in their work.

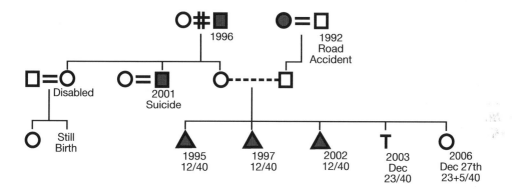

FIGURE 18.1 One simple format of the family tree

On examination of the tree in Figure 18.1 it becomes clear that there will be a large number of losses that may be re-opened by the admission of a 23+5 baby into NICU. It is possible that the previous grief has not been processed and that the grief has become 'frozen'. Any grief distress in the frozen state will become internalised and 'distracted' from. On admission to the Neonatal Critical Care, loss feelings may be reactivated from the past and influence the parents' ability to handle the present loss situation. The consequences of this relatively common situation may mean that there is serious impairment to be able to listen and understand. There may be changes in behaviour and the ability to attach and bond with the baby may be seriously affected.

If all of these factors are known then it is it reasonable to consider the use of a risk assessment tool to identify the parents who may be at a higher level of risk. Identifying the risk in this way could mean that proactive work in trauma and grief support would be highly beneficial to the mental health of the parent and the relationship between parent and their baby.

Box 18.4 A possible Risk Assessment Tool[7]

Referral Rating

Points (please circle)

1 Age of baby at birth _____ (if <28weeks please tick box).	15
2 Did the baby require significant resuscitation at birth?	20
3 Any medical problems other than pre-term?	
Specify _____ .	20
4 Caesarean section (unplanned).	15
5 Previous miscarriage(s) >12 and <20 weeks.	
Specify gestation _____ weeks.	10
6 Previous death of a baby/child.	
Specify gestation _____ weeks.	30
7 Death of family member or significant other within last three years.	10
8 Twin/triplets transferred to NICUs elsewhere in the UK.	15
9 More than 30 miles from home.	5
10 Other children <12 years.	
Specify ages _____ .	5
11 Father of child self-employed.	5
12 Visible signs of trauma/distress, either one or both parents.	15
13 Social issue documentation in Care Plan.	15

Add points for boxes ticked

TOTAL score

Scores over 50 require a formal Priority referral to psychological support (sticker in referral book).

Name of parents: _____

Mother: _____

Tel. no: _____

Father: _____

Tel. no: _____

NB. Please place this assessment in the box. Thank you.

Baby's addressograph label

TEAM WORK TO LESSEN THE SENSE OF HELPLESSNESS

It would hardly surprise the reader to know that the author of this part of the chapter makes a case for well coordinated and thought through team work around the psychological issues that surround pre-term parents.

It would be helpful if the medical or nursing staff were part of the risk assessment by being part of the early documentation completed on admission to the NICU. Similarly the drawing of family trees by the nurses or some appointed other person would contribute to the understanding of the loss history of the parents.

Any small action to stimulate bonding and attachment that the staff can encourage the parents to be involved with is potentially very important. Parents respond with enthusiasm feeling that in the midst of their helplessness they can do something. Asking a mother to sleep with a small piece of cloth in her breast cleavage, which can be placed on the incubator so that smell bonding can continue can be so liberating for a mother. Asking mothers and fathers to be fully involved in their baby's care is essential. It may be that gentle encouragement from the staff is needed. Parents (often especially fathers) are very frightened of all the wires and the fragility of the tiny pre-term.

Parents are often frightened (for the same reasons as above) to ask for cuddles and kangaroo care. Neonatal services have to acknowledge that often important bonding moments are lost for parents on the basis that there are not enough staff to cover the event and care for the other babies. Parents may not feel confident to ask for cuddles and kangaroo care as part of their fear or because the service so institutionalises parents to the extent that their helplessness is compounded.

Parents are excluded from ward rounds in some places giving rise to a sense that there may be information about their baby that they are not party to. How helpful is that, given the psychological map that we have already drawn from the parents' experience?

Within post-death grief work the use of memory boxes has been acknowledged. It needs to be recognised that no research evidence has been produced to show that the use of such boxes is helpful although comments from parents indicate that they are invaluable. At Addenbrookes Hospital in Cambridge the use of the box has been very successfully extended to include the loss and trauma time from the beginning.

A 'Journey Box' is given to all parents on day two of their stay in NICU.[7] The box contains significant objects selected by the parents. Such objects include the syringe that was used for the first meal, the first size (clean!) nappy, hats, any pieces of medical equipment that can be safely kept, photographs, etc. The clear rationale of the project is that the significant objects will give an opportunity for a chronological sequence and a life history for the baby, which can be explained by the parents later, thus continuing bonding into the future.[16] If the baby were to die, a 'Memory Box' is already in place. It is suggested that such significant objects may aid the grief process for many years. More evidenced-based research is needed on this subject.

There is often a family unit that surrounds the parents. That unit may include grandparents and siblings. It would be reasonable to recognise that both grandparents and siblings will react to the pre-term birth.

Grandparents often suffer in silence as they go into supporting roles for their daughter- and son-in-law. There is a place within the caring strategy to consider the grandparents with special grandparent coffee mornings or meetings. If the baby dies, bereavement support for grandparents should be a serious consideration.

'It should have been me' is an expression often made by grandparents that demonstrates the perceived unfairness of the unnatural death of a baby. That is not how the generational death sequence is understood.

NICUs may be fascinating places for siblings who have a concentration time span of two nanoseconds. There may need to be allocated provision for sibling work both for the sibling to understand the environment and to address the attention deficit that may exist from parents.

A Unit would do well to consider the active involvement of siblings in the NICU. A creative play therapist might save the health services money by attending to the issues when they arise on the Unit. There should be no reason why the parent's already difficult life should be made more difficult by the behaviour of a sibling who has not been given the opportunity to express, in an age-appropriate manner, the feelings that have been created by having a baby on the Unit and an absent mother.

CONCLUSION

The acknowledged experiences of parents who have trodden the NICU path should inform the planning of support. There will always be arguments about money and questions about the necessity of the support that should be available. It is, however, clear from listening to the case loads of counsellors working in the field of neonatal loss and grief that early intervention is helpful to the well-being of the family unit. More research is needed to underpin the perception.

The future may be a little brighter for families if coordinated psychological support is part of the provision from conception through to the community. That may prove to be a cost saving development, for the facts are known about the trauma experience and we owe it to the parents to deliver coordinated care based on the rationale of the trauma reaction experienced by parents. Only then can we ever dare use the phrase 'family-centred care'.

STAFF

It is not within the remit of this chapter to write fully about staff support. However, it would be negligent not to point out that working alongside families who exhibit such trauma and loss is exceedingly demanding. Compassion, fatigue and burnout are well acknowledged psychological concepts.[17] The staff may need support in various ways and at least it needs to be acknowledged that it is not possible to work in such areas of trauma without it having an effect on the staff member. There is, here, another area of duty of care that employers need to take seriously.

N.I.C.E. analysis

Please reflect on the issues raised in this chapter in relation to your own practice.

Needs

- Counselling/psychological support for all families with a baby in NICU and SCBU.
- Understanding and recognition of the emotional loss that parents may suffer within neonatal services.
- Strategic planning and policies to be written for psychological support within neonatal services.
- Regional strategies for the future development of psychological support on a national basis.
- Specific training for professionals to work with loss in neonatal services should be included in neonatal training courses.

Interests

- Parent involvement in decision making and policies within neonatal services.
- More research needs to be carried out on the emotional cost on relationships/bonding between parents and a pre-term baby.
- Loss issues within families when a premature baby is born into the family.

Concerns

- That emotional/psychological issues within neonatal medicine are considered to be an expensive luxury.
- Psychological 'talk the talk' is not reflected in resources provided to parents for support.
- That multidisciplinary working within neonatal services is not planned to include psychological support for parents.
- Counselling/psychological support workers are deemed to be too expensive within the service provision.

Expectations

- Families of pre-term babies and early pregnancy death should have support for their losses and for any future anxious pregnancies.
- That all staff have information about parents' previous pregnancy history and support parents with appropriate sensitivity: attitudes, language, waiting areas, clinic times, etc.
- National Neonatal Services resource and plan for the provision and the development of psychological support.
- That the pain and loss of parents is listened to, understood and acted upon and documented in neonatal care plans.

From the above analysis please reflect on:
- On your NICU/SCBU who has responsibility to focus on the losses for parents?
- If nobody has time and no support post exists, what do you think happens to all the trauma that parents may experience?
- Why do you think pre-term losses are less important than post-death bereavement? (This is asked because many support posts only work with post-death losses.)

- Within your Unit how could parent involvement improve psychological support?

Action plan: next steps

- To map psychological support posts within national neonatal services. (Psychological service provision before and after pre-term death.)
- Production of strategies to support parents.
- To discharge parents, or transfer them to another hospital without a developed psychological care plan clearly developed is a failure of duty of care.
- Seek resources nationally to support parents after neonatal/birth trauma.
- Establish a national association for staff who deliver psychological support to parents.
- The association would communicate examples of excellence and seek to develop improvement of services with reference to international practices.

REFERENCES

1 Department of Health. *Better Care: Better Lives*. 2008. Available at: www.dh.gov.uk/en/Publicationsandstatistics/Publications/PublicationsPolicyAndGuidance/DH_083106 (accessed 17 February 2010).

2 Kauffman J, editor. *Loss of the Assumptive World: a theory of traumatic loss*. New York: Brunner Routledge; 2002.

3 American Psychological Association. Diagnostic and Statistical Manual of Mental Disorders DSM-IV. New York: American Psychological Association; 2006.

4 Rothschild B. *The Body Remembers: the psychophysiology of trauma and trauma treatment*. New York: Norton; 2000.

5 Herbert M. *Psychology for Social Workers*. London: BPS and McMillan; 1998.

6 Bowlby J. *Attachment and Loss*. Vol 1. London: Hogarth Press; 1980. Volume 3. Available at: http://pep.gvpi.net/document.php?id=ipl.079.0001a (accessed 23 February 2010).

7 Woodroffe I. Multiple losses in neonatal intensive care units. *J Neonatal Nurs*. 2006; **12**: 144–7.

8 Van der Kolk BA, McFarlane AC, Weisaeth L, editors. *Traumatic Stress*. New York: Guildford Press; 1996.

9 Holditch-Davis D, Bartlett TR, Blickman AL, *et al*. Post trauma stress symptoms in mothers of preterm infants. *J Obstet Gynecol Neonatal Nurs*. 2003; **32**: 161–71.

10 www.birthtraumaassociation.org.uk

11 Kastenbaurn R. Death and bereavement in later life. In: Kutscher A, editor. *Death and Bereavement*. Springfield: Thomas; 1969.

12 Wigert H, Johansson R, Berg M. Mothers' experiences of having their newborn child in a neonatal intensive care unit. *Scand J Caring Sci*. 2006; **20**: 35–41.

13 Bowlby J. The making and breaking of affectional bonds. *Br J Psychiatr*. 1977; **132**: 201–10; 421–31.

14 Simos BG. *A Time to Grieve*. New York: Family Service Association; 1979.

15 Worden WJ. *Grief Counselling and Grief Therapy*. London: Brunner-Routledge; 2001.

16 McGoldrick M, Gerson R, Shellenberger S. *Genograms in Family Assessment*. New York: Norton; 1985.

17 Klass D, Silverman PR, Nickman SL, editors. *Continuing Bonds: new understandings of grief.* London: Taylor & Francis; 1996.

18 Figley CR. *Treating Compassion Fatigue.* New York: Brunner-Routledge; 2002.

19 Bowlby J, Parkes CM, editors. Separation and loss within the family. In: Anthony EJ, editor. *The Child in His Family.* New York: Wiley; 1970.

20 SSRU. Foretelling futures: dilemmas in neonatal neurology: a social science research project 2002–2004. Available at: www.ioe.ac.uk/study/departments/ssru/222.html (accessed 17 February 2010).

21 Goldson E, editor. *Developmental Interventions in the Neonatal Intensive Care Nursery.* New York: Oxford University Press; 1999.

22 Jotzo M, Poets C. Trauma-preventive psychological intervention. Helping parents cope with the trauma of premature birth. *Pediatrics.* 2005; **115**: 915–19.

23 Mattiesen A, Ransjo-Arvidson A, Nissen E, *et al.* Postpartum maternal oxytocin release by newborns: effects of infant hand massage and sucking. *Birth.* 2001; **28**: 13–19.

24 Parkes CM. Acquainted with grief. *Illness Crisis Loss.* 2003; **11**: 37–46.

25 Rossi E. *The Psychobiology of Mind-Body Healing.* New York: Norton; 1993.

26 Speece and Brent cited by Corr CA. Children's understandings of death – striving to understand death. In: Doka KJ, editor. *Children Mourning, Mourning Children.* Hospice Foundation of America. New York: Routledge; 1995.

19

Managing transitions to hospice care: the hospice consultant's perspective

Mike Miller

INTRODUCTION

Due to the nature of the cases admitted, a majority of inpatient childhood deaths occur on the Paediatric Intensive Care Units (PICU).[1] However, similar to a children's hospice the mortality rate is lower than in adult practice. Despite all attempts to maintain or replace organ function, either the disease processes lead to an organ failure or the chances of a worthwhile recovery are so unlikely that care is withdrawn. Recent guidelines help with such considerations.[2] Decisions about maintaining or withdrawing treatment have to be reached in relatively short time periods. Although it is possible to provide good palliative care on an intensive care unit, privacy is limited and there are often insufficient facilities for the family. A recent examination of the PICAnet database showed that only a very small proportion of children were deemed to be transferred to palliative care as determined by the completion of the discharge form.[3] This raises known concerns about the understanding that staff working in PICU may have about the role of palliative care.

Children known to palliative care

Children with life-limiting conditions often have reduced reserves and so are more likely to deteriorate quickly with inter-current illnesses and need care on an intensive care unit. It is very difficult to be certain which chest infection is likely to be the last. If these children have had stays at a children's hospice and their parents are aware of the facilities there, they may ask to be transferred to the hospice for the child's last few hours or days. They may have had contact with the staff at the hospice who may then suggest the option of transfer. This is relatively straightforward, as the child and family will be known to the hospice; managing terminal care is a hospice's core business and the Paediatric Intensive Care Team should be happy to support this in the knowledge that the family and child will receive the most appropriate care. Even so the PICU will have to have confidence in the hospice and knowledge of the level of support they will provide.

Children not known to palliative care

Once links are established, the intensive care unit is likely to identify children and families who may benefit from hospice support but are not known to the hospice. This might be sudden, severe neurological damage following trauma or infection in a previously healthy child. When discussions are held with the family about future options it can be helpful to include the option of transfer to a hospice. This helps to reinforce the severity of the illness, acknowledge the difficulties of the family in coming to terms with this and to be seen to offer continuing support. The hospice will be rung to check that a bed is available; however, mostly the family will not wish to take up this offer. Distance from relatives, getting to know another team and uncertainties about a hospice are all reasons given.

MANAGING LINKS

At least two consultants in paediatric palliative care have attended regular ward rounds on an intensive care unit. Both intensive care consultants and palliative care consultants share the care of the child with colleagues, yet may have to make difficult decisions about that care. Good communications, including with primary care, are important. The palliative care consultant may take the opportunity to stay abreast of current acute paediatric thinking as well as experiencing what can and cannot be achieved on the PICU. They are then able to speak with authority to families when having end-of-life discussions. At times those discussions may lead to families wishing their child to have full intensive care and the palliative care consultant can then negotiate with their intensive care colleagues to ensure that admission takes place as smoothly as possible. Most parents do not wish their child to have a long stay and the palliative care consultant can be present to help with discussions about care.

Hopefully the intensive care unit gains from having a recognition of the presence and purpose of palliative care and the relatively frequent transfers of children to the hospice suggest that the service is appreciated.

ARRANGING THE TRANSFER

The timing of transfer may be able to be controlled, but often the illness dictates that events move swiftly.

The hospice will need to know:

1   that the parents accept that options for further treatment in the hospice are limited. In particular it is unlikely that any electronic monitoring will take place in the hospice
2   that the parents know that there will be no attempts at resuscitation should the heart or breathing stop
3   there may be risks that the child dies in transit
4   they will have to have some details of the family and family structure, including who will wish to stay
5   whatever treatment will be continued in the best interests of the child, e.g. IV infusion pumps, IV drugs (including antibiotics) and IV fluids may all need to be transferred with the child

6   what the plan is for withdrawal of care and in particular the timing of events
7   if death occurs, will the coroner be involved or will there be a doctor who can sign the death certificate?

If there is time, it is helpful to have contact between the family and the hospice before the child is transferred. For children who are not known, it may be that staff from the hospice are able to visit the child and family on the PICU or that the family come to view the hospice supported by PICU staff.

In the rush of arranging the transfer it is very easy to forget to communicate this to the GP and community nursing teams, even though any transfer of a patient is a good prompt to ensure that primary care is informed of progress. Passing information on at this stage will make future communication easier.

TRANSFER

Arranging the ambulance is an important, often rate-limiting step. Once the nature of the transfer has been explained, the fact that a doctor will be accompanying the child helps manage the risks, although the ambulance crew will be reassured by seeing a written and signed care plan that includes treatment limitations and expectations. Almost all children will need a doctor to ensure the safety of ventilation during transfer. Allowing a parent to accompany the child in the ambulance is important as is reassuring the parent who is likely to follow that the ambulance may stop if things need to be rearranged in transit. Before transfer discussions should take place to ensure that electronic monitoring and drug treatment is reduced to a minimum and the rationale for this explained to parents.

Details about whether the child will be ventilated by bag or on a mechanical ventilator and the level of sedation involved will depend on individual circumstances. Minimal monitoring may be used during transfer but all monitoring is usually withdrawn on arrival at the hospice. Family and staff can then focus on the child and the needs of the child, not the output of the monitors.

TIMING OF WITHDRAWAL

In some circumstances, no treatment may be being withdrawn. A child with peritonitis and severe cerebral palsy was admitted urgently to a hospice from a surgical ward, having relapsed after four days on PICU. The hospice was able to provide privacy and support for her and her family. The oxygen, IV fluids and IV antibiotics were all continued and to everyone's surprise she recovered over the next 10 days.

For most children there is an expectation by all concerned that treatment (usually extubation) will occur very soon after arrival in the hospice. It is important that the family should have some time to catch their breath, and adjust to their surroundings before extubation (this can be done in 20 minutes) if possible. Sadly some children are so severely ill that extubation on arrival and acceptance of their death is the only right option.

One family, whose son had suffered severe hypoxia following an attempt at self-strangulation, expressed the view they were not ready to withdraw treatment then but would be in a few days. It was arranged to ventilate the child in the hospice for three nights and then withdraw treatment. There were some concerns that when the time came the family would wish there to be further delays, and other concerns that the hospice nurses did not feel qualified to be in charge of a comatose, ventilator-dependent child. It was agreed between parents, hospice and PICU that PICU would provide nursing support for the first 36 hours to help train the hospice staff on the ventilator. Hospice nurses would provide care for the remaining time. After only two nights, the family decided that the time had come to stop treatment. In future it may become easier to allow the families this little bit of control. I feel that this is an example of the duty of care to the child becoming secondary to the duty of care to the family as the child declines.

MANAGING THE WITHDRAWAL OF TREATMENT

For most families, the hard work of coming to a decision about withdrawal and the timing of withdrawal will have occurred on the intensive care unit. The family can then take the lead with hospice staff ensuring that the child has sufficient sedation and pain relief to prevent any suffering. At this stage the primary aim will be to prevent any pain or distress, the secondary aim is to treat the child with dignity and to be seen to be not taking any chances away from them. All hospices and intensive care units will have tales of children who have continued to breathe after withdrawal of mechanical ventilation. Often the use of sedation is sufficient to remove anxiety so the child does not develop increasing distress. Sadly the respiratory effort is usually not sufficient to support life more than a few hours. The family will need considerable support during this uncertain time.

This process allows the family to focus on the child and their needs. Discussions can be framed in terms of allowing the child the dignity of making their own decision and not having a decision imposed on them. This helps avoid the conflict of parents wishing everything done.[4]

MANAGING CONTINUING SURVIVAL

Some children will have enough respiratory drive to survive and then questions of when to start giving fluids and nutrition arise. Almost invariably these children will have severe neurological impairment and it is likely to be appropriate that they continue to be cared for in a hospice even though all medical techniques are not available. Any techniques started in a hospice are usually able to be continued at home.

Managing suffering and uncertainty is said to be a function of palliative care. If a child continues to breathe there will need to be further conversations with the family about the level of support provided to the child. Withdrawal of care will only have taken place if the child's future quality of life is thought to be unbearable. It may therefore be reasonable to continue to ensure the child is comfortable but provide no extra oxygen nor treat intercurrent infections with antibiotics.

Some children will survive to transfer home and then the earlier good communications with the primary care team will be seen to have been very helpful.

TRANSFER FOR BREAKS FROM INTENSIVE CARE

Children's hospices are known for providing high-quality short breaks. However, they are unable to deliver this service (often free of charge) to all children with complex needs. Therefore acceptance criteria involving prognosis and progression will be developed by all hospices. Occasionally there are children who need high levels of support but are thought to have a good long-term prognosis. They may need to stay for many months on PICU while home-care packages are organised and there will be pressure on a hospice to accept such children for short breaks. Often nursing support will be provided from the PICU. This will help to improve links so that provided care of other children is not compromised. Such stays may be encouraged.

It is then possible for the occasional child who has a sudden loss of respiratory function of unknown cause to spend time at a children's hospice without the parents blocking transfer because of fears about the nature of a children's hospice. The space and time available during the stay will enable correct decisions to be made about future care. Hospices are one place where it is possible to talk about death and what happens after death in a calm and considered manner.

ADVANTAGES OF TRANSFER FOR THE PICU

Staff on a PICU may have little time to get to know and support the families of critically ill children. Being able to understand and support the family will help develop trust between strangers and allow open discussions about the best interests of children. Knowing that the family will have this continuing support at all stages of their child's life as well as in bereavement, enables clear discussion about death. Often bereavement support will only be readily available from a hospice if they have been involved in a child's care. Hopefully the intensive care unit will value the end-of-life care provided by the hospice and recognise that they are best able to focus on ensuring the child's comfort while supporting the family.

ADVANTAGES OF TRANSFER FOR THE CHILDREN'S HOSPICE

The transfer of a previously unknown, severely ill child and their family can create great uncertainty for a hospice. Generally, decisions are taken by both teams and a consensus reached. However, providing high quality end-of-life care should be the principal function of a hospice and being confident that this can be achieved in all circumstances can be very rewarding. The hospice then becomes a stronger part of the care community with a recognisable set of transferable skills and knowledge to the benefit of the day-to-day care of children with complex needs, including those with life-limiting illnesses.

N.I.C.E. analysis

Please reflect on the issues raised in this chapter in relation to your own practice.

Needs

- To use the facilities of the hospice to the full to benefit children and families.
- To support families at this difficult time.
- To make sure that families know we continue to support and care, come what may.
- To work and support decisions made on the Paediatric Intensive Care Network.

Interests

- Decision making at end of life.
- Providing the right care in the right settings.
- Keeping a promise of full support to families.

Concerns

- Overloading staff in the children's hospice, with very challenging work.
- Managing the expectations of parents.
- Working to get it right for children and their families.

Expectations

- Managing expectations of families.
- Understanding that death is one part of life.
- Recognition from intensive care of the part a hospice can play in the support of a life-limiting illness.

From the above analysis please reflect on:

- How to balance the needs and expectations of families with the needs of the intensive care unit and the resources of the hospice.
- The training needs of the staff.
- When is the right time to discuss this choice with parents?
- How to disseminate this course of action to other groups and reassure them that it is appropriate.

Action plan: next steps

- Make sure that we continue to offer the choice and work hard to get it right when we do.
- Publicise these possibilities.
- Maintain good working relationships with intensive care units.

REFERENCES

1 Pearson GA, editor. *Why Children Die: a pilot study 2006; England (South West, North East and West Midlands), Wales and Northern Ireland.* London: CEMACH. 2008

2 Royal College of Paediatrics and Child Health. *Withholding or Withdrawing Life-sustaining Treatment in Children: a framework for practice.* 2nd ed. London: RCPCH; 2004. Available at: www.rcpch.ac.uk/Publications/Publications-list-by-date (accessed 17 February 2010).

3 Craig F, Comac M, McCulloch R, Rajapakse CD. Will the families of children dying on

Picu choose to transfer their child's care to a palliative care service and leave Picu? Cardiff International Conference on Paediatric Palliative Care: *Speaking of Dying: what are we saying?* 2008, July 7–9.

4 Gillis J. We want everything done. *Arch Dis Child.* 2008; **93**: 192–3.

20

Supporting transitions: effective palliative care teams

Stefan Friedrichsdorf, Jody Chrastek and Stacy Remke

Paediatric palliative care teams come in many different forms and variations; to provide excellent comprehensive care it is essential to have a strong team, since no one professional group can provide the care alone.[1] Sims and Jassal describe a team as being a group of individuals who share goals and work together to deliver services for which they are mutually accountable.[2] The team works in a coordinated, cohesive way to reach shared goals. Paediatric palliative care emphasises a family-centred approach to care which includes the family and child as key team members, an approach essential to the development of an appropriate individualised palliative care plan. Our challenge is that it is only when there is a cohesive and collaborative palliative care team in place that the child and family can be fully served.

Communication is an essential ingredient for the success of any team and this includes communication both within the team and of course with the family and child. The importance of communication cannot be underscored; for example, research has demonstrated that in some situations, families of deceased patients felt that with improved team communication they would have experienced more comprehensive care both for themselves but most importantly for their child.[3] Teams change and evolve over time, increasing in both capacity and complexity. This will be highlighted throughout this chapter, where we will share 15 years of experiences gleaned through working within an interdisciplinary team.

THE GOAL: TRANSDISCIPLINARY CARE

Sims and Jassal describe different styles of team functioning.[2] Many programmes will evolve from a multidisciplinary approach to care where several disciplines are involved in the care of a child and his/her family; to interdisciplinary care where several disciplines work together and actively interface to collaborate, plan and coordinate care; to transdisciplinary care in which, an interdisciplinary team frequently working with children with life-limiting conditions addresses issues outside their classic roles – in the interests of meeting the total care needs of the child and family as these arise.[1] In our team's experience, transdisciplinary care has included our chaplain identifying a poor analgesia regime or a physician attending to the spiritual needs of the family because of an immediate or specific need in a given encounter. That practitioner then uses the trust the child and family have in them to enlist the assistance of the other team member with the most appropriate skill set for the identified concern. This interweaving of skills and relationships seeks to leave families confident that they have been well attended to throughout their child's illness course and beyond. This also requires the team members themselves to develop a comfort level in asserting their own roles and skills, talking openly with colleagues about needed referrals and respect for existing relationships.

In Minnesota, we now have a large interdisciplinary team, but it has not always been this way. Initially, dying children were cared for by whichever home care nurse was available to see them. Clearly, this was not ideal. There were issues of continuity both in terms of the medical care of the patient and in building trust with the family. The effectiveness of the service varied, based upon the level of comfort the visiting nurse had with caring for a dying child. There was no identified programme or team working together. Psychosocial and spiritual issues were addressed in a hit or miss pattern as the nurse focused on the nursing needs of the child, and social work needs were ill defined.

Later, financial support was applied for through a US-based childhood cancer foundation and a fledgling programme was now able to become better organised with the inclusion of a part-time nurse, chaplain and social worker now defined as the hospice team. Gradually nurses who were skilled at, and wanted to provide care at the end of life became part of the team. Development of the team continued over the next 10 years and the programme was shaped and grew under the leadership of a social worker and a nurse with a medical director providing back-up as needed. The development of the programme was based on available literature about palliative care principles and service options about five years after it first became organised as a home-based hospice. It was not until another five years after the palliative care programme was formally organised that a medical director was hired and became an active part of the team on a daily basis, involved in patient care from a palliative care perspective.

As we evolved with limited available resources and insurance boundaries, which we will discuss later, team members utilised familiar networks for the development of the team. A few years ago, we became aware of the work of ACT in the UK. What was clear is that we had in fact utilised a similar type of pathway and there are now many examples where we have overlapping principles. It was unfortunate, perhaps, that at the time we were developing we were not aware of the work of ACT, but we now are able to utilise the ACT principles to make changes or complement our programme.

As the programme developed there were growing pains both internally in the team and externally for individuals and the institution as the team grew in size and acceptance. These challenges can be expected, and can be managed with good communication, flexibility and a strongly connected team.

Teams often start by putting together parts of positions from the hospital or the community. This can help establish relationships and develop stakeholder investment in the programme. Often additional resources can come from outside the healthcare community in schools or religious institutions. However the team is structured, it is essential to have excellent communications and shared understanding of the goals and strategies for care provision within the team from the outset. Such practices will also help the team orient and acculturate new members as growth occurs.

Collaborative teamwork has positively improved patient care[3] and is an essential part of any palliative care programme's effectiveness. A review of the literature underscores the value of the interdisciplinary team, yet offers little insight into how effective teamwork is accomplished. The concept that a team is essential to the provision of care is inherent to palliative care, and especially in paediatric palliative care. It is often considered as a component essential as any specific skills provided by any individual discipline in the holistic care of the patient. However, what that means, and how it looks in practice, is much more difficult to determine. Periyakoil identifies the importance of collaborative versus cooperative teams, and the critical support of the administrative structure behind the team as components of success.[4]

Clarity of purpose, a supportive environment, and factors like trust, conflict management skills, and effective communication have been cited as key components of effective teamwork.[4,5] The tendency for teams to function in an interdisciplinary or multidisciplinary fashion more often, working in parallel or in cooperation; and the challenges for achieving true transdisciplinary effectiveness, often due to the lack of a shared approach, are also highlighted.[6,7] Changing roles and leadership patterns as the field develops, leading to frustrations among palliative care professionals, have also been described.[5,6] The importance of casting a critical eye on team functioning and examining how each discipline contributes to optimal care needs further examination.[6]

TEAM DYNAMICS

Team dynamics and considerations affect multiple levels of our work in paediatric palliative care. On the one hand, it is critical to operate from an intention to meet the needs of our patients and their families. Flexibility and responsiveness are important aspects of this work. The family is the unit of care, and our respect for the diversity of needs and interests that we encounter require that we adapt ourselves to a variety of service patterns, needs and requests.

Yet, the healthcare system that we work within has its interests, too. Concern for sustainable, productive service models that allow us to meet the needs of children and their families while at least addressing the need for a practical business foundation is a significant tension. Whether the team works within the context of a national health service or a more diverse, American style healthcare marketplace, the need to demonstrate productivity, utility to the mission and positive outcomes for key stakeholders is essential.

It is clear that the American healthcare system, which is dependent on private insurances, is in desperate need of re-modelling. It is a system that is largely dependent on private insurance, which can be problematic, as reimbursement for care is not always forthcoming. Like many others, our programme never refuses to provide care for a child and family due to a lack of reimbursement for services. However, reimbursement is an issue that does influence how paediatric palliative care is provided for across the US. The focus does remain on the child and integrating other resources that are not in the healthcare field. Presently there is a great movement to legislate improvement of this part of the system. It is an ongoing challenge.

Our interdisciplinary team straddles these tensions as it serves patients and families, and in addition has a few needs of its own. Clinical capacity development is dependent upon the accumulation of experience and skill, as well as effective collaborative relationships within the team.[8] The capacity of the team to meet the demands of the patients and families, as well as the conditions set by the healthcare system, and to also create an effective and sustainable group dynamic is directly related to the ability of the programme to grow, increase volume capacity and thrive over time. If team members move in and out too quickly, and experienced caregivers are burdened with unrealistic expectations or inadequate resources for care delivery, the team can be adversely affected. Often, inadequate internal and external resources for helping the staff to cope will also challenge the ability to sustain a team capable of doing the work. As the members of the team move in and out of the system, it is important to address the training and support needs of each person so that the team as a whole functions with a shared set of knowledge and expectations for each other's performance.

In situations where a team is made up of parts of positions it is essential to have regular meetings not only for continuity of care and assurance of holistic care planning, but also for support and guidance to the front line workers. A preventative intervention strategy that is also consistent with those outlined within Standards 3 and 4 of ACT.

These interdependent aspects of care delivery each need to be identified, addressed and planned for as programme development occurs. Each aspect is also prone to its own sets of challenges, like complex, escalating and unpredictable patient care challenges, budget crises and financial constraints of the organisation, or episodes of short staffing. Some of these occur simultaneously, which is not an infrequent occurrence with our team. It is therefore increasingly essential for teams to consistently work on individual and team dynamics, and in these added stressful situations, need to deconstruct the issues and plan how the team can provide the best quality care in this often very intense environment.

Eight-year-old Anna had been through months of chemotherapy and treatments only to find her cancer had spread aggressively. After much discussion and deliberations with the extended medical team the family said they just wanted to go home and focus on comfort. They lived in a small town two hours from the children's hospital. The local hospice home care agency had not taken care of children before. When our team approached them about this, they were willing but nervous. With the family's permission, the hospital's palliative care team discussed with them how they might adapt and expand their traditional adult hospice model of care to meet the needs of Anna and her family. The hospice primary nurse had some paediatric experience in her past and was identified as the lead person for this case. The social worker was interested in learning more and contacted the local school district to engage their help. The whole staff had in-service training from the children's hospital's palliative care team. These 'just in time' trainings can be done in person or over a secure Internet connection or even by teleconference that includes a PowerPoint presentation. PPC care staff provided the community hospice team with a 24/7 number to call for questions. In places where this is not available, often the oncologist or even a familiar physician from a paediatrics floor will offer to answer questions for the home-based team. The family was ready to go home. The hospice home care team began visits, got to know the child and family, and everything was going well.

Anna seemed so much better, she was even going to school. The family began to second-guess their decision and began looking for alternative therapies. Grandmother, who had never accepted that they should stop treatment, became a moving force in suggesting that they resume aggressive therapies. The parents who once had been united in their decision now were in disagreement about how to move forward. The extended team members from the school and the parish also began to express a variety of views. The nurse began to get frustrated and said, 'I thought we had already been through this.' She called our team in frustration.

In a case like this, teams can expect these kinds of changing tensions and plan accordingly, or become impatient with these very common patterns of coping under stress. The capacity of the team to adapt itself to the family is closely associated with the eventual success of the care plan, but takes time and creativity, as well as an understanding of the nature of the process for many families. There is more going on than a simple educational or cognitive process: families need to assimilate complex information under stressful, highly emotional circumstances. In our experience, we have found, over time, that team members who frequently become frustrated with these types of family processes often burn out and become unproductive members of the palliative care team.

Essential at the beginning of each case is that these conflicts and feelings be identified and discussed so they do not split the team or cause confusion for the family. The coordinators of care need to specifically articulate the family objectives and ensure the explicit understanding on the part of all the team members. In many cases, assumptions can arise that in fact work against well-intentioned efforts to assist the family. Many times these are the result of unarticulated goals and expectations. Other times providers may need to step off the case if their feelings or personal values affect the way they are present to, or care for the family. This becomes an ongoing process of clarifying and communicating the goals of care over time[9]. This process can be quite time-consuming and complex. Repeated collateral communications between the team members, including the family, can be needed to achieve consensus and clarity.

As this case illustrates, there are significant challenges to providing care across sites of care, and over time. Team dynamics affect multiple levels of work. In Anna's situation, the once-clear goals and care objectives became unclear as the team expanded, different players joined and left the team, and the family gained more experience and processed their situation over time. One group of caregivers may be centrally involved in one phase of care (the hospital team, for example) while another is more primary at another (in the home, for example). The child's condition and the family's experience with their situation are also changing over time. There are multiple variables in play, and in dynamic tension. While this may be frustrating for some on the team, it is important for the palliative care perspective to expect and plan for this kind of evolution in any case. During those episodes of frustration, one team member can help another identify the issues and take a step back to regain perspective. It can be particularly helpful to have expectations for these kinds of reflections normalised, and built into team tasks, like weekly patient rounds, or other team meetings. In Anna's case, the extended team was called together to discuss the situation. The family were invited but decided that the team should figure things out and then they would join in the discussion later. They said they would get all the information from the nurse: 'she is just like family anyways'. The extended team met and reviewed goals and coping processes. A smaller team met with the family to discuss what the larger team recommended and to review the family's goals. As the family meeting progressed many fears and misunderstandings were aired. The professionals provided solid ongoing support for the family, led by the nurse as the family's identified key worker, but only possible because of the cohesiveness and trust within the team itself. Background discussions amongst involved team members enabled the nurse to be effective in this role, confident she was representing the concerns and insights of her colleagues.

As you see, it is essential to maintain effective and frequent communication with all members of the circle of care. From the family's point of view, these providers and others all comprise the 'team' for their child's care. Learning more about the family, checking with them to see if any previously unidentified or 'silent' members are influencing care decisions, can be critically important. As seen in Anna's situation, communication must be continuous and collaborative, flowing to and from each member of the expanded team. This task of coordinating the system dynamics often goes unaddressed or unplanned for, yet can make a great difference in improving care delivery when managed well. We have found that the palliative care social worker is often in a good position to adopt this role.

As Anna's situation also illustrates, the fact is that paediatric palliative care team dynamics and considerations affect caregivers on multiple levels. Generally individuals who become involved in paediatric palliative care do so because they want to help within their professional capacity and so, on a personal level, compassion and caring is evoked. This is natural but at times can challenge appropriate boundaries that are protective of both families and caregivers, while at the same time on a professional level, a high degree of objective skill and expertise is warranted. Both must be kept in balance. A team becomes most effective when enough trust can develop that colleagues can discuss these issues with each other directly and the team leader needs to be prepared to identify and assist in debriefing and intervening as necessary. To minimise or prevent this situation from a common occurrence, it becomes necessary for the team to articulate the performance expectations associated with these behaviours, and support them with policies and behavioural guidelines.[10]

Care providers also have obligations to the professional associations and organisations they work for. Productivity, reporting guidelines and procedures must be followed and documented while maintaining the family as the centre of care. Thus in order for the team to meet all the patient and professional demands, there is a need for ongoing planning and support for the team on a number of levels: as individuals, as teams and as an organisation.

NURTURING THE TEAM

> On any given day, someone on the team is feeling psychologically overwhelmed. During any given month, someone on the team is suffering symptoms of burnout for several consecutive days. During any given year, someone on the team is suffering a major burnout episode . . .
>
> David Weissman[10]

How does the team cope personally and as a team to provide holistic comprehensive care for children with palliative care needs and their families without burning out?

Team dynamics affect multiple levels of our work. How we manage patient and family-centred care objectives and how we address the demands of stressful work that includes considerations as to how we sustain ourselves, develop increased capacity to provide care, and continually improve our functionality in an ever-changing healthcare environment are questions we must grapple with. It is essential to take time to choose, build and nurture the team. This work is essential to do, beginning with the team's formation. In our work across the US we have spoken to many teams who did not incorporate this important step and then have regretted it, often left with an inflexible, fractured team. This not only does a disservice to the children and their families that they sought to serve, but damages the acceptance of the team in the institution and perhaps even into the community. The team is the foundation of the work. We have learned an important lesson through trial and error that you must build your team carefully even if it means slowing the work down to learn what you need to learn and find best fit of staff.

As a team we are constantly challenged to provide excellent care efficiently and cost effectively within an often emotionally charged context. As well we are cognizant of system considerations like business models, service models and accountability to productivity expectations that are just as important as skilful and compassionate care at the bedside. If we are not careful, those providing care can be caught in the middle of these essential but sometimes seemingly competing priorities

It can be argued, however, that balancing the team's needs for time, resources and support can actually prove to be an effective and sustainable business model. Staff turnover, patient dissatisfaction, poor coordination, and medical re-work or errors can be very costly to any healthcare organisation over the long term. Thus it becomes imperative that an investment in a compatible staff with clear working objectives can and should be considered an investment in resources that pays off well over time.

Our interdisciplinary team straddles many tensions as it serves patients and families, and in addition has needs of its own. The ability to provide comprehensive paediatric palliative care is something that has developed and grown within each individual, and in the team as a whole. Our success has been dependent upon the accumulation of experience and skill, as well as effective communication and collaborative relationships within the team. The capacity of the team to meet the unique demands and care needs of patients and families as well as the boundaries and limitations prescribed by the healthcare system, creates an ongoing dynamic situation from which our team has grown and matured. Over time we have come to appreciate that if demands and expectations overwhelm staff then we are left working short, due to turnover of staff – a situation that will adversely affect the work of the team and their impact on families. While it seems so obvious that support for the team is an imperative, it is too often forgotten. Needless to say, if there is not a consistent investment in the team, their efficacy is seriously compromised.

PROFESSIONAL SELF-CARE

It is clear that compassionate care, individualised approaches to situations, and managing the intensity of emotions and relationship dynamics are essential components of care delivery.[12] These require a great deal of skill and relational capacity on the part of care providers and we feel that the emotional and psychological resilience of the team is directly related to their success in this field.

Over time we have come to learn that it is a very different experience for a professional caring for a single child in palliative care at a given moment in time versus one who manages, as the sole focus of their work, simultaneously a case load of 20, 30, or more children receiving palliative or end-of-life care. Capacity for care is developed over time, and with experience. Protective measures to prevent burnout and to ensure one's skills are available not only to this child and family, but also to future children, are essential to both the individual and the whole system of care. It is important that teams are aware of this issue and establish the idea that self-care is an integral part of the everyday life of the team and the individuals in it. There are a variety of practical ways to do this and how it is done is perhaps not as important as that it is done.

Healthcare workers are familiar with care plans for patients, but few have them for themselves. In order to care well for children with palliative care needs and their families, it is important to have a plan for self-care. This self-care plan may be rather simple. For example, it may start by listing two ways that one will care for one's spiritual, emotional, social and physical health while doing this work. Such plans can be individualised and informal, or done as a structured team exercise that helps to establish norms for self-care. This simple planning step will help encourage staff to actually follow through by creating positive peer pressure, and expectations for behaviour.

Throughout the palliative care world there is ongoing discussion about the best way to provide staff and team support. Many approaches have been attempted with varying degrees of success depending on numerous factors such as the individuals in the team, the support of the institution and the importance given it by the leadership. We have learned from colleagues that regular support groups facilitated by internal or external professions, offering individual support from specific team members or having a psychologist available for appointments have been met with some levels of success. Another team has shared that they found that monthly sessions providing mandatory 'clinical supervision' for all staff with an offsite psychologist have been successful.

Improved team communications, morale, productivity and effectiveness are some of the benefits reported by this team. In our team, clinical staff members meet with their discipline leader for clinical mentoring, case discussion, problem solving and debriefing. This approach has been well received, but the message we want to impart is that every team must choose the best form of support for themselves but effective teams will ensure that action plans are developed for addressing these important issues. The 'group culture' can be encouraged to affirm such practices.

TEAM CONFLICTS

In Anna's case there was conflict between what the nurse felt needed to be done and what the community support worker felt. This situation was splitting the team and could begin to affect the family.

Facilitation of the team's group dynamic is often something that gets attention only when problems and conflicts arise. By then, much damage may have occurred to impede the team's functioning. There is an essential 'group process' that evolves in teams, and can be managed consciously or unconsciously. When recognised and facilitated, the team and its individual members can grow in their skills and resiliency but if left unattended, the dynamics can be destructive, painful for workers, and have a negative impact on care delivery.

In Anna's case team workers began to be in disagreement with each other on how aggressive to be. The physiotherapist began to push physiotherapy, while the nurse was encouraging, using her energy for what gave Anna pleasure.

By incorporating mechanisms for fostering positive team dynamics, much can be done to improve the effectiveness and job satisfaction of the group. For example, in our programme, a nurse and social worker that have office-based clinical supervisory responsibilities have incorporated team support into their roles. They check in with staff as individuals, but also as a group, raising concerns as needed, and supporting staff in self-care and conflict management tasks. The focus is on issues that interfere with personal effectiveness or care of the child and family. They also model the interpersonal skills and processing of tensions that they encourage throughout the team. By making this an intentional part of their roles, they have helped to create a group culture where these types of occurrences can be resolved. In our team, those in leadership positions have picked up this role, and it has been an important process to establish some structures where issues can be reflected upon as needed, for example within clinical supervision, or facilitated meetings between those with conflicts. Such situations we have found need to be distinguished from performance issues, and also from 'therapy', so that trust in team colleagues can develop. Staff leaders have also been able to use their positions within the organisation to advocate for appropriate productivity expectations and needed supports for the team. Improved trust and increased effectiveness in managing complex care has been a positive outcome.

The provision of high quality paediatric palliative care often requires sophisticated interpersonal skills. Team members must to be able to interact effectively with children of different ages and abilities, listen to families under great stress and help find mutually agreed solutions to difficult problems. While some disciplines, for example psychologists, social workers, chaplains, may have more advanced training in these or other areas of practice, the reality is that all team members must be prepared to manage complex communication and problem solving dilemmas on a daily basis, and so often in our situation team meetings also become team learning events, where those with additional expertise assist and coach those who require some further assistance – a very important function of a team. The art and science of palliative care is something that grows with increased personal capacity. It can be modelled through observation and role play. In our department, new nurses role-play difficult conversations and discuss how they could approach them in different ways. This same role modelling is done for non-palliative care staff so that they can apply it to difficult situations within their own practice. A common example in palliative care that we have found is when a physician is telling the family that no further curative treatments are available and says 'I am sorry. There is nothing more we can do.' The palliative care worker can interject 'I think what doctor meant was "there is nothing further we can do with these medications to cure the disease but there is always something more we can do to provide comfort and improve quality of life".' This type of rehearsal allows for skill development and professional growth while educating others about the practice of paediatric palliative care.

BOUNDARIES IN CARE PROVISION

> Professional boundaries are easy to cross when you are sharing families' most vulnerable times and spending long periods of time in close proximity. This issue is one that every team must address. As a professional care team, it is important to establish early the expectations for how these relationships will be conducted. We have found that clarity regarding expectations can also be helpful for families. It is important for professionals not to fall into the belief that while families will describe them as 'just like family', they are not family and what they have is a professional role with that family. We, like other teams, have found that both in the home or in the hospital, intense situations can cause boundaries to blur.

The complexity of care demands, and the strong emotional, spiritual and psychological dynamics that arise in paediatric palliative care, can predispose staff and families to blur boundaries. Factors contributing to such dilemmas include the unavoidable inequity in caregiving relationships, the compelling nature of these situations, potential ethical considerations, the vulnerability of the ill child and their family, the potential for caregiver burnout and the importance of family empowerment. Boundary dilemmas can become burdensome to both caregivers and families.[10] Sometimes, no harm is done. At other times, real suffering, errors and burnout can occur. Through the promotion of more effective team collaboration, we can minimise the potential harm to the children we care for, their families and our colleagues.

Another case in point:

Jay is a six-month-old baby with a slowly progressing degenerative neurological condition. A paediatric palliative care nurse follows Jay's family at home. Jay has been medically stable for several months. The nurse has grown fond of him as he is charming and the family is delightful. Jay's family has told her 'no one understands us like you do . . .' and they decline involvement of other team members. The nurse, drawn in by her emotional attachment, goes outside the policy that all telephone calls go through the central system and tells the family just to page her directly. The family was very grateful and appreciative. The nurse feels confident she can manage the needs of this child and family alone. One day, Jay's nurse went out of town for a family event and had her phone and pager turned off. She was tired and the child had been very stable. The nurse didn't expect a sudden change in events. Unfortunately Jay had a crisis event related to changes in his breathing. The family tried to page and call the nurse without success. They became quite distraught and felt they could no longer trust the nurse. The nurse felt terrible when she realised what had happened. In her effort to be flexible and kind, she over-extended herself and did a disservice to the family.

We can look at this example and empathise with all the different perceptions in the case. Yet the problem for care provision is also evident and suffering has inadvertently resulted from this boundary dilemma. Had the nurse gently pressed the family to use their trust in her to enable the involvement of her colleagues, their child's needs may have been better served by the broader care system. The system structure is there for a reason, to protect family and support staff. It needs to be respected and followed.

Because there are inherent and compelling pressures on boundaries between professionals and family members in these situations, it is important to develop structures that support good interpersonal relationships and protective boundaries for all parties. These can be accomplished through education aimed at increasing awareness. Our experience has also demonstrated the need for clear guidelines, policies and performance expectations to reinforce the importance of attention to good boundaries. Well-intentioned individuals can easily extend themselves to help or meet needs in the short run, but over time, and as providers care for an increasing volume of children and families, the burden of this kind of behaviour becomes more problematic for both the caregiver and the family and resentments, unclear expectations, and disappointments can occur on both sides. These results can be further emotionally draining for families and caregivers, and contribute to burnout in professionals. Destructive team dynamics can also evolve when one nurse is seen as a 'helpful friend' for offering a ride for example, and another social worker is seen as 'cold and uncaring' because she refuses to babysit on a day off.

As a team, when we consider strategies to improve the care to more and more children with life-limiting conditions, we need to consider the concentric circles within which our staff delivers care: they are individual caregivers, belonging to teams, and work within organisations and systems of care. Each of these interdependent aspects of care delivery need to be identified, addressed and planned for as programme development occurs. Each aspect is also prone to its own sets of challenges, including complex, escalating and unpredictable patient care challenges, budget crises and financial constraints of the organisation, or episodes of short staffing. When some of these occur simultaneously, which can be the case more often than one might suppose, they can affect the quality and stability of service delivery.

Another common scenario that we are faced with as our caseloads increase and our capability does not match demand is the reluctance of adult services to take on paediatric palliative care patients. Our colleagues have expressed some real concerns and fears of taking children on their caseload and this is very evident when young adults are often more likely to be picked up by an adult service rather than an infant. Their issues usually focus on the perception that paediatric palliative care is seen as more demanding and specialised on many levels of care than adult palliative care. The numbers of involved professionals, the patterns of communication, emotional intensity, pressures for decision-making, and the need for collateral coordination often increase the complexity of care. Teams that care for children frequently do seem to have an increased capacity to carry larger paediatric caseloads. In the beginning our team felt overwhelmed if there were more than 10 patients on service. As the capacity of the team members grew along with our census, a daily census of over 80 patients became a manageable norm.

We have found that adult programmes that started to take children, like Anna's home-care agency, while hesitant and in need of a lot of support, are increasingly able to take children with more comfort and skill. They too have grown in capacity. Other scenarios that we are not encountering too often but are aware of the trend, is what to do when the child survives to adulthood. At the current time this has not been a significant issue for our team since half of the children in service are under five years. Fortunately in our practice environment there are specialty clinics that have been able to provide continuity of care to this population and collaborate with adult services to assume care, thereby helping ease transitions between systems of care. However, we are aware that we perhaps are not the norm when it comes to issues of transition care between child and adult services.

EFFICIENCY IN PAEDIATRIC PALLIATIVE CARE

The problem of creating efficiencies and productivity expectations within the complex system of paediatric palliative care, which also demands a high level of personal effectiveness, is one that many programmes seek to address. While no easy answers exist yet, we can try to visualise a sustainable model of care that emphasises time, costs, skills and human beings in a dynamic tension. Taking the time at the outset to develop rapport, establish expectations, and plan for the peaks and valleys that occur in paediatric palliative care can actually save money, energy and frustrations over time because trust and more efficient communications result. A team that works well together, understands the problems at hand and available resources, accurately anticipates needs, and effectively communicates with each other, as well as with the children and families they serve, becomes productive and uses resources effectively. This continues to be our challenge within a complex healthcare environment.

TEAM CONSISTENCY

There are a number of models for the provision of paediatric palliative and hospice care around the world. The location of care may vary from inpatient hospitals to freestanding children's hospices providing respite and end-of-life care, to palliative home-based services, or indeed a combination of the above.

The authors of this chapter work in the United States of America in a children's hospital-based Pain and Palliative Care Program. The programme provides care for hospitalised children, as well as through an outpatient clinic, and home-based care in the community. A range of services is provided by a multidisciplinary team of practitioners including acute, complex and chronic pain management, palliative care, hospice care and perinatal hospice care. The core team consists of 21 professionals including nurses, social workers, physicians, advanced practice nurses, a psychologist, child life specialist, chaplain, volunteers and support staff. However, every programme's needs regarding staffing will be very different depending on their scope of service and the population served. As paediatric palliative care programmes emerge worldwide, many of them will likely begin with a 'core team' of one to two professionals. While one provider does not a team make, new technologies and other options for creating a virtual team are available. Practitioners can partner with local resources and obtain consultation from colleagues at a distance through tools like email, phone or as secure web-based programmes. In our practice over 15 years we have found that having a core mission, vision and clear boundaries are tools for a successful team and can enhance capacity development and nurture further growth.

N.I.C.E. analysis

Please reflect on the issues raised in this chapter in relation to your own practice.

Needs
- Staff development and training.
- Capacity development.
- Staff support: resources of time, expertise.
- Clarity of roles and boundaries.

Interests
- Staff coping.
- Capacity development.
- Recruitment and retention.
- Team effectiveness.
- Excellent care delivery.
- Efficiency.
- Staff morale and enjoyment of work.
- Staff retention.

Concerns
- Staff coping with stressful work.
- Team experience of losses.
- Cost containment and productivity.
- Staff retention.
- Team morale.

Expectations
- Productive work habits.
- Effective team collaboration.
- Excellent patient and family care.
- Adequate resources available.
- Open communications.

From the above analysis please reflect on:

What is already known about your concerns?

- This work is stressful for the staff members and requires high degrees of interpersonal and technical skills.
- To date, there has been little in literature re: how to facilitate team effectiveness.
- Impact of this specialisation on workers/teams over time is largely unknown given the rapid and recent development in the field.

Are there any misconceptions contributing to barriers of delivering care?

- That individuals can manage all these requirements and challenges without support.
- Resource issues: time, money, and unclear/undefined productivity expectations.

Are there advantages/disadvantages with the required changes you have highlighted?

- Disadvantages: There is a significant commitment needed in both time and resources to effectively support teams.
- Effective strategies are unclear.
- Advantages: Allows for individualised approaches to participation and coping.
- Provides a way to look at issues that are often not well addressed.

How ready are the various parties involved for change?

- Unclear: resources and motivations are undefined. Newness of the field creates unclear expectations, as these parameters are not yet defined.
- Productivity vs coping pressures challenge team support strategies.

Are there any barriers to this change?

- Financial and productivity pressures.
- Lack of clarity re: needs and best practice approaches.
- Need to define goals for team collaboration and patient-care strategies.

What is the most effective way of communicating with the people who can effect change?

- Data: define best practices and benchmark data as available.
- Define consequences of lack of attention to these issues.
- Offer a plan to address deficiencies.

REFERENCES

1 Hall P, Weaver L, Gravelle D, *et al.* Developing collaborative person-centered practice: a pilot project on a palliative care unit. *J Interprof Care.* 2007; **21**: 69–81.
2 Sims J, Jassal S. Working as a team. In: Goldman A, Hain R, Liben S, editors. *Palliative Care for Children.* London: Oxford University Press; 2006.

3 Parker-Oliver D, Bronstein L, Kurzejeski L. Examining variables related to successful collaboration on the hospice team. *Health Soc Work*. 2005; **30**: 279–86.

4 Periyakoil V. Growing pains health care enters the 'team' age. *J Palliat Med*. 2005; **11**: 171–5.

5 Hermsen M, Henk AMJ. Ten Have. Palliative care teams: effective through moral reflection. *J Interprof Care*. 2005; **19**(6): 561–8.

6 O'Connor M, Fisher C, Guilfoyle A. Interdisciplinary teams in palliative care: a critical reflection. *Int J Palliat Nurs*. 2006; **12**: 132–7.

7 Bruce A, Boston P. The Changing landscape of palliative care: emotional challenges for hospice and palliative care professionals. *JHPN*. 2008; **10**: 49–55.

8 McNeilly P, Price J. Interdisciplinary teamworking in paediatric palliative care. *Eur J Palliative Care*. 2007; **14**: 64–7.

9 Hays R, Valentine J, Haynes G, *et al*. The Seattle Pediatric Palliative Care Project: effects on family satisfaction and health-related quality of life. *J Palliat Med*. 2006; **9**: 716–28.

10 Weissmann, D. Verbal comment. *Annual Conference of Center to Advance Palliative Care*. 2008 Oct 23. Grapevine, TX.

11 Remke S. Boundary issues in pediatric palliative care. Poster. *International Congress on Palliative and End of Life Care*. Montreal, QC: 2006 Sep.

12 Browning D. To show our humanness: relational and communicative competence in pediatric palliative care. *Bioethics Forum*. 2002; **18**: 23–8.

SECTION 5

Evidence/knowledge transfer into practice

Susan Fowler-Kerry

Within Section 5, we leave you with many thoughts and ideas to ruminate on and think through. There is no doubt that a better world for these children and their families is possible. But as Brazilian educator Paulo Freire said: 'Hope . . . does not consist of crossing one's arms and waiting.'[1]

Healthcare is a complex system and unfortunately there is too often a disconnect between what is known and what is practiced. Bringing change to this very complex system can appear to be a rather daunting challenge, but looking back in time the growth of social activism in health arose out of workers' collective daily experiences resulting from the impact of social inequality. Civil society activists have partnered academics, scientists to bring about social change. Examples include: on local levels, parents have joined forces to regulate fast food from infiltrating schools, communities have united to ban alcohol at sporting events and thousands of grassroots organisations around the world work tirelessly to bring about change at community level. So how do we raise the consciousness of communities, governments and global institutions about the universal need of paediatric palliative care?

Not an easy question, but in this final section it becomes clear that change cannot be solely addressed by an infusion of funding capital. Rather what is needed includes targeted or strategic investment directed to enhance or develop new services for these children and families, an approach that will require healthcare professionals to work together in new and novel ways to support children and their families in their homes and communities, to support parents to care for their kids, to build stronger community capacity, and to use existing resources more efficiently and effectively. Strategies which are consistent throughout basic civil liberties, highlighted throughout myriad international, national documents and tenets of law. These children, like all others, must not be denied a fair chance at a standard of living that includes good education, protected environments, economic opportunity and healthcare including paediatric palliative care, because every child is, after all, a citizen of the world.

REFERENCE

1 Freire P. *Pedagogy of the Oppressed*. Sao Paulo, Brazil: Continuum International Publishing Group; 1970.

21

Knowledge transfer within the general paediatric setting

Paula Dawson

How do general children's nurses feel and act when a child with palliative care needs is admitted for care and support to a general children's ward? This is a question worth exploration as, although in some areas it may not be a frequent occurrence, it is an occurrence which requires particular skills, sensitivities and insights that will challenge even the most experienced generalist practitioner.

It is worth discussing some of the issues, dilemmas and choices faced by children, families and health professionals when a child with a life-limiting condition is being cared for in an acute, general setting. We should consider how the profile of palliative care needs to be raised with general nursing practitioners, so that it becomes a key part of whole lifecycle care for all for whom it is relevant. There is a need for palliative care to be a part of all pre- and post-registration nursing curricula, in order that its concepts are understood by, and embedded within the practice of, the existing and future nursing workforces.

General children's wards tend to be busy, some would say 'frantic', places. We see an increasingly rapid throughput of patients as services strive to adhere to recommendations that children should spend as little time as possible in hospital.[1] In acute care areas the majority of children will recover and be discharged with limited follow-up requirements. However, a significant number of children who spend time in acute care settings will have, by virtue of their life-limiting condition, a longer-term relationship with an area and the professionals who spend their working hours there.

Many children with palliative care needs, who are not yet at the 'end-of-life' stage, will experience episodes of hospitalisation at one time or another. How important it is that these care experiences are not approached as isolated, acute 'moments', but as part of a holistic, progressive process of learning together on the part of child, family and health professional, with the aim of finding the best way forward for the child.

Children continue to die in substantial numbers in the acute setting rather than at home or in a hospice setting. Many of these children die with little documentation of palliative or end-of-life care.[2] If the death of an infant or child does not occur on the day of admission, the length of stay should be sufficient to provide the opportunity for the provision of palliative and end-of-life care. The number of childhood deaths in both general and children's hospitals after the day of admission[3] makes it clear that all inpatient institutions providing care to infants and children need to be able to provide palliative and end-of-life care. However, what constitutes the 'best way forward' for the child may often be a contentious and difficult issue to address.

Palliative care of course includes so many elements – not only symptom management, comfort care and family services, but also the timely delivery of information regarding diagnosis, prognosis and treatment effectiveness. Offering palliative care to infants and children who are continuing to receive curative therapy is a challenge for the healthcare provider team and family because it may be perceived as 'giving up hope' for recovery or cure. It is clear that the term palliative care is often used by healthcare providers as synonymous with end-of-life care. With the increasing use of technology and treatments that can save lives, healthcare providers may offer and even push these options hoping for success. Families, on the other hand, are almost invariably seeking any hope they can find that their child will not die. This dichotomy can result in a high degree of burden and internal conflict for both families and healthcare providers, not least in general care settings where 'cure' is generally the expected care outcome.

The complexity of the technological advances available to care for infants and children in the twenty-first century requires a complex approach to the provision of palliative care. Any one model is unlikely to be sufficient for children cared for in diverse unit environments with diverse life-threatening illnesses. The range of ages and illnesses associated with infant and childhood deaths indicates that all providers would benefit from a working knowledge of and access to expertise in the provision of end-of-life and palliative care. The creation and use of the ACT Care Pathway,[4] has made it possible for some standardisation and structure to be available for all – perhaps not before time.

In order for advance care planning to be possible and seen as acceptable, everyone involved in discussion and decision making needs to be aware of realistic prognosis. This can be difficult. Some studies have shown that parental recognition of there being no hope of a cure tends to occur much later than that of health professionals.[5,6] These studies found that earlier recognition of poor prognosis by parents was associated with earlier discussion of hospice care, better parent ratings of home care, earlier DNR orders, less use of active therapies in the last month of life and a better chance that both parent and physician would identify comfort as the primary therapeutic goal.

In a study undertaken by Meyer et al.,[7] more than half of families reported feeling they had little to no control during the child's final days. Nearly 25% reported that they would have made different decisions had they been given more information. A study by Kreicbergs et al.[8] demonstrated that dying children tend to know that they are dying and that adult denial and/or refusal to discuss 'the truth' makes little difference to a child's own ability to perceive the reality of their situation. This would imply that parents' and health professionals' difficulties with approaching the 'big' questions of how best to prepare for the end-of-life are ill-founded and need to be surmounted. Dying children need honest answers and unconditional love and support.[5] How very important it is, therefore, that staff are trained to be both physically and emotionally prepared to tackle these issues in order to prevent them being overwhelmed and ultimately left with the knowledge that they have provided less than holistic care when a child has died.[9]

In exploring the experience of nursing children with palliative care needs within the general paediatric setting, I offer some examples.

EXAMPLE 1

A nurse arrived on a night shift to discover a child with severe special needs whose condition was seriously deteriorating. His parents were not with him and lived some distance away. There was no evidence of forward planning and no detail in his medical notes as to how it might have been decided to respond in the event of a respiratory arrest – which was clearly imminent. He was being nursed in a four-bedded bay of a general children's ward. His parents were called. He was moved to the high-dependency ward where it was possible to provide a quieter, more private environment for him. However, procedural guidelines being adhered to, he was subject to attempts at full resuscitation and intubation when he ceased breathing. These attempts were unsuccessful but, again due to procedural guidelines, the tubes had to remain *in situ* after his death as he would need a post mortem examination. Hence, when his parents arrived, deeply distraught, they had to witness their beloved child in this parlous state.

EXAMPLE 2

Another child with special needs, whose parents had left him in hospital as they took a short, much needed holiday, deteriorated and died in their absence. Despite frantic attempts being made to reach them, in order that they might get back to be with him when he died, they did not arrive at the hospital until several hours after his death. They were devastated. Little forethought had been given to the possibility of the child's death in their short absence.

Compare the experience of these examples with the third scenario.

EXAMPLE 3

A child with a life-limiting congenital condition was being cared for. Her parents had decided they wanted to care for her at home and for her to die at home. But when she started to deteriorate they found they were unable to cope with the practical elements of her care, their other children and their own feelings, and decided that they wanted her to die in hospital. Careful plans were drawn up, with clarity about how much active participation in care they wanted. In contrast to the earlier examples I gave, although it was a painful process, in this instance there was a pervading sense of acceptance and almost of peace – all people involved were doing what the family and the healthcare team had together determined was 'the best' they could do for the care of this child and family.

These cases, and the preceding discussion, cannot but help lead to the conclusion that there is an undeniable need for all healthcare professionals working within any setting where children with life-limiting conditions may attend, to be aware of, understand and feel confident with, the provision of care which addresses the full spectrum of life's (and death's) activities. If we are committed to child and family-centred, negotiated care, we must be committed to this end. It is therefore imperative that all pre-registration nursing curricula and further professional development programmes have these issues interwoven into them at every point. I would argue that healthcare students need to be introduced to the needs of the child or young person with a life-limiting condition and their family, and to the principles and concepts addressed by the ACT Care Pathway[4] at an early stage, so that its standards become an accepted and integral part of their practice when dealing with any child and their family.

Currently, at the University of Nottingham, while nursing students' are encouraged to focus particularly on the full content and implications of the pathway during complex and critical care modules of study, their learning experiences include references to the needs of these families and to the standards and use of the pathway throughout the pre-registration branch programme. Clinical practitioners, including a variety of professional disciplines and experts in relevant fields, are invited to share with students their own experiences of working with the pathway, as are service users and carers whenever possible. Involving such personnel in the learning process for students is essential, particularly due to the rapid evolvement of our approaches to palliative care – students need to hear from people who have current and relevant experience to share in this field. We should acknowledge that teaching staff who may not have recent clinical experience, or who may only recall instances when palliative care was inadequate or non-existent, will probably not be the best facilitators of student learning. Knowledge of, and preparedness to discuss, the ever-developing moral and ethical issues associated with palliative care are vital in opening students' minds to the truth that in this area, as of course in many others, we are 'at the cutting edge' of promoting quality care, and we are all learning together. Information sharing and discussion at this early career point for students is essential. We should also note that those students who will ultimately practice in general care settings may join a team where their colleagues have limited experience, skills and/or confidence in assessing, planning and contributing to the delivery of the most appropriate palliative care, due to a focus on acute care and expected recovery. When determining staff development and training needs, managers should be encouraged and supported to seek appropriate additional education access for staff, and consider including palliative care experience and education as an essential or desirable attribute within a team's establishment.

N.I.C.E. analysis

Needs
- Development of skills, sensitivities and insights in teams.
- Addressing fears and lack of knowledge in teams and individual professionals.
- Considering the needs of staff working in 'general' settings.
- Raising the profile of palliative care.
- Making palliative care a part of all pre- and post registration nursing curricula.
- Early discussion of end-of-life issues where indicated.
- Dissemination of knowledge of ACT pathway.
- Appropriate use of the ACT pathway.
- Honest communication with children and families.
- Making palliative care education an essential element of a team's establishment requirement.

Interests
- Involving children, young people and families in the education of health professionals.
- Inter-professional learning.
- Involving practising professionals in the education of health workers.

Concerns
- Time factors with drive for children to spend as little time in hospital as possible – could encourage 'ducking' of the issues.
- Limited and untimely communication between agencies and teams.
- Limited documentation of issues.
- Limited forward thinking and planning.
- The challenge of offering palliative care in conjunction with curative therapy.
- Out-of-date education and support on this rapidly evolving area of care.
- Ethical issues, such as individual philosophical and/or religious values impacting on information sharing and decision-making.

Expectations
- Increasing acknowledgement of the need for children's palliative care to be an integral part of learning programmes and service developments.
- Improving communication and collaboration between professions and agencies.
- Increasing numbers of practitioners trained in palliative care for children.

Action plan: next steps

- To work towards the inclusion of palliative care issues as a central theme in all nurse education programmes.
- To encourage the involvement and children, young people and their families as well as practising professionals in the delivery of children's palliative care education.
- To develop holistic nursing and multi-professional assessment and planning care documentation that acknowledges palliative care issues.
- To include the need for personnel trained in children's palliative care in training needs analyses and establishment setting in appropriate areas.

REFERENCES

1 Department of Health. *The National Service Framework for Children, Young People and Maternity Services.* London: Department of Health; 2007.

2 Brandon D, Docherty SL, Thorpe J. Infant and child deaths in acute care settings: implications for palliative care. *J Palliat Med.* 2007; **10**(4): 910–18.

3 www.statistics.gov.uk

4 Elston S. *Integrated Multi-agency Care Pathways for Children with Life-threatening and Life-limiting Conditions.* Bristol: ACT; 2004.

5 Himelstein BP. Palliative care for infants, children, adolescents and their families. *J Palliat Med.* 2006; **9**(1): 163–81.

6 Wolfe J, Klar N, Grier HE, *et al.* Understanding of prognosis among parents of children who died of cancer: impact on treatment goals and integration of palliative care. *JAMA.* 2000; **284**: 2469–75.

7 Meyer EC, Burns JP, Griffith JL, *et al.* Parental perspectives on end-of-life care in the pediatric intensive care unit. *Crit Care Med.* 2002; **30**(1): 226–31.

8 Kreicbergs U, Valdimarsdottir U, Onelov E, *et al.* Talking about death with children who have severe malignant disease. *NEJM.* 2004; **351**: 1175–86.

9 Sumner L. Staff support in pediatric hospice care. In: Armstrong-Daley A, Zarbck S, editors. *Hospice Care for Children.* 2nd ed. New York: Oxford University Press; 2001.

22

Supporting learning in paediatric palliative care

Joanne Griffiths and Rita Pfund

INTRODUCTION

Professionals working with children who have life-limiting or life-threatening illness and their families need appropriate knowledge and ongoing support. Continuing education is a fundamental need for all those involved, including not only nursing and medical staff, but also all of the wider multi-agency team. Any programme of education must be able to meet the challenge of tailoring resources to the learning needs of professionals who may have very different backgrounds and work experiences as well as varying levels of knowledge. This means that education and service providers need to collaborate to develop and set educational standards and develop appropriate means of accreditation, monitoring and re-validation appropriate to a variety of settings and professional groups.

This chapter examines issues in continuing education for those currently working in the field and issues in educational preparation for those undergoing professional training. To begin with, we discuss the wider issues that influence the learning needs of diverse professional groups who come into contact with children and young people who have life-limiting or life-threatening illnesses and their families. This will be linked to the current challenges of children's and young people's palliative care. From there we then examine two case study examples of programmes currently available in the UK.

PRINCIPLES OF EDUCATION IN RELATION TO PALLIATIVE CARE

Education has been described as the process through which learning occurs and in which learning is analogous to a journey to a different, hopefully better and more interesting place.[1] Motivation, energy and engagement with real experiences are necessary to fuel the journey of education. In contrast, training more narrowly is about the acquisition of knowledge or skills to deal with a particular type of event. Wee and Hughes[1] examine the role of education within palliative care. They explain that training can be achieved through repetitive practice, whereas education is value-based and involves a process of active thinking and reflection. In education, an 'informal curriculum' emerges from the unscripted interactions that take place between the teacher and learners and between learners themselves.[1] These informal interactions are profoundly influenced by the cultural milieu in which education is delivered.

The European Association for Palliative Care (EAPC) has published guidelines which provide a framework for European curricula.[2] These recognise a country's right to diversity dependent on local custom and practice and the huge variation in resources for palliative care across Europe. The guidelines were targeted for nurse education and suggest that educational templates should have the following key features:

➤ a reflective structure
➤ using a multidisciplinary approach to education in which working together and sharing responsibilities is valued
➤ based on the principles of adult education, thus reflecting the process of self-directed and problem-based learning to produce the benefits of clear critical thinking and problem solving.

In addition, the following factors have been identified as critical in the preparation of professionals for palliative care practice by De Vlieger *et al.*:[3]

➤ clinical competence
➤ sharing learning
➤ partnership
➤ the ability to function effectively within a multidisciplinary team
➤ integration with the existing healthcare services
➤ self-awareness and coping skills.

Promotion of the latter depends on the quality of partnerships between service providers and educationalists. With this in mind, in the UK, a framework for commissioning education has been promoted by ACT[4] for different levels of service involvement.

CHALLENGES SPECIFIC TO PAEDIATRIC PALLIATIVE CARE EDUCATION
Outgrowing its own brief: transition
In the UK, palliative care services for children and young people emerged in the 1980s as predominantly nurse-led initiatives through the children's hospice movement.[5] Much campaigning work focused in the early days on achieving a distinction between adult and children's services, since campaigners argued that palliative care for adults seemed synonymous with care in the last days of life, with hospices seen as places for the dying. In contrast, the emerging context for children was that palliative care started at the point of a diagnosis of life-limiting illness and hospices were places for living. The contribution that children's hospices make, according to Brown,[6] is ensuring quality care for life-limited children and their families, potentially over many years.

Nearly 30 years later and as illustrated in previous chapters in this book, it is clear that the needs of palliative care for children and young people have expanded beyond the original principles on which care provision was based. Meticulous attention to symptom control and involving technological supportive treatment as part of the palliative care management is extending both the quality and length of life for some young people. Many will now live into adulthood, with support being provided from recognition of the life-limiting illness throughout childhood. Challenges then occur when the young adult must leave paediatric services.[7]

Adult palliative care services have also undergone dynamic processes of change. There is now a much greater emphasis on the role of a palliative care approach for all adults with life-limiting conditions, not just cancer, and on the value of introducing a palliative care approach much earlier in the disease trajectory. Adult providers are needing to learn how to manage young adults with complex disability and adults with the cognition of children. However, some major differences remain. These are illustrated by ACT.[8]

There is a growing recognition from both adult and paediatric sectors that transition must be an active process, with each group learning from the other. This exposes learning needs in both the paediatric and adult carers. Learning works best when teams collaborate over the transition of their patients as there is presently little formalised education available. In some parts of the UK the children's hospice sector provides a 'bridge' between children's and adult services. Indeed, many of these hospices now provide separate facilities for young adults, some for service users of up to 40 years of age. It can be argued that this merely creates another transition stage at a later date.[5]

International perspective

Many of the educational needs are shared by the international community. Given the commonality of many of the issues, and the mutual support to be gained by exchanging ideas to aid problem solving across the globe, it makes good sense to aim for collaboration beyond individual countries. In many parts of the world there will be comparatively small numbers of individuals working in paediatric palliative care. They can easily feel isolated and struggle to access both the formal and informal teaching that continuously improves practice. If these practitioners can access education programmes they can then disseminate this knowledge on a larger scale across their local teams. Chambers *et al.* (*see* Chapter 2) has given a glimpse of the provision currently available in Germany and Uganda, whilst Millington and Marston (*see* Chapters 5 and 6) expand on the issues of provision in resource-poor countries. One such programme is in place through Hospice Africa Uganda.[9]

The core principles of good care are the same irrespective of disease process, but the means by which they can be delivered and the underlying pathology will vary greatly across the globe. Any programme purporting to provide education on a global scale must have the flexibility to encourage the student to diversify and share knowledge gained in their own countries.

Multi-professional education

Good multidisciplinary working is reliant on differing professions who not only bring their own skills to the workplace but also recognise the contributions of others (*see* Figure 22.1). There exists therefore, the need to develop education and training that is complementary for all of the following:

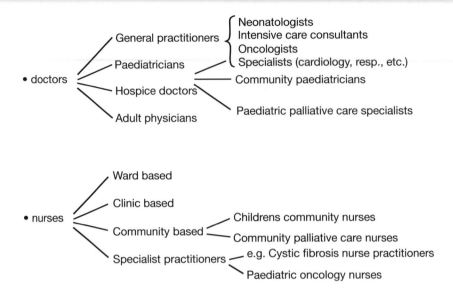

- counsellors
- psychologists
- chaplains
- therapists
- lay workers
- volunteers/NGOs
- teachers
- social workers
- parents
- respite carers
- police
- youth workers
- bereavement services
- Child and Adolescent Mental Health Services (CAMHS).

FIGURE 22.1 Multi-professional education

Education also needs to be available to all agencies whether community or hospital-based, health, social services, education or the voluntary sector.

If one acknowledges that the numbers of people working in this field will be small and that most learning in paediatric palliative care will occur post graduation, it might seem sensible to design larger multi-professional programmes which can utilise newer teaching tools such as the Internet. These will, however, have implicit challenges.

1   Who should have detailed knowledge of palliative care of children and young people?

It could be argued that many practitioners only dip in and out of contact with these children and therefore need not be experts in the field, but unless all practitioners have sufficient basic understanding of the nature of the issues these children and young people face, they will not be identified and appropriately referred to palliative care services. Earlier chapters are compelling evidence for this assertion. The authors therefore welcome the multi-layered approach to education for all exemplified by both ACT[3] and the UK curriculum in paediatric palliative medicine[10] as described on p. 306.

2   Can large-scale programmes cater for very diverse needs, a diverse range of professional backgrounds, and deliver both a local and international context? Such programmes will indeed have problems, but are they more likely to be effective than trying to establish many smaller programmes in specialist settings where resources are poor?

3   How can adult and paediatric palliative care services amalgamate established and evolving patterns of care? Over time each has evolved differing policies and frameworks guiding practice. For example, in the UK children's services follow the ACT Care Pathway as themed through this book,[11,12] whilst adult services follow the Liverpool Pathway[13] and the Goldstandard Framework for Palliative Care.[14]

In the following section we will first examine the educational needs of non-medical practitioners followed by medical practitioners. Whilst examining the different philosophies guiding medical and non-medical education provision, it soon becomes obvious that a clearer path for medical education in palliative care is starting to emerge compared to other professions. For children's nursing courses, there is some data with regards to breakdown of hours taught of palliative care content.[15] On the other hand, for dietetics, physiotherapy and occupational therapy, there might be no discreet paediatric palliative care content at all. However, through personal communication with colleagues of these disciplines it became obvious that there are many elements relating to palliative care that are very workable starting points to build on.

Nursing and allied professions

In the same timeframe that palliative care for children and young people has emerged as a new speciality in the UK, nurse education moved to diploma level education, and currently towards an all graduate profession.[16] This has brought nursing into line with other specialities, such as physiotherapy, occupational therapy and dietetics, providing a common academic starting point for multi-professional programmes. This is important since it has been argued that shared and overlapping roles are desirable for achieving good outcomes for patients and their carers in palliative care.[17] In terms of collaboration, Eva et al.[17] state that to understand one another's roles sufficiently in order to foster the trust and respect required to enable cooperation and compromise, requires confidence in one's own expertise and skills, and clarity about boundaries. Giving an overview of the way that physiotherapy, social work and occupational therapy interlink and retain their own individual areas of practice, Eva et al.[17] identify a detailed template for the knowledge and skills that are required to be taught by each professional group. They do not specify the content for particular areas of practice, such as palliative care.

Personal communication with lecturers in physiotherapy, occupational therapy and dietetics by the authors identified some general input on adult palliative care interlinked with various topics and consolidated in practice. Due to the diversity of practice areas students will experience a range of different situations where patients have palliative care needs, for example, physiotherapist students will meet children with cystic fibrosis or children with neuro-degenerative problems.

Furthermore, lecturers[18] identified that dieticians have no particular paediatric training in palliative care skills. Specific skills, such as nutritional support, are acquired depending on the professional role they take post-qualifying. Eva *et al.*[17] believe that on balance only a small minority of students will have had any pre-qualifying palliative care experience.

On considering closer how learning is structured in these programmes, it is important not to underestimate the 'informal' curriculum as illustrated earlier by Wee and Hughes[1] and the skills and knowledge developed by these means rather than an explicit palliative care content. For example:

➤ dietetics students work on integrated case studies
➤ students have contact with (adult) patients with palliative care needs
➤ coping skills are nurtured in practice by a mentor and the multidisciplinary team
➤ a 'buddy' is provided in college as students come to grips with communication skills and learn about emotional care.

Many transferable skills are learnt that can easily be drawn on, but not taken for granted. One aspect identified in personal communication[18] with a physiotherapy colleague is that therapists often are not included in staff support that clinical staff such as doctors and nurses access when a patient is terminally ill or has died, yet the therapist might have known the patient and family for many years.

HOW CAN THESE FINDINGS BE USED TO SUPPORT MULTI-PROFESSIONAL EDUCATION?

Patterns of practical work

Common to palliative care, whether adult or child, is that all patients have either life-limiting, life-threatening or life-shortening conditions. Whilst practical learning in terms of role modelling is desirable, it is not always easily achievable, because so many professionals work in isolation or across huge geographical areas. One such example are specialist nurses working with caseloads of families with children with comparatively rare disorders, such as epidermolysis bullosa.

Generic issues, such as working in small teams or in comparative isolation, are encountered globally, and sharing each other's good practice in courses that can cater for a global audience can be one way forward.

Level of delivery

One implication for nursing of an all-graduate profession will be a progression to cater for the educational needs of specialist practitioners by delivering post-graduate palliative care education at Master's degree level. This is the level of educational achievement currently stipulated by Macmillan Cancer Relief[19] and increasingly other practice settings.[20]

Lifecycle approach

Taking the changing face of children's and young peoples' palliative care into account, education programmes in palliative care should ideally not only focus on the paediatric spectrum which traditionally is 0–18 years, but provide an overarching programme taking a whole lifecycle approach.

Recognising the need for education at various levels throughout the health service and across disciplines and grades, the ACT education pathway[4] suggests a training framework in a tiered format. This pathway features four levels of learning, and four core skills and knowledge areas: communication skills, assessment skills, symptom control and role development. They consider skills at a 'universal', 'targeted' and 'specialist' level. A similar multi-tiered approach has been used by the medical profession in the UK.[10]

Medical profession

Undergraduate medical training across the globe requires students to assimilate a huge amount of information on many topics but the luxury of exploring any in depth is rare. Palliative care may fall in the curriculum under oncology or care of the elderly, but is rarely considered in the child health section. Many of the generic skills that underpin good paediatric palliative care, however, will be acquired and can later be shaped to children's care; communication skills, a grounding in ethical principles and the psychosocial impact of ill health on family functioning being examples.

As physicians progress through early training, management of the core symptoms experienced by the dying should be learned through both theoretical and practical experiences. The basic principles of good pain management and nausea/vomiting being examples of those which are central to good care.[21] The experience of working with families provides professionals with not only the hands-on experience of symptom control but enables them to experience the importance of the wider multi-disciplinary team and the nature of palliative medicine in children, components that are less readily assimilated in taught courses.

The structures of medical hierarchy vary geographically with practitioners choosing generalisation or specialisation at varying points. All paediatricians will be expected to have some knowledge of paediatric palliative care: What it is, how to deliver care in their own setting, basic symptom control and who to refer to in more complicated cases. Only small numbers will choose to specialise and be expected to manage complicated symptoms, acting as a referral centre for other professionals. Between these two lie a large number of doctors who utilise day-to-day palliative care skills to care for children and families in oncology, neuro-disability, community and specialist cardiac, respiratory and neonatal settings. It is also important to remember that not all paediatric palliative care is delivered by paediatricians. GPs, both those caring for identified families in their practice and those working in children's hospices, have educational requirements as do those adult palliative care physicians who have contact with children, either because of a local lack of paediatric facilities or through joint working around transition as noted above. The differing needs of these groups can be seen to fit in with the 'universal', 'targeted' and 'specialist' services as defined by ACT.[4]

Defining a curriculum in paediatric palliative care

Understanding the differing needs of doctors in the UK and the increasing recognition and value placed on doctors who have specialist training in the field led to the development of a 'Curriculum in paediatric palliative medicine'. Published in 2008, the British Society for Paediatric Palliative Medicine and the Association of Children's Hospice Doctors combined to document the minimum set of paediatric palliative medicine skills that they felt should be achieved by doctors, whether GPs or paediatricians, at four different stages in their development:

Box 22.1 Curriculum in paediatric palliative medicine: levels of competencies

Level 1: A doctor just completing a medical degree.
Expectation: An understanding of the basic principles of palliative care.

Level 2: A Paediatric trainee who has completed core training prior to choosing specialisation.

or

A children's hospice doctor after one year of experience.
Expectation: Ability to apply basic principles of palliative medicine to the care of children specifically. Recognise reversible causes of symptoms in children, whether with a life-limiting condition or not.

Level 3: A consultant paediatrician who has gone on to general or subspecialty training in a related field and developed a special interest in paediatric palliative medicine.

or

A children's hospice medical director or other established children's hospice doctor who has gained a validated qualification (e.g. Cardiff University diploma in palliative medicine).
Expectation: To be able to manage most common symptoms safely and effectively. Be prepared to recognise need for specialist help and access it where necessary.

Level 4: A consultant in specialist paediatric palliative medicine.

or

A few hospice medical directors.
Expectation: Able to manage uncommon symptoms; understand principles in order to develop a logical approach even where there is no evidence basis. Considerable emphasis on leading and developing services within and beyond the local hospice, and on supporting and teaching other professionals involved with children with life-limiting conditions who are not trained in palliative medicine. This level will probably only be seen to be achieved if the doctor has obtained FRCPCH or similar distinction.

(adapted from Curriculum in Paediatric palliative medicine[10])

The curriculum organises competencies into knowledge, skills and attitude and then considers 'testable skills', e.g. technical skills, interpersonal skills and intrapersonal skills. Technical skills such as symptom control are defined as techniques relating to the practice of palliative medicine. Interpersonal skills include communication skills and teaching skills whilst intrapersonal skills include coping mechanisms and one's own ability to learn.

The curriculum has been designed with UK graduates in mind and relies on existing evaluation tools such as the MRCPCH and Cardiff University's postgraduate diploma in palliative medicine. Tools to evaluate skills acquired include those traditionally used by GPs and in the Cardiff University course; structured reflective portfolios, written exams, direct observation in practice, case-based discussion, use of audit and communication skills evaluation through video recording of both simulated and actual patient consultations. All of these are increasingly being encouraged by bodies such as PMETB for practitioners to use in revalidation and certification, often combined in individual e-portfolios.

Whilst the curriculum provides a balanced framework of competencies it does not purport to be a comprehensive document. There remains scope for individuals to consider their own needs according to differing settings, e.g. the neonatal practitioner or paediatric intensive care trainee. The curriculum and assessment tools need validation and whilst the document has been endorsed by the RCPCH it would benefit from further research.

Exemplar 1: The Cardiff experience

Cardiff University (UK) has a well-established programme in palliative care education. It was adapted to develop first a paediatric component (2000) and subsequently a multidisciplinary pathway for nurses and pharmacists (2008). Current programmes, offered in both adult and paediatric subspecialties, lead to post graduate qualifications in palliative medicine for doctors and in palliative care for non-medical healthcare professionals.

It is structured over two years leading to a qualification in its own right, or contributes academic credits towards the award of an MSc. Short courses are in development for those who require less in depth knowledge but recognise gaps in their professional development, particularly subspecialists in allied branches of paediatrics and general practitioners.

In originally designing the paediatric material, the structure and much of the adult content was retained, recognising the valuable lessons that can be learnt from the adult field. A large percentage of the material shares common principles, e.g. the pharmacology and science of pain management, ethical principles and grounding in communication skills. How this is put into practice within children's care can be very different. The main premise of learning is that students select patients from their own clinical practice for detailed study forming the basis of written reflective work. They can then review the similarities and differences in their own practice through case reflections, learning summaries and communication skills workshops. Other work-based reviews on aspects of palliative care including service provision and the role of audit also need to be relevant to students' own clinical settings.

Where adult taught content is inappropriate for paediatric practitioners (e.g. prostate cancer), sections are replaced with topics more applicable to paediatric practice. Reflection on developmental issues, more in-depth discussions around neurological symptoms (seizures, spasms) and consideration of unique settings in which care is provided, such as neonatal units, are included. The course has been delivered in a modular format from 2009 and the latest paediatric modules have been aligned carefully with those outlined in the BSPPM/ACHDox curriculum. Offering the course through a modular route will allow the addition of further modules in the future to meet any new developments in palliative care or the specific requirements of different healthcare professional groups.

Students are encouraged not only to change their own clinical practice to improve patient care, but also to positively influence behaviour throughout their working environment. It is hoped that they are empowered to act as local facilitators for subsequent education and research developments in palliative care. The multidisciplinary approach is stressed throughout.

Exemplar 2: The Nottingham experience

A further example of an educational programme, but not targeted at medics, is the Master's degree in Palliative and end-of-life care at Nottingham.[22] This programme currently offers one freestanding learning module on palliative and end-of-life care in childhood and on transition to adulthood.

It is situated in a Master's programme, which mainly caters for students involved in adult palliative care. It allows for dialogue between adult/children's services and emphasis of similarities (i.e. neuro-degenerative illnesses) whilst exploring the different needs at different stages of development and disease trajectory for the infant, child, adolescent and young adult.

It welcomes a global audience by working with reflection, encouraging students to explore principles and relate them to their own working environment. By means of creating cartoon images (avatars) of all participants we have created a 'virtual class' for the discussion forum. Students informally meet the other course participants, and have opportunity to discover a little of their backgrounds, their work in palliative care and the challenges they encounter.

Scenario work allows tailoring the module to students' individual requirements and work context acknowledging the diversity of specialisation. It is possible to focus around the younger, critical care or technology dependent group of children and their families in a variety of settings, as well as the other end of the spectrum more relevant to individuals working with young people. A common knowledgebase is developed through core material that once covered is reflected upon in the student's individual working environment.

Delivering learning material electronically opens up learning beyond geographical boundaries. This also allows inclusion of pre-recorded material developed with user and carer involvement and in different settings. It allows to explore different ways of presenting material through animation and inclusion of available web-based material. Links to such material and pdf files on a very practical level ensures that students with no access to library facilities or databases can access relevant material.

WHERE DO WE GO FROM HERE?

These are exciting times. The Internet and faster broadband speeds have enabled education to create a global classroom and enable learning from each other's good practice at the click of a mouse. Both access and the scope for developing supportive evidence-based material is significantly easier than even a couple of years ago. On the Nottingham course at present, avatars symbolise students in their virtual class, but the possibility of conducting discussions via desk to desk videoconferencing allowing students to have face to face contact is now a real possibility. This is relevant in terms of the informal curriculum, and presents openings in terms of practical skills teaching, e.g. technical skills and communication skills. A further possibility is the linking up of educational institutions globally, each bringing to a programme its particular expertise, sharing commonalities and being able to provide content specific to its particular context.

These possibilities come with responsibilities, too: The need of educationalists, be this in higher education institutions or based in practice, to stay abreast of the dynamic state of both palliative care and educational technology knowledge to remain credible in their field of practice and to remain accountable for providing the best possible learning environment.[23] Currently there is a wealth of study opportunities, many leading to accreditation of prior learning, in principle allowing for the compilation of a very specific portfolio of skills.

Herein lies a danger, that with diversity could come a fragmentation of key areas studied. It will be necessary to maintain a core knowledge which forms the basis of individual professional development. Pathways can provide a tool to achieve this. Even within the programmes examined in this chapter we found that questions arise, such as 'can we teach communication skills via distance learning?' Other practicalities include consideration of language and time zone differences when encouraging face to face discussions using technology.

Perhaps the way forward both in clinical practice and in education lies in how we approach the questions we are asking and attempting to address: then maybe the question is not 'can we?', but by necessity becomes 'how can we?', given the challenges posed and the means at our disposal.

There is no doubt that much debate around education is generated worldwide, as well as examples of good practice. Developing a clear curriculum on both national and international levels might be seen as the gold standard. But have we got the evidence currently to have a definitive content for such courses? As demonstrated throughout this book there is still much confusion as to the definition of palliative care for children and young people. We can see the changes the field of palliative care, both paediatric and adult, has undergone over the years in everyday practice. The stark differences seen many years ago have blurred,[24] so has the interpretation of symptom control in both specialties to include an often 'high tech' solution to improve quality and quantity of life. None of these were components when the term 'palliative care' was coined. However, we can also see how there is still a struggle with the very same issues that posed problems many years ago, for example clear communication with families, or getting the right equipment before the child physically outgrows it (*see* Brunton, Chapter 11). These are not issues for specific palliative care education but must be anchored in the initial preparation for professionals. Practice education and mentoring here play an important part. It is the setting where students first have the opportunity to observe skilled negotiation and advocacy for the child by experienced members of the multidisciplinary team. It also is the setting where, if consequent action is lacking, the impact of failure to implement appropriate care will become obvious. Skills of reflection acquired at this stage will serve as the foundation for life-long learning.

It may be that one answer to the question 'how can we?' is addressed in the UK by the creation of the first Chair in palliative care of children and young people with a number of key areas to address, but within that a brief of the

> development and delivery of education and training opportunities across the spectrum of disciplines and levels of expertise ensuring the development of leaders in the field.[25]

Another answer to 'how can we?' is the creation of 'networks'[26] discussed in Chapter 23. These can serve informally to raise the profile of palliative care education by empowering individuals to give clear consideration to team requirements at local level.

None of these elements can be seen in isolation, but all contribute to an overall picture of how a formal, informal and hidden curriculum come together on the journey of learning, leaving us in this different, and hopefully better place from which we started off.

CONCLUSION

This chapter has attempted to tease out the challenges currently encountered in providing education in the palliative care of children and young people for a multi-professional audience on the path of life-long learning. This has been found to be a process that allows for learning in both formal and informal curricula and to assist individuals to reach their full personal and professional potential. We all follow a common goal: to ensure that:

> patients with palliative care needs, and their families, receive high quality care because –
> * those involved in their care know what to do and
> * how to do it well and
> * are able to exercise wise judgement when doing this and
> * have the ability to teach others about palliative care and to learn from them in return.[1]

We have explored with the aid of two exemplars how this can be achieved in the UK. Some of the challenges that might be experienced in resource-poor climates have been considered along with the strengths and weaknesses of applying single educational programmes across the globe using technology.

There is a climate of change in the world at present. It is the authors' hope that through education, for the good of the children, young people and their families involved, we cannot only move forward from 'can we?' to 'how can we?', but also to 'yes, we can!' (Obama 2009).[27]

N.I.C.E. analysis

Please reflect on the issues raised in this chapter in relation to your own practice.

Needs

- Professionals working with children and young people who have a life-limiting or life-threatening illness and their families need appropriate knowledge and ongoing support.
- Continuing education is a fundamental need for all those involved.
- Being cared for by staff with appropriate experience and knowledge is a fundamental right of children, young people and their families.
- Collaboration between service providers, service users and carers and education to establish and formulate appropriate educational programmes.

Interests

- Continuing education for professionals working with children, young people and their families who have palliative care needs.
- To develop programmes in collaboration between education, service providers, and service users and carers.
- To develop programmes utilising the full range technology available within education.
- This will also enable collaboration between institutions each contributing local expertise to a virtual global classroom.

Challenges

- Meeting the learning needs for a wide range of professional contexts both within paediatric and adult settings.
- Meeting the needs for an international audience and facilitate learning across geographical boundaries.
- Viability of programmes delivering educational material to comparatively small numbers of professionals with diverse learning needs.
- Cost of continuing education, both in terms of release of staff to attend programmes and the cost.

Expectations

- Education is based on the principles of adult education, reflecting the process of self-directed and problem-based learning, has reflective structure and uses a multidisciplinary approach.
- Education reflects the educational needs identified by the various stakeholders.
- Meeting the needs for an international audience and facilitate learning across geographical boundaries.

From the above analysis please reflect on:

- What are the specific issues around education in your working environment?
- How can individuals best meet their professional requirements both to keep professionally up-to-date and to share their specific expert knowledge within a wider forum?
- How can education best meet these leaning needs?

Action plan: next steps

To develop a wide range of accessible opportunities for palliative care education both formally and informally to ensure children, young people and their families have the best possible evidence-based care worldwide.

REFERENCES

1 Wee B, Hughes N. Introduction: learning and teaching palliative care. In: Wee B, Hughes N. *Education in Palliative Care: building a culture of learning.* Oxford: Oxford University Press; 2007.

2 De Vlieger M, Gorchs N, Larkin P, *et al. A Guide for the Development of Palliative Nurse Education in Europe.* Milano: European Association for Palliative Care; 2004. Available at: www.eapcnet.org (accessed 17 February 2010).

3 De Vlieger M, Gorchs N, Larkin P, *et al.* Palliative nurse education – towards a common language. *Eur J Palliat Care.* 2004; **11**(4): 135, 137–8.

4 Association for Children's Palliative Care and Children's Hospices UK (2008) *A Practical Guide to Commissioning Children's Palliative Care Education and Training: planning and developing an effective and responsive workforce.* Draft consultation document. Bristol: Association for Children's Palliative Care; 2008.

5 Bence A. (2009). A first from Oxford. NMC News; February 2009.

6 Brown E with Warr B. *Supporting the Child and the Family in Paediatric Palliative Care.* London: Jessica Kingsley; 2007.

7 Pfund R. *Palliative Care Nursing of Children and Young People.* Oxford: Radcliffe Publishing; 2007.

8 www.act.org.uk

9 www.hospiceafrica.or.ug/index.php?mod=article&cat=educ&article=13

10 www.act.org.uk

11 Elston S. *Integrated Multi-agency Care Pathways for Children with Life-threatening and Life-limiting Conditions.* Bristol: ACT; 2004.

12 Association for Children's Palliative Care. *The Transition Care Pathway.* Bristol: ACT; 2007. Available at: www.act.org.uk/ (accessed 17 February 2010).

13 www.mcpcil.org.uk/liverpool-care-pathway/

14 www.goldstandardsframework.nhs.uk/

15 Ferguson L, Fowler-Kerry S, Hain R. Education and training. In: Goldman A, Hain R, Liben S, editors. *Oxford Textbook of Palliative Care for Children.* New York: Oxford University Press; 2006. p. 513.

16 www.dh.gov.uk/en/Publicationsandstatistics/Publications/PublicationsPolicyAndGuidance/DH_4138756

17 Eva G, Percy G, Chowns G. Occupational therapy, physiotherapy and social work education. In: Wee B, Hughes N, editors. *Education in Palliative Care: building a culture of learning.* Oxford: Oxford University Press; 2007.

18 Personal communication with lecturers in physiotherapy, dietetics, occupational therapy during February and March 2009.

19 www.macmillan.org.uk/About_Us/Specialist_healthcare/How_to_become_a_Macmillan_ Health_Profess/How_to_become_a_Macmillan_Nurse.aspx

20 Dixon L. Nurse education. In: Wee B, Hughes N, editors. *Education in Palliative Care: building a culture of learning.* Oxford: Oxford University Press; 2007.

21 Frager G, Collins J. Symptoms in life-threatening illness: overview and assessment. In: Goldman A, Hain R, Liben S, editors. *Oxford Textbook of Palliative Care for Children.* New York: Oxford University Press; 2006. pp. 231–47.

22 www.act.org.uk

23 Costello J. Welcoming the development of an end-of-life e-learning initiative. *Int J Palliat Nurs.* 2009; **15**(1): 5.

24 Payne S, Seymour J, Ingleton C. *Palliative Care Nursing Principles and Evidence for Practice.* Buckingham: Open University Press/McGraw Hill; 2008.

25 www.sfct.org.uk/pdfs/chairinchildrenspalliativecare.pdf

26 www.act.org.uk/index.php/networks.html

27 www.youtube.com/watch?v=Fe751kMBwms

23

The path to excellence

Rita Pfund

Compiling this book has been an amazing journey.

On the way we have met many amazing people who willingly shared with us their lived experiences of the current state of palliative care of children, young people and their families. Whilst we can only provide a snapshot, we have had first-hand accounts from a cross-section of stake holders, namely a young person himself, parents, siblings and professionals working either independently or in teams, in countries with varying degrees of resources. Their stories speak for themselves, but it remains for the editors to highlight some of the common issues identified.

Our project was ambitious: we started out with two editors – both working in education, one based in Canada, the other in the UK – and an Internet phone, allowing for some pretty long and pretty deep discussions. We both started out sharing ideas of where we thought palliative care of children and young people was at today.

We both shared a curiosity as to how the evolving evidence base, and service development through pathways, which have now been available for nearly five years, is translating into practice.

Soon multiple conversations were going on. We were anxious to move with the material that was coming in to be able to give a reflection of what the issues are that families and professionals are currently dealing with. As this project progressed new writers came on board. For example, the parent who wanted us to hear her story about the transitions families experience on the life path of their child. We felt deeply privileged that so many so willingly shared some very painful and often private thoughts.

Reassuringly we found commonalities upon which to build. Where pathways are firmly on the agenda, implementation is progressing well, although there are hurdles to overcome – not least that following a different path may bring you to new crossroads that may need some manoeuvring. Another new writer we welcomed was the generalist, who is going to strengthen her input on 'early support' in her general nursing programme prompted by our dialogue.

In areas where individuals have an awareness of children's palliative care, but are not required to take the principles on board, there seems some misconception and resistance. Much re-invention of wheels that are already turning elsewhere can also be observed, the problem is often rooted in not having a meaningful dialogue with others. This might be due to discrepancies that still exist in the way palliative care is interpreted and developing, even within our own field of education.

This is why further dialogue is needed:

➤ to learn from each other's good practice and adapt it so it is fit for purpose in individual environments

➤ to continuously reflect on issues past present and future, so that systems put into place are pro-active and not reactive.

Palliative care for children and young people has evolved for nearly 30 years, and will continue to evolve. However, extraordinarily, there are some issues that come up consistently both in publications and at professional meetings, which as a speciality we have not yet managed to resolve. Yet these issues are crucial to overcome the challenges to implement the care to which children, young people and their families have an entitlement:

➤ working with an evidence base

➤ data collection

➤ service user and carer involvement

➤ transition to adult services

➤ collaboration between adult and paediatric services

➤ meeting educational needs.

But why are we having such trouble in these areas?

EVIDENCE-BASED PRACTICE

Is it possible that in our quest to find and utilise evidence we are losing sight of what this evidence is and who generates it? Much anecdotal evidence exists of parents' and young peoples' accounts of their experiences. Direct quotes from families are utilised in 'Better Care: Better Lives',[1] as well as a number of research reports by New Philanthropy capital.[2,3] The use of narratives is not new; examples can be found freely on the Internet,[4] and within texts such as 'Shelter from the storm'.[5] Bryckzynska (*see* Part Two) demonstrates how the philosophical context of narratives can help us to reflect, and Greatrex-White (*see* Chapter 7) explains how narrative research is validated as evidence. Whilst all areas of research, qualitative and quantitative need to be utilised, this type of qualitative research adds to a more complete body of knowledge. It has also been demonstrated that the body of knowledge within children and young people's palliative care is fluid and will continue to be so by the very nature of its being a rapidly developing field.

DATA COLLECTION

It would be inconceivable that any field of science or industry could not underpin their work with up-to-date statistics.

Yet to date the only statistics existing in palliative care for children and young people are 'guesstimates'. These will not be repeated here, as they are easily accessible and have often been quoted. Oncology has slightly more robust data, however, even there no accurate statistics exist for young people contacting malignancies: as this age group falls between children's and adult services, statistics are split between these different healthcare sectors and not considered as an overall total.

But why has this been discussed since the early 1980s with little discernable progress made?

Perhaps adding voices of real people to the hard data that in a clinical context for many count as 'statistics' will prompt some reflection. We have heard their voices, and their stories show that behind every statistic are real people, with real issues they are struggling with. Professionals involved in caring for families cannot devolve this to researchers or academics. This information should be compiled by all practitioners and is vital to provide the ammunition for good service provision. Brunton (*see* Chapter 11) speaks of the gasps when a father told a group of professionals at a conference that his daughter had outgrown her wheelchair before she even had it – yes, we need the number crunching, yes, we need accountability. At every level. Stories like these add to the evidence base. One that is uncomfortable. The gasps in this context symbolised that we have still not resolved the very same problems we were dealing with nearly 30 years ago.

Whilst differences between adult and children's services are the subject of much debate, there appears also to be a somewhat uncomfortable separation with oncology. Perhaps some of it stems from different and confusing terminology, for example much debate is currently centred in the UK around key workers, a concept named 'navigator' in oncology. As Brunton (*see* Chapter 11) illustrates, her son had a level of disability before the diagnosis of a brain tumour, but was left with complex needs in the aftermath of cancer treatment. Whilst it does not matter whose term gets adopted, it potentially adds a sphere of confusion where different sub-specialities need to work together following the same pathway to benefit the child and his family immaterial of the root cause of the health problem.

A national mapping exercise of children and young people currently living with life-limiting illnesses is being undertaken in the UK, initiated by ACT and with partners within the NHS and Children's Hospices UK.[6] (For further details www.act.org.uk/index.php/mapping.html) This is a very positive step, and early indications of this project are encouraging.

Concurrently children's palliative care networks[7] across the UK developing over the last couple of years, are proving to be a successful vehicle for the dissemination of information and ensuring collaboration and more informed commissioning across the multidisciplinary workforce.

However, the implementation of data mapping is less than straightforward: whilst there are clear systems of the information that needs gathering, this is proving difficult due to incompatible computer systems and databases. Current safeguards around data protection, especially where voluntary and state sector need to share data to ensure a comprehensive system need re-evaluating to allow the gathering of these vital data whilst ensuring the maintenance of individual rights.

COLLABORATION BETWEEN ADULT AND PAEDIATRIC SERVICES AND EDUCATIONAL PROVISION

Palliative care for adults has been evolving since the 1960s. Much effort has been spent to establish the differences between our counterparts in adult services and those in children's palliative care services. However, on closer consideration it becomes obvious that adult, just like paediatric palliative care, has undergone the same dynamic process, and has also evolved over the years. This might be more obvious in the UK, where duration of care is not limited by funding. Whilst there are obvious differences between services, and a merger is neither feasible nor desirable, there is significant overlap between the two services, and dialogue, collaboration and shared imaginative educational provision are a must as outlined in Chapter 22. Whilst there is evidence of poor experiences where content of children's palliative care has simply been 'tagged on' to adult programmes, this is not what is suggested here. What is suggested is to develop programmes that cater for the learning needs of both specialities in the light of how both have evolved.

TRANSITION TO ADULT SERVICES

The collaboration between adult and children's services is nowhere more obvious than for the increasing numbers of young people outliving children's services with no clear pathway into adult services. We have heard from Gill (*see* Chapter 9) and Wilford (*see* Chapter 8) of the difficulties when young people reach the chronological age of maturity. Strikingly both the young people in our chapters have had parents with the ability, vision and tenacity to achieve the best possible outcomes for their children.

Transition, according to ACT[8] and the Department of Health in England,[9] begins early and flexibly around the age of 14. Yet as we have seen in the case of Jamie systems were not put into place until very close to his 18th birthday (*see* Gill, Chapter 9). This is daunting for families, not knowing how health and social care will be provided for their children, rapidly realising that for each of the usually multiple health problems a young person may have, within adult services this is likely to be dealt with by individual consultants according to the speciality required for each problem. What these have in common is that they are unlikely to be familiar with the type of complexity these young people present.

It is equally daunting for other professional groups, as they are unlikely to regularly care for young people, and young people and families might arrive with expectations borne out of precedents set in the children's services. For example, in children's hospice care the experience for many children receiving a short break (respite care) is synonymous with a holiday – a break from the routine care that provides an outlet for new and fun experiences. Professionals working within children's palliative care provision must therefore be prepared to actively engage with their adult counter parts to facilitate the development of similar short breaks within adult hospices.

Whilst this is one of the challenges currently dealt with in the UK, in the informal dialogue we had with chapter contributors, and visiting colleagues from other countries, on a number of occasions we heard the response 'we have no problems with transition'. During discussion it became obvious that this is due to the way that services are organised and funded in some countries. If end-of-life care funding cannot exceed six months of a patient's life in many countries then the way this is addressed needs to be creative. In practical terms this means a new referral for each crisis point that may not exceed six months. For example, the child diagnosed with muscular dystrophy is discharged once the 'crisis' of diagnosis is over, or when the child is 'stable'. This approach to care delivery continues at each crisis point, i.e. when the child stops walking and needs a wheelchair, when he needs scoliosis surgery, when he needs night time ventilation. The next episode is likely to be dealt with under the adult services and so on transition is needed. But does this fragmented approach provide the continuity of care and emotional support through transition, which is in the spirit of the WHO[10] or ACT[11] definitions of paediatric palliative care?

STRENGTHENING USER AND CARER INVOLVEMENT

In compiling this text much informal discussion has also taken place. One such discussion at the start of this book in 2008 focused on user and carer involvement, both in an educational and in a service development context. Clear guidelines such as those laid down in the National Children Bureau (NCB) Participation Charter[12] are intended to make it easier for families to participate in service development activities. Yet families often find it difficult to do this, as their actual situation is not always taken into consideration. Ability to participate can depend on avoidable obstacles, such as geographical distances to travel to meetings, which affect the organisation of care for their child whilst attending such meetings. Cancellations or relocation of meetings might be a day-to-day reality professionals have to accept, but easily becomes an expensive and logistical nightmare for a parent who has arranged babysitters for a technology-dependent child. Likewise where appropriate arrangements have been made the unpredictability of the child's condition might prevent the parent from attending. Whilst such basic issues are not adequately resolved, it is unlikely that we can move forward to explore user and carer involvement in areas where their input and experience means so much. Whilst there is evidence of consultation with parents and young people in some areas pertaining to care, which will be strengthened through the 'Aiming High Agenda' for disabled children in England[13] it is clear that there is a need not just to give voice, but clearer awareness of entitlement. It also needs to be recognised that not all parents feel able to be involved. It is recognised that the more complicated and involved the care for a child or young person is, the more flexible we need to be in the ways with which we engage with families. For example, using focus groups, web-based chat lines, inviting parent representatives to meetings and including parents on the distribution list of minutes of meetings. It is important to many organisations to hear the voices of children and young people and there is an increasing use of specialist consultancy to provide expertise with communicating with children and young people in an age appropriate way and to overcome specific communication difficulties.

Examples of areas that do not invite user and carer involvement are ethics committees, who often decide that it is inappropriate and insensitive to conduct research with bereaved parents on palliative care issues. This statement was quoted at a conference to which parents were invited, and prompted one parent to get up and ask whether anybody had actually asked the views of the parents on this.

A second situation was encountered, again at a conference during a presentation explaining the child death review process in the UK[14] and again it transpired that parents had been excluded at the planning stage of the process because it was thought to be too upsetting for them. Parents being faced with this statement and whose children have end-of-life plans felt very strongly that they should have been consulted from the outset.

Two issues emerge from this observation: First, it takes courage to attend a meeting largely geared at professionals and stand up and ask questions. This might reflect the motivation of families to be involved with service development for their children. It also reflects how strongly they might feel around certain issues.

Second, in relation to the child death review process there is clearly the need for guidance to be followed which enables the process to investigate suspicious child deaths appropriately and with the necessary police investigations, but which also enables families of children with life-limiting or life-threatening conditions to circumvent the process, so that they can care for their child's body as per their end-of-life care plan.

When making decisions to 'protect' we need to be clear it is indeed the families that are being protected, not an avoidance of conversations that might be uncomfortable to the professionals.

BEING INCLUSIVE

Throughout the book we have highlighted the need for professionals, not just the ones specialising in palliative care to have a working knowledge of the issues involved and where to get the information they require. The multi-agency aspect of the child death review process, for example, serves as a further illustration of this.

Other sub-specialities who also do not see themselves as providing palliative care, but who provide either universal services or target services need to be reached proactively. Networks[7] play a pivotal role in reaching out and making themselves known to the regional services that will benefit from their support.

WHERE DO WE GO FROM HERE?

It would be over simplistic to attempt to draw hasty conclusions from our findings. Our discourse took place over a timeframe of just eight months, and has taken place through individuals either known to the editors, or recommended by individuals that we approached, or who approached us. We have been anxious to recruit a diverse group of writers, some of whom are well known in the field, but also some who are highly experienced and in key positions, but who have not necessarily shared their expertise with a wider audience. What we found speaks for itself.

From the snapshot we have captured it appears that the concept of the ACT Care Pathway[15] has been embraced and can work well as evidenced in one of the areas we sampled in the UK (*see* Wolff and Browne, Chapter 16), and is also found to be considered in terms of service development in resource-poor countries (*see* Millington, Chapter 5).

No doubt that with the implementation of the Strategy 'Better Care: Better Lives'[1] and the implementation of the 'Aiming High Agenda' in England[13] this will gain further momentum.

In a field as diverse as palliative care of children and young people, the development and professional collaboration of 'children's palliative care networks' advocated in the UK[7] hopefully will address some of the gaps that currently exist. The potential for these networks is immense in terms of service development, collaboration and sustainability of resources. 2010 will see the appointment of the first chair in children's and young people's palliative care in the UK, who will hopefully develop and cement an emerging research and development agenda.

So many positive developments are happening in the field of palliative care for children and young people, yet the global crisis we are currently experiencing is likely to pose a threat to these tender shoots that are developing. Brennan (*see* Chapter 1) has clarified how an entitlement to palliative care can be extrapolated through legislation, especially the United Nations Convention on the Rights of the Child.[16] Whilst 193 countries have signed up to this, neither Somalia nor the US have ratified it; the difficulties for the US explained by former President George W Bush as:

> The Convention on the Rights of the Child may be a positive tool for promoting child welfare for those countries that have adopted it. But we believe the text goes too far when it asserts entitlements based on economic, social and cultural rights . . . The human rights-based approach . . . poses significant problems as used in this text.[17]

Ling[18] observes that tough measures are likely to be taken to deal with tough times, and the impact on future provisions will not be known for some time. Firm evidence will be needed to advocate for our client group to prove effectively and convincingly that the provision of palliative care services not only improves care, but is also cost efficient.

We are therefore finishing by highlighting yet again that palliative care is one of the human rights to be preserved for all the children and families in our care.

REFERENCES

1 Department of Health. *Better Care: Better Lives*. 2008. Available at: www.dh.gov.uk/en/Publicationsandstatistics/Publications/PublicationsPolicyAndGuidance/DH_083106 (accessed 17 February 2010).
2 Joy I. *Valuing Short Lives: children with terminal conditions*. London: New Philanthropy Capital; 2005.
3 Langerman C, Worrall E. *Ordinary Lives: disabled children and their families*. London: New Philanthropy Capital; 2005.
4 www.staceyfoster.co.uk/
5 Hilden J, Tobin D, Lindsey K. *Shelter from the Storm*. Cambridge, MA: Perseus Publishing; 2003.
6 www.act.org.uk
7 www.act.org.uk
8 ACT. *The Transition Care Pathway: a framework for the development of integrated multi-*

agency care pathways for young people with life-threatening and life-limiting conditions. Bristol: ACT; 2007.

9 www.dh.gov.uk/en/Publicationsandstatistics/Publications/PublicationsPolicyAndGuidance/DH_4132145

10 www.who.int/cancer/palliative/definition/en/

11 www.icpcn.org.uk/page.asp?section=0001000100080004&itemTitle=What+is+Children%92s+Palliative+Care%3F

12 www.ncb.org.uk/dotpdf/open%20access%20-%20phase%201%20only/partposter_participation052006.pdf

13 www.everychildmatters.gov.uk/socialcare/ahdc/

14 www.londonscb.gov.uk/files/resources/cdop/rcpch_guidance_on_child_death_review_process.pdf

15 ACT. *Integrated Multi-agency Care Pathways for Children with Life-threatening and Life-limiting Conditions.* Bristol: ACT; 2004.

16 www.unicef.org/crc/

17 www.wnd.com/news/article.asp?ARTICLE_ID=21590

18 Ling J. Palliative care in changing economic times. *Int J Palliat Nurs.* 2008; **14**: 523.

Index